THE
MAYO CLINIC
BREAST
CANCER
BOOK

Lynn C. Hartmann, M.D.
Charles L. Loprinzi, M.D.

Medical Editors

This book is made possible by the generosity and philanthropy of Karen L. Vierk.

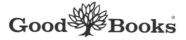

Good Books

Intercourse, PA 17534 • 800-762-7171 • www.GoodBooks.com

The Mayo Clinic Breast Cancer Book provides reliable, practical, comprehensive, easy-to-understand information on issues relating to breast cancer. Much of its information comes from physicians, research scientists and other health care professionals at Mayo Clinic. This book is intended to supplement the advice of your personal physician, whom you should consult about your individual medical condition. *The Mayo Clinic Breast Cancer Book* does not endorse any company or product. MAYO, MAYO CLINIC and the Mayo triple-shield logo are marks of Mayo Foundation for Medical Education and Research.

Published by Good Books

Photo credits: Photos on pages 9, 33 and 303 are from Getty Images. The individuals pictured in these photos are models, and the photos are for illustrative purposes only. There is no correlation between the individuals portrayed and the condition or subject being discussed.

© 2012 Mayo Foundation for Medical Education and Research (MFMER)

ISBN 978-1-56148-772-1

Library of Congress Control Number: 2012940469

First Edition

1 2 3 4 5 6 7 8 9 10

If you would like more copies of this book, contact Good Books, Intercourse, PA 17534; 800-762-7171; *www.GoodBooks.com.* For bulk sales to employers, member groups and health-related companies, contact Mayo Clinic, 200 First St. S.W., Rochester, MN 55905, or *SpecialSalesMayoBooks@mayo.edu*

Printed in the USA

Editorial Staff

MAYO CLINIC

Medical Editors
Lynn C. Hartmann, M.D.
Charles L. Loprinzi, M.D.

Managing Editor
Karen R. Wallevand

Product Manager, Books
Christopher C. Frye

Director, Content Services
John (Jay) W. Maxwell

Art Director
Richard A. Resnick

Illustrators
Joanna R. King
Michael A. King
Kent McDaniel

Photographers
Joseph M. Kane
Jodi O'Shaughnessy Olson
Rebecca Varga
Randy Ziegler

Editorial Research Manager
Deirdre A. Herman

Editorial Research Librarians
Anthony J. Cook
Amanda K. Golden
Erika A. Riggin

Proofreaders
Miranda M. Attlesey
Donna L. Hanson
Julie M. Maas

Indexer
Steve Rath

Administrative Assistant
Beverly J. Steele

Contributors and Reviewers
Jamie N. Bakkum-Gamez, M.D.
Rachel Bartony
Brent A. Bauer, M.D.
Judy C. Boughey, M.D.
Barb Boyer
Kathleen R. Brandt, M.D.
Karen Canzanello
Matthew M. Clark, Ph.D.
Fergus J. Couch, Ph.D.
Amy C. Degnim, M.D.
Matt A. Derechin
Sean C. Dowdy, M.D.
Shawna L. Ehlers, Ph.D.
Karthik Ghosh, M.D.
Katrina N. Glazebrook, M.B.
Matthew P. Goetz, M.D.
Tufia C. Haddad, M.D.
James N. Ingle, M.D.
Jennifer L. Jacobson
James W. Jakub, M.D.
Aminah Jatoi, M.D.
Valerie Lemaine, M.D.
Noralane M. Lindor, M.D.
Harry J. Long III, M.D.
Margie D. Loprinzi, R.N.

Anne Mehnke
Linda K. Miller, M.D.
Timothy J. Moynihan, M.D.
Sheryl M. Ness, R.N.
Prema P. Peethambaram, M.D.
Edith A. Perez, M.D.
Ivy A. Petersen, M.D.
Sandhya Pruthi, M.D.
Effie Psimos
Derek C. Radisky, Ph.D.
Carol Reynolds, M.D.
Deborah J. Rhodes, M.D.
Paula J. Schomberg, M.D.
Deanne R. Smith, C.N.P.
LeAnn M. Stee
Keith M. Swetz, M.D.
Daniel W. Visscher, M.D.
Janet Vittone, M.D.
Katherine M. Zahasky, C.N.P.

GOOD BOOKS

Publisher
Merle Good

Executive Editor
Phyllis Pellman Good

Assistant Publisher
Kate Good

Administrative Assistant
Tony Gehman

Designer
Cliff Snyder

Preface

If you've picked up this book, you've likely been touched by breast cancer. So many women have been. *The Mayo Clinic Breast Cancer Book* can provide you with information you need to face a cancer diagnosis and the challenges of treatment, or to prevent the disease if you're at high risk.

What does this book add in today's information-rich age? It contains the most accurate and reliable information available, reflecting improvements in both the understanding and treatment of breast cancer. It also provides "the why" behind the facts.

The Mayo Clinic Breast Cancer Book is rich in hope, with stories of women who've successfully navigated similar waters. It's also realistic. When a cure may not be possible, the book provides guidance for redirecting hope and priorities toward other goals.

Each chapter was reviewed by multiple experts at Mayo Clinic. We've tried to provide you with a balanced account of where things stand — similar to the guidance Mayo Clinic doctors give their patients. Nonetheless, the information in this book isn't a substitute for the one-on-one relationship between patient and doctor. The purpose of this book is to allow you to discuss treatment options with your doctors in a more informed manner so that together you can make the best choices for your medical care.

This book is a tribute to many, especially the extraordinary women who've taught us about breast cancer.

Lynn C. Hartmann, M.D.
Charles L. Loprinzi, M.D.

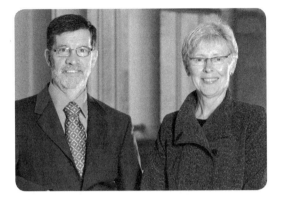

Charles L. Loprinzi, M.D., is a medical oncologist and the Regis Professor in Breast Cancer Research at Mayo Clinic Cancer Center, Rochester, Minn. He is a past chair of the Division of Medical Oncology at Mayo Clinic. Dr. Loprinzi has authored more than 350 scientific publications. His primary areas of research involve doctor-patient communication and the control of cancer-related symptoms. Dr. Loprinzi is also a recipient of two Susan G. Komen Foundation awards: the Brinker International Award and Komen Foundation Professor of Survivorship Award.

Lynn C. Hartmann, M.D., is a medical oncologist and the Blanche R. and Richard J. Erlanger Professor of Medical Research at Mayo Clinic Cancer Center, Rochester, Minn. Dr. Hartmann led the effort to develop a Women's Cancer Program at Mayo Clinic to advance the scientific understanding of breast and gynecologic cancers and to educate professionals, patients and the public about these cancers. With funding from the National Cancer Institute, Department of Defense, American Cancer Society and the Susan G. Komen Foundation, Dr. Hartmann has authored more than 200 research articles. Her focus is on the identification and management of women at high risk of breast cancer.

Contents

Preface .... *iv*

Part 1: Cancer Basics

Chapter 1: When Cancer Strikes...11

Chapter 2: Understanding Cancer 17
What Is Cancer?
How Does Cancer Occur?
Causes
Advancing Our Knowledge of Cancer

Visual Guide... 33

Part 2: Breast Cancer

Chapter 3: An Overview.. 43
Your Breasts
Breast Cancer
What Causes Breast Cancer?
How Common Is Breast Cancer?
Advancing Science

Chapter 4: Making Sense of Risk Statistics 61
What Is Risk and How Is It Measured?
Quantifying Risk
Risk Factors

Chapter 5: Hereditary Breast Cancer...75
Is it Hereditary?
Inheriting a Genetic Mutation
Genetic Counseling and Testing
Making a Decision

Chapter 6: Preventing Breast Cancer 91
Lifestyle Factors
Women at High Risk
Future Directions

Chapter 7: The Latest on Screening 111
Ongoing Controversies
Screening Recommendations
Breast Self-Awareness
Clinical Breast Examination
Mammography
New Approaches

Chapter 8: Diagnosing Breast Cancer 127
    Signs and Symptoms
    Medical History
    Physical Examination
    Imaging Tests
    Biopsy Procedures
    Pathology Report
    Staging

Chapter 9: Precancerous Conditions 149
    Atypical Hyperplasia
    Lobular Carcinoma *In Situ* (LCIS)
    Your Options

Chapter 10: Ductal Carcinoma *In Situ* (DCIS) 153
    Diagnosis
    Key Factors
    Treatment Options
    Making the Decision

Chapter 11: Treating Invasive Breast Cancer 161
    Treatment Options
    Surgery
    Radiation Therapy
    Decision Guide: Lumpectomy vs. Mastectomy
    Additional Treatment
    Therapy Options
    Decision Guide: Adjuvant Systemic Therapy
    Clinical Trials

Chapter 12: Breast Reconstruction 203
    Immediate vs. Delayed
    Types
    Issues to Consider

Chapter 13: Special Situations 211
    Locally Advanced Breast Cancer
    Women at High Risk of a Second Cancer
    Bilateral Breast Cancer
    Unknown Primary Cancers
    Metaplastic Breast Cancer
    Lymphomas and Sarcomas
    Paget's Disease
    Breast Cancer and Pregnancy
    Breast Cancer in Men

Chapter 14: Follow-up and Surveillance 225
    Understanding Recurrent Cancer
    Follow-up Care
    Dealing With Uncertainty

Chapter 15: If the Cancer Comes Back 235

    Types of Recurrence
    How Cancer Cells Spread
    Local Recurrence
    Regional Recurrence
    Metastatic Recurrence

Chapter 16: Treating Advanced Breast Cancer 247

    Determining Prognosis
    Treatment Options
    Monitoring Treatment
    Localized Treatments
    When Treatment Stops Working

Chapter 17: Ovarian Cancer: What You Should Know 271

    Your Ovaries
    What Is Ovarian Cancer?
    How Common Is It?
    Risk Factors
    Preventing Ovarian Cancer
    Screening Methods
    Early Warning Signs
    Spread of Ovarian Cancer
    Diagnosis and Treatment

Chapter 18: Uterine Cancer: What You Should Know 287

    The Uterus
    Uterine Cancer Basics
    Risk Factors
    Can It Be Prevented?
    Warning Signs
    Diagnosing Uterine Cancer
    Determining the Extent of the Cancer
    Treatment Options

Part 3: Life After a Cancer Diagnosis

Chapter 19: Feelings and Emotions 305

    Making the Journey
    Tips for the Trip
    Communicating With Family
    Communicating With Children
    Communicating With Friends

Chapter 20: Treatment Side Effects 323

    Fatigue
    Nausea and Appetite Problems
    Hair Loss
    Decreased Arm and Shoulder Mobility
    Lymphedema
    Sudden Menopause

Sexual Changes
Osteoporosis
Neuropathy
Joint Aches and Pains
Weight Gain
Cognitive Changes

Chapter 21: Complementary Therapies 351
Getting the Most of Complementary Therapies
Types of Therapies
Finding Reliable Information

Chapter 22: Survivorship...365
Moving Forward
Taking Care of Your Health
Support Groups
Public Events

Chapter 23: Making the Transition to Supportive Care..379
Accepting Your Situation
Maintaining Hope
When You and Your Family Disagree
Managing Signs and Symptoms
Hospice Care

Chapter 24: For Partners..395
Dealing With Your Loved One's Diagnosis
How You Can Help
Talking to Each Other
Maintaining Sexual Intimacy
Caring for Yourself
Dealing With Incurable Cancer
Resources
A Time of Growth

Additional Resources *413*
Glossary *417*
Index *433*

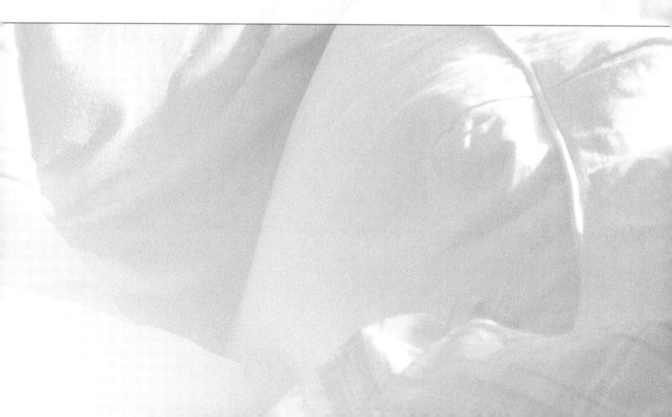

PART 1:
Cancer Basics

Chapter 1: Cancer Basics

When Cancer Strikes

"When I was not only called back for more mammogram films, but scheduled for an ultrasound, my anxiety began to skyrocket."

Mary Amundsen
Breast cancer survivor

A cancer diagnosis can be a lightning bolt. Once the word *cancer* is spoken, life stops — or seems to. Normal routines unravel. Emotions are laid bare. Concentration is lost. Things that once were so important no longer are.

With the lightning comes the rain — a pelting of information, statistics, questions and tests. At a time when all you may seek is warmth and shelter, you can't get out of the storm. Appointments need to be scheduled. Decisions need to be made. Steps need to be taken.

Sometimes, it's difficult to know where to begin or which way to turn for guidance. This book was written to provide reliable and easy-to-comprehend information to help you better understand your cancer, make informed decisions regarding your care, and cope with the emotional and physical effects of cancer treatment.

The focus of this book is on the most common and serious cancer to affect women — breast cancer. Each year in the United States, more than 200,000 women are told they have breast cancer. The good news is, deaths from the disease are declining, due in large part to ongoing research and continued advances in diagnosis and treatment. You'll also learn key facts about two other cancers that affect women,

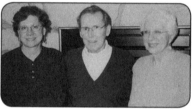

Mary Amundsen, right, with her daughter and her husband.

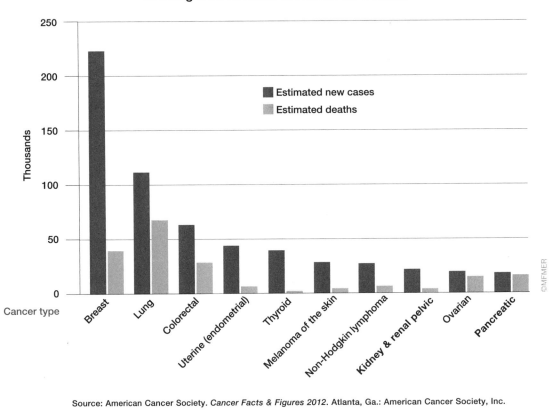

Leading new cancers in American women

Source: American Cancer Society. *Cancer Facts & Figures 2012.* Atlanta, Ga.: American Cancer Society, Inc.

ovarian and uterine cancer. These cancers are included because they're more common in breast cancer survivors.

The book is divided into three sections. Part 1 provides an overview of cancer in general: What it is, how it develops, and how it spreads. Part 2 focuses mainly on breast cancer. The chapters in this section provide a comprehensive discussion of all aspects of the disease from risk and prevention to the latest in diagnosis and treatment. Part 3 discusses strategies for dealing with the emotional, social, spiritual and physical challenges that accompany cancer treatment and survival.

The book also contains personal stories from women who've been diagnosed with cancer. They talk about the decisions they faced, the choices they made and their lives today.

We begin with Mary's story. Mary Amundsen is a registered nurse and licensed psychologist. Not only has Mary confronted — and weathered — cancer herself, she has witnessed firsthand the fears, concerns and courage of many women facing the same struggle. Mary offers her story and shares her advice, to reassure you that you aren't alone in your journey.

Mary's Story

My annual mammogram. I didn't feel particularly anxious, although in the past I had been called back for additional films, which had reassured me that the radiologists were very precise. Because I was over age 50, I was at increased risk of breast cancer, even though I didn't have a family history of it. No one in my family had had breast cancer, but our daughter had been treated for ovarian cancer. So, when I was not only called back for more mammogram films, but scheduled for an ultrasound, my anxiety began to skyrocket.

Summoning my husband, to give me support and to provide an extra listening ear, we met with the radiologist. He explained the finding of clustered microcalcifications on my mammogram and suggested that I could get another mammogram in six months. No one, not even I, could feel a lump, and the mammogram films didn't show a suspicious mass. But did I want to wait until a lump developed? The questions, ambivalence and fear were just beginning. We asked for a second opinion. The second radiologist explained that the microcalcifications had been present on previous films but now were clustered, suggestive of cancer. He recommended a biopsy, although I still had the choice of waiting six months for another mammogram. That was decision point No. 1.

Fear and uncertainty

At the time I was faced with this decision, I thought of my years as a nurse and of my leadership of a breast cancer support group. The stories of others waiting too long for a biopsy and not having enough information to make an informed decision gave me a sense of urgency. It suddenly felt like my life was spinning out of control once again. It had been only six years since our daughter, at age 30, was diagnosed with ovarian cancer. At that time, I had desperately wished it were me instead of her. Four years after that, my husband had gone through extensive surgery and radiation for a sinus cancer. I felt our family had paid its dues to the "Big C," and I was angry that we might be facing this ordeal again.

The radiologist tried to assure us that most breast biopsies are benign, but the experience with our daughter and my husband, whose cancer shocked even the surgeon, made us very uneasy. The biopsy wasn't an emergency requiring an overnight decision, so I had some time to gather information and talk with supportive people, but by now I knew I didn't want to wait six months for another mammogram.

A possible cancer diagnosis seems to bring up every emotion and bad outcome you've ever heard. I knew literally hundreds of women who had had breast cancer and were still alive, but my mind jumped to those who had died of it.

An even stronger reaction was the grief and guilt that I felt in putting our family through this again. Our daughter was doing very well after her two surgeries and her chemotherapy treatment, and we were anxiously waiting out each checkup for my husband. My reactions felt familiar, and although I knew I could get through this, my heart was heavy.

Once I made the decision to have the biopsy sooner rather than later, I was faced with another decision point.

Choices and more decisions

If the biopsy did show cancer, what type of surgery would I want, if I had a choice? Did I want the surgeon to proceed with a mastectomy, if indicated, and what about reconstruction? By this time I had talked with two radiologists, a surgeon and my personal physician. What I found, and now tell others, is you must be your own advocate and gather as much information as you need to be comfortable with your decisions.

Although it may feel like a burden to be involved in the decision-making process, we're fortunate that there are choices. You likely will be given treatment options that will require you to make decisions. As much as you might wish for the old days when a doctor made all of the decisions, times have changed.

If you're feeling overwhelmed by the information you receive from your doctors regarding treatment for your cancer, take some time to process what you've learned and don't be afraid to ask questions.

My surgeon was very patient with all of my questions and my desire to be involved in the decision making. Even though I preferred to keep my breast, I wasn't going to put my future at risk. We discussed the research findings of lumpectomy and radiation versus mastectomy. This information conflicted with my gut reaction to have my breast removed and be done with it.

I was very lucky. My cancer was discovered early, which increased my chances of a good outcome. Surgery showed a small, slightly invasive cancer, and the surgeon removed only a small part of the breast. A lymph node dissection was negative, so only radiation, not chemotherapy, was recommended as part of my treatment.

After I was finished with radiation, I wondered what was next. I wasn't comfortable doing nothing, so I contacted an oncologist to discuss the possibility of using tamoxifen or a similar drug. I knew others who were taking these types of medications, and I felt like I needed to pursue every avenue. The oncologist, after reviewing my records, didn't recommend any additional treatment, because my prognosis was extremely favorable without it. At this point, I needed to trust the opinion of my doctor but also keep myself informed as new research results were published.

The decision of whether to have additional treatment once your primary treatment is complete is another major decision point for many women. Learning more about possible therapies is essential to prepare yourself for this phase of your recovery. If your doctor recommends additional treatment, knowing why he or she is recommending that particular treatment can help to alleviate the anxiety. During this time, your relationship with your medical team needs to be one of support, understanding and patience by all individuals involved. Your physical recovery may be progressing, but the emotional aspects of cancer now are beginning to surface. The changes cancer has brought to your family and your life are now being realized.

Dealing with loss

When cancer involves the reproductive and sexual organs, it strikes at the very core of a woman's identity. Your physical appearance and physiology may be very abruptly and significantly altered. The gradual changes that come with adolescence and menopause allow a woman to adjust psychologically over a period of time. Cancer, however, often brings sudden changes. And not only are they sudden, they're unwanted and uncomfortable. Your feelings of femininity may be challenged, and you may feel insecure about your most intimate relationships. Future dreams and plans may never be realized in ways you had hoped.

It's a time of grief and loss and a time of coping, often in new ways. Cancer can bring out a creativity never realized. A friend of mine started to write a poem about her breasts and what they had meant to her. The poem became many poems as her feelings poured out onto the paper. Other women have used art and sculpture to evoke their deepest emotions, and music to ease some of the difficult times during sleepless nights or chemotherapy treatments. My daughter played meditation tapes during her chemotherapy treatments. Quilting or fiber art can express our darkest times and our birth of hope. To view one of these artistic creations is to know the deeper connection with others who have walked this path of cancer.

Keeping a journal of your experience is a way to express fears and feelings that are difficult to speak aloud. Humor can provide some relief to the seriousness we live with every day. I keep a folder of cartoons for those times. Just the physical act of a smile changes the way I feel, for a short time at least. You can choose how you deal with this crisis in your life.

A changed life

Is cancer a life-changing event? You may read about those who radically altered their lives after a cancer diagnosis and you may wonder if you need to think about major changes. Cancer does change your life in many ways as you learn a new language (medical), meet new people (the medical team), fill up your calendar (with appointments) and, perhaps, see a different body in the mirror. Many women in my support group have expressed feeling a sense of urgency to do things now, instead of later. As a cancer survivor, you become very tuned in to news reports of cancer research, new treatments and statistics of survival. Every ache and pain is viewed with new concern, and checkups are approached with anxiety. So, yes, cancer is a life-changing event. But then, any major life-threatening diagnosis will change a person's life. You are face to face with your vulnerability. The illusion of an open-ended future has been shattered and reality can be harsh.

One of the biggest fears, of course, is that of recurrence — that the treatment didn't get rid of everything. It's a fear all people who've had cancer live with and don't want to think about. However, some preparation can help you cope if that day comes. Think about what information you would want to know, who would be most helpful to you and how you coped with your initial diagnosis. The courage and strength of those I have known with cancer is a continuous source of hope and inspiration for me during anxious times. If others can get through it with grace, then so can I.

In addition to my daughter, husband and me, cancer has been diagnosed in my brother (melanoma) and in my daughter-in-law (bladder). We are now all considered cancer-free, or in remission, although we know that at any time our status could change.

MYTH vs. FACT

Myth: **If we can travel in outer space and put people on the moon, we should have a cure for cancer by now.**

Fact: Cancer is a large group of diseases, and each type of cancer may be associated with many different factors. Researchers are still learning about what triggers a cell to become cancerous and why some people with cancer do better than others. In addition, cancer is a moving target. Cancer cells continue to mutate and change during the course of the disease. This can cause cancer cells to no longer respond to medications or radiation treatments that initially worked well when the disease was first diagnosed.

Finding a "cure for cancer" is, in fact, proving to be much more complex than mastering the engineering and physics required for spaceflight.

Being proactive

What factors made a difference in our outcomes? There was no doubt some luck and other factors beyond our control that contributed to our successful treatments. But we also did some things that probably made a difference. I had a routine mammogram, which found the cancer at a very early stage. My daughter had some unusual abdominal discomfort and had a checkup. My husband pursued the increasing pain in his sinus area, which he considered unusual. I noticed a mole on my brother, and I urged him to see a dermatologist. Our daughter-in-law sought attention for intermittent episodes of urinary bleeding. In other words, we were aware of body changes, and we were persistent in having those changes evaluated. When you feel that something is physically wrong in your body, you do have to be assertive and be an advocate for yourself. No one else can truly know how you feel.

Support and strength

Many people made a difference in the quality of our lives during those months and years, for those of us with cancer and for our family as a whole. Cancer is a family affair and everyone needs support and understanding. It's not a journey to travel alone. A burden shared is easier to carry.

No doubt you've experienced other difficult times in your life, and you've managed to get through them. Think back now to those times and what you did that was the most helpful. Draw on those strengths now. Educate yourself, select a skilled medical team, find support and proceed with hope.

Chapter 2: Cancer Basics

Understanding Cancer

What Is Cancer?	18
Normal cell behavior	18
Cancer cells	19

| How Does Cancer Occur? | 23 |
| A long process | 23 |

| Causes | 24 |
| Risk factors | 24 |

Advancing Our Knowledge of Cancer	26
Basic research	27
Epidemiologic studies	27
Clinical trials	28

It's been more than 40 years since the U.S. government declared war on cancer, and the disease remains a formidable foe. Each year in the United States, more than 1.5 million people are diagnosed with cancer. It's the second-leading cause of death after heart disease. More than 500,000 Americans die of cancer annually.

Yes, those are sobering statistics, but there is cause for optimism. Much has changed since President Richard Nixon signed the National Cancer Act, providing federal funding for cancer research. At the time, cancer was poorly understood and usually deadly. Today, thanks to improvements in the detection and treatment of many forms of cancer — and even prevention of some — the death rate from all cancers combined is declining. In 1974, the five-year survival rate for women diagnosed with breast cancer was approximately 75 percent. Today, it's nearly 90 percent.

Scientists now have a far better understanding of how cancer develops and progresses. Unprecedented growth in the area of biomedical research along with an explosion in sophisticated technologies such as gene sequencing and supercomputing has resulted in a new era of molecular oncology — the study of cancer at its core, at the submicroscopic, molecular level.

Although total elimination of all cancers likely isn't possible, some cancers are increasingly being seen as longer term, manageable conditions, such as heart disease and diabetes. Regular screening can result in early detection of many types of cancer. Most cancers are curable if found early. With prompt treatment, regular monitoring, and social and psychological support, many people with cancer can live productive, satisfying lives for many years. Today, there are about 12 million cancer survivors in the United States.

Scientific discoveries of the last few decades have given researchers a better understanding of just how complex cancer is. They know more about what makes cancer so challenging to detect and treat — and have developed better approaches.

This chapter is an overview of what's known about the biology of cancer and how that knowledge has been gained. The chapter goes into a fair amount of scientific detail and, therefore, might provide more information than you wish to learn right now. Feel free to move on to other chapters that follow, and then come back to this chapter in the future.

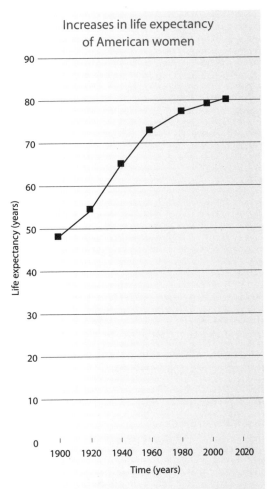

Due to improved sanitation and medical advances, including advances in cancer detection and treatment, American women are living significantly longer than did their grandmothers and great-grandmothers.

Data from *National Vital Statistics Reports*, vol 60 no 4; National Center for Health Statistics, 2012.

©MFMER

What Is Cancer?

Although cancer is often thought of as a single disease, the term actually refers to a group of related diseases that begin in cells, the body's basic units of life.

The human body is made of trillions of cells, categorized into about 200 different types that combine to form human tissues, such as skin, muscle, bone, breast and blood. To understand how cancer develops, it's helpful to know something about how healthy cells behave.

Normal cell behavior

Normally, cells grow and divide to produce more cells only when the body needs them. This process takes place according to genetic programs and instructions that are unique to each type of cell. As a cell grows, it takes its proper place among other cells. When the cell matures, it performs the task it's genetically programmed to do. After a certain number of divisions, the cell is programmed to die — a process known as apoptosis — and it is replaced by a new, younger cell. This orderly process keeps the body healthy and functioning.

Cells are also equipped with controls designed to prevent them from making too many copies of themselves or from making flawed copies of themselves.

No cell, however, is an island unto itself. The body's cells are regularly bombarded at their surfaces by nutrients and by hormonal and chemical signals, including signals from neighboring cells. To remain alive and healthy, cells must decode, filter and respond properly to many such molecular "conversations." For example, normal cells are stimulated to multiply by molecular messages called growth signals. They also receive antigrowth signals when it's time to stop multiplying. If you cut yourself, skin cells around the wound multiply to replace the injured cells. When the gap is filled properly, cell growth is turned off.

Some researchers compare this intricate network of cellular signaling pathways to a computer chip, in which the interconnected components are each responsible for receiving, processing and sending signals according to specific rules. Cellular pathways involve interactions among thousands of diverse molecules within and outside the cell. These interactions regulate cell growth.

Cancer cells

Cancer results when there's a loss of control in this intricate system of normal cell growth. Cancer is characterized by the overgrowth of abnormal cells. The development of these abnormal cells is a complex, lengthy, multistep process called carcinogenesis. It starts with the transformation of one normal cell into an abnormal cell. Over time, the abnormal cells multiply out of control and accumulate into a mass of tissue — called a growth, or tumor — that can invade and destroy nearby normal tissue. Cancer cells can also spread throughout the body.

Even though cancer cells arise from normal body cells, they change so that they don't look or act like normal cells. Normal body cells, like law-abiding citizens, follow the rules set out for them by their genetic instructions. They multiply when told to and stop multiplying when they get a signal to do so. Cancer cells, however, are biological anarchists. They stop following the rules. Not only are there too many of them, but they develop new and different characteristics. Their growth is disorderly, and they don't mature properly. Unlike normal cells, which tend to form exact copies of themselves when they divide, cancer cells are more likely to change when they divide. Tumor cells often look different from one another, and they can be highly disorganized. These abnormal cells tumble over each other, and they stack up on neighboring cells.

Characteristics of cancer cells
Cancer cells have many genetic differences from normal cells. In cancer cells, important regulatory genes become

Cancer development and progression

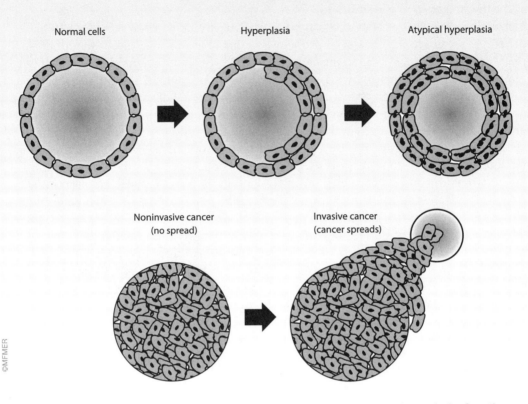

©MFMER

Cancer development first begins with excess production of cells. This is known as hyperplasia. Over time, the excess cells may begin to change in appearance and become abnormal. This is known as atypical hyperplasia. As the cells continue to change and multiply, cancer develops. If the abnormal cells stay contained within normal borders and they don't invade neighboring tissue, the condition is known as noninvasive cancer. When the cells invade deeper into surrounding tissue, it's called invasive cancer.

mutated or lost. Genes that slow growth in a normal cell are shut off in cancer cells. Just the opposite, genes that stimulate growth in a normal cell may be duplicated many times in cancer cells. Cancer genes often become unstable, meaning they can change rapidly, and as they multiply, they can acquire additional deadly features.

By studying the molecular makeup of cells, researchers have identified specific characteristics that cancer cells acquire as

they develop that allow them to grow out of control.

For example, cancer cells:

- **Supply their own growth signals.**
  Normal cells receive growth signals mainly from neighboring cells or hormones, but cancer cells generate many of their own growth signals. They also coerce their neighbors to make growth factors that stimulate their growth.
- **Stop responding to anti-growth signals from neighboring cells.** Cancer cells

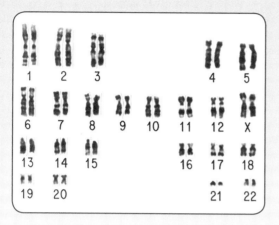

Normal chromosomes

The extent of genetic changes in cancer cells can be seen in this comparison of the chromosomes in a woman's normal blood cells (left) and in her ovarian cancer cells (below).

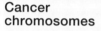

Cancer chromosomes

don't obey the molecular messages that normally stop cell growth to maintain a balanced cell growth cycle.

- **Develop their own blood supply.** A tumor gets the nutrients and oxygen it needs by developing new blood vessels in a process called angiogenesis. Normally, angiogenesis is tightly regulated, but cancerous tumors don't always follow this regulation.
- **Don't self-destruct.** Normal cells have a natural life cycle — they age and

eventually they die in a process called programmed cell death. Cancer cells become seemingly immortal and resist the process. This resistance is a hallmark of most, if not all, types of cancer.

Although the life-threatening properties cancer cells acquire may seem daunting, keep in mind that these properties can serve as targets for treatment. The illustration on page 29 shows how scientists are taking advantage of certain cancer cell characteristics in designing new drugs.

Genetics 101

Each cell in the body, except for mature red blood cells, has a control center called the nucleus. The nucleus houses your DNA, a long, double-stranded structure composed of sugar and phosphate molecules that are joined together by paired chemicals called nucleotide bases. DNA is tightly packed into structures called chromosomes. There are two sets of 23 chromosomes in the cell nucleus, for a total of 46 chromosomes. One set comes from each parent. The only cells that don't contain two sets of chromosomes are the sex cells — eggs and sperm. These contain only one set of chromosomes. Thus, when an egg and sperm join together to form what's called a zygote, the zygote contains a new, complete set of 46 chromosomes.

A gene is a defined segment of DNA on a chromosome. Genes are the blueprints for the cells of your body. They provide instructions for making proteins that, in turn, do the business of a particular cell. Many kinds of proteins play various roles in the body. They control how cells divide, grow and function.

Genes determine characteristics such as how tall you are and what color your eyes are. They tell your body to repair tissue that has been injured and to keep tumors from growing. Your genes also influence your susceptibility to diseases such as cancer.

Genetics is the study of genes and the diseases caused by genetic defects.

When a cell divides, each gene must be copied so that each of the two resulting cells has a complete set of genes. Mistakes in this process can and do occur. Quite often these mistakes are harmless and easily repaired, but sometimes they can lead to the development of cancer or other diseases.

Not all genes are active all the time. Some genes continuously produce proteins for basic cell function, and other genes are switched on (activated) only when their protein-coding information is needed. Each cell's function is largely determined by which of its approximately 25,000 genes are activated.

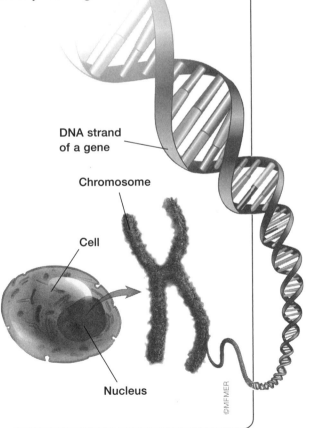

DNA strand
of a gene

Chromosome

Cell

Nucleus

©MFMER

How Does Cancer Occur?

A key question for scientists studying cancer is to understand what causes the transformation of a normal cell into an abnormal one. How does cancer begin?

Major progress in understanding this process came in the 1950s with the discovery of the structure of deoxyribonucleic acid (DNA) and the advent of molecular biology. Since then, powerful new technologies for studying DNA and genes have led to breakthroughs in understanding the biology of cancer.

All cancers involve the malfunction of genes that control cell growth and division. The order (sequence) of molecules in each gene spells out instructions for producing the proteins that carry out a cell's activities. When the chemical sequence of a gene is altered, it's like a genetic misspelling that can cause problems. These errors (mutations) can result in a cell either losing an important regulatory function or gaining an abnormal function.

Over time, as more cell divisions occur, the chance for errors increases. Although there are genes that control orderly cell division (replication) and others that check for errors, these too can become damaged, allowing cells to pass along genetic defects. In fact, the change from a normal cell to a cancerous cell requires several separate, different genetic alterations.

Alterations in the following genes important to cell growth play a critical role in the development of cancer:

• **Tumor suppressor genes.** These genes are responsible for restraining cell growth. They can slow cell division, increase programmed cell death and repair DNA. Defects (mutations) in these genes can make them inactive, allowing a cell and its offspring to divide rapidly and grow out of control. The gene defects may be passed on from one generation to the next (inherited) or develop during a person's lifetime.

• **Oncogenes.** Oncogenes are genes that normally stimulate cell division but in a properly regulated way. When these genes become abnormally active, they allow for excessive cell growth.

• **Mismatch repair genes.** When DNA is duplicated — a part of the normal process of cell division — errors can occur. There's a complex apparatus, known as the DNA mismatch repair system, that's designed to detect and repair these mistakes. Individuals who inherit defects in this mismatch repair system have a higher likelihood of developing certain cancers, such as colon, uterine or ovarian cancer.

A long process

Cancer development is a process. It has a beginning and a number of steps that must occur for the cancer to progress and become a lethal threat. The first stage, called initiation, involves damage to critical areas of a cell's DNA. The cell can then reproduce abnormal versions of itself.

As cancer cells reproduce, they can become very adaptable. New generations acquire properties that give them an advantage in growth, helping them compete with normal cells for nutrients, so the tumor becomes larger and more destructive. This is the second stage of cancer development, known as progression. The cancer cells are able to evade recognition by the immune system, develop their own blood supply and spread to distant areas.

Several years often pass between the time a single abnormal cell divides and a cancer is detectable. By the time a tumor is large enough to be felt as a lump or seen on an imaging test, it probably contains at least 1 billion cells.

Causes

The exact causes of many cancers aren't yet known. And for most cancers, it's likely that a complex interplay of factors is involved, rather than a single cause. These factors can be divided into two groups:

- **External factors.** These are outside influences on the body, including lifestyle and environmental factors. External factors associated with cancer include tobacco use, excessive use of alcohol, an unhealthy diet, a sedentary lifestyle, radiation from the sun and other sources, and exposure to certain chemicals, such as benzene or asbestos. Some cancers are caused by infections. For example, the human papillomavirus (HPV) contributes to cervical, vaginal and vulvar cancers.
- **Internal factors.** These include hormone levels, inherited genetic factors, immune conditions and lifestyle factors.

Researchers estimate that 50 to 75 percent of all cancers in the United States result from lifestyle factors. Those most commonly associated with cancer include tobacco and alcohol use, an unhealthy diet, lack of physical activity, and sexual behaviors that may lead to certain sexually transmitted infections.

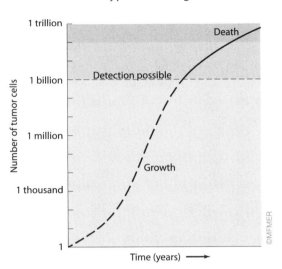

Typical tumor growth

Initially, cancer cells grow rapidly. But it still takes several years before a tumor is large enough to be detected. When it contains approximately 1 billion cells, growth may slow because the tumor is outgrowing its nutrient or oxygen supply or the cells are so abnormal they can no longer divide properly.

Data from Alberts B, et al. *Molecular Biology of the Cell*. 5th ed. New York, N.Y.: Garland Science; 2008:1205.

Risk factors

Features that increase a person's chance of developing cancer are called risk factors. Identifying risk factors points the way to possible causes of cancer. For example, the observation that lung cancer occurs more frequently among smokers led to research that identified cancer-causing agents (carcinogens) in cigarette smoke.

A number of risk factors for cancer have been identified, although it's not known exactly how some of these factors cause cells to become cancerous.

Having a risk factor or a combination of risk factors means you have a greater than average chance of getting cancer, but it doesn't mean that you'll definitely get it. Many people who develop cancer don't have any of the known risk factors for that specific cancer, while other people who do have risk factors never get cancer.

Following are some of the common risk factors for cancer.

Age

For the large majority of cancers, age is the most significant risk factor. Simply stated, the older you are, the more likely you are to get cancer. People older than age 55 develop 80 percent of all new cancer cases. Age might contribute to cancer for several reasons:

- The natural process of aging leads to changes in the body's cells. Over time, as cells divide, problems with the replication of genetic material may occur. Some genes may mistakenly be turned off, and others may be altered in a way that changes how they function, allowing cancer cells to form and take hold.
- Another theory suggests that immune function declines with age, so people may lose some of their natural ability to fight cancer.
- Yet another factor may be that as people live longer, they're exposed to cancer-causing substances for a longer period of time.

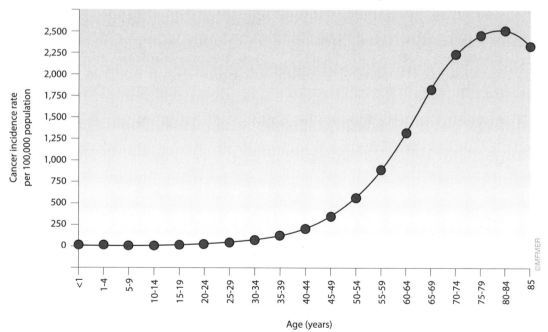

Increasing cancer risk with age

Cancer is relatively uncommon in young adults. It becomes considerably more common once people reach age 70.

Source: Surveillance, Epidemiology, and End Results (SEER) data, National Cancer Institute, 2011.

Family history

People who have close relatives with cancer may be at higher risk of the disease. For example, a woman whose mother or sister had breast cancer is about twice as likely to develop the disease.

In some families, cancer is linked to an inherited mutation in a specific gene, such as BRCA1 or BRCA2 (see Chapter 5). But families with such gene mutations are uncommon. Cancer risk is more likely to be familial than inherited. Familial means that something occurs more commonly in a particular family, but it isn't related to passage of a single cancer-causing gene. Familial cancer may be due to environmental or lifestyle similarities shared by family members, more subtle genetic effects, or a combination of these.

Others

Other risk factors associated with cancer include tobacco use, obesity, a sedentary lifestyle, exposure to radiation, excessive alcohol use, use of hormones after menopause, exposure to certain chemicals, race, socio-economic status, certain health conditions, and reproductive and sexual behaviors. Risk factors for cancers discussed in this book are described in more detail in subsequent chapters.

Advancing Our Knowledge of Cancer

"Without research, there is no hope," wrote Paul Rogers, sponsor of the legislation that launched the war on cancer in 1971. Since the passage of the National Cancer Act that same year, endless hours have been spent learning more about the disease. This growing body of scientific knowledge has resulted in major strides in our understanding of cancer and its detection and treatment, offering hope for more discoveries in the future.

QUESTION & ANSWER

Q: **Does *genetic* mean the same thing as *inherited*?**

A: The words *genetic* and *inherited* are often used interchangeably, but the two words have different meanings.

Genetic refers to a cell's genes, or DNA. Inherited means something that's passed from one person to his or her descendants. A gene can have a defect (mutation), and that mutation can be inherited. About 5 to 10 percent of cancers are clearly hereditary, with the inherited susceptibility passing from parent to child. An individual born with a defective gene inherited from a parent is generally at a much higher risk of a particular cancer than is the general population.

More commonly, though, gene alterations associated with cancer development aren't inherited. Rather, the mutations develop in the body's cells over the course of a lifetime.

Many different types of scientists are engaged in cancer research. They include individuals who study the molecules that make up living matter (molecular biologists) and scientists who study the chemical makeup of living matter (organic chemists). Physiologists study the functions and vital processes of organisms, and biochemists conduct research in the chemistry of life processes. Epidemiologists examine the frequency and distribution of cancer within populations along with certain factors that appear to influence those particular patterns. Pharmacologists study how drugs work. Clinical researchers move basic fundamental discoveries into the clinical setting.

The research process is complicated, time-consuming and costly, and the outcome is never known at the outset.

Basic research

Basic research lies at the heart of scientific discovery. Research independently conceived and developed by scientists has often been the driving force behind medical advances. Basic research provides insights into how cancer starts, and it offers clues regarding key steps involved in cancer progression.

Through basic research, scientists can:
- Explore how errors in genes and proteins disrupt normal cellular communication and regulation and lead to uncontrolled growth of abnormal cells
- Learn which genes and proteins play key roles in cancer invasion and spread
- Identify the ways neighboring cells and tissues contribute to tumor growth
- Develop and test new approaches to prevent, detect and monitor cancer

QUESTION & ANSWER

Q: What types of radiation exposure contribute to cancer?

A: Some forms of radiation exposure are linked to a higher risk of cancer. One familiar example is ultraviolet (UV) radiation from sunlight or tanning lamps. UV radiation exposure is a risk factor for skin cancer, especially in light-skinned people.

Being exposed to large amounts of X-ray (ionizing) radiation also can increase cancer risk. For example, women who received radiation to the chest area to treat Hodgkin disease or tuberculosis have an increased risk of breast cancer. This is particularly true for women who received radiation to their chests during their teenage and young adult years when breast tissue was developing.

In comparison, the small amount of X-ray exposure you get from occasional dental exams or ordinary diagnostic exams, such as chest X-rays or mammograms, doesn't appear to pose a significant health risk.

- Develop new drugs and technologies for treating cancer
- Conduct laboratory and animal tests of new drugs

Epidemiologic studies

Epidemiologists look at trends in cancer frequency (incidence) and death (mortality) rates, and they study patterns of cancer in the population to identify risk factors and protective factors. They compile statistics, such as the number of estimated new cases of cancer, annual deaths from cancer, the most common cancers in men and women, cancer rates among various age groups, and cancer occurrence in various racial and ethnic groups. The findings from this research provide important clues about what contributes to the development of cancer.

Epidemiologists conduct studies that may be either retrospective or prospective in nature. A retrospective study goes back in time and evaluates a group of people who previously had a procedure or a type of exposure. A prospective study evaluates participants going forward in time and follows them for certain outcomes of interest. Both types of studies have different strengths and limitations.

Clinical trials

Clinical trials are research studies in humans that test new approaches for diagnosis, treatment and prevention. These studies are used in all areas of medicine.

Today's cancer treatments are based on the results of past clinical trials. Doctors all over the world conduct many types of clinical trials to study ways to prevent, detect, diagnose and treat cancer, as well as to understand and treat the psychological effects of the disease and to improve comfort and quality of life.

The importance of clinical trials can be seen in how surgery is used to treat breast cancer. In 1970, the treatment for virtually all women with localized breast cancer was the same: radical mastectomy. Clinical trials then compared that approach with less extensive surgery

combined with radiation therapy. The results were comparable, and women had another option for treatment. Clinical trials also showed that shorter durations of chemotherapy were just as effective as the yearlong treatment that women with breast cancer used to receive.

All clinical trials begin with a basic ethical question: Do the potential benefits of a particular treatment outweigh the potential harm from it? When researchers believe that a treatment or prevention approach may be valuable to the patient, a clinical trial is conducted.

Phases of clinical trials
A clinical trial involves a long and careful process. Before a new treatment or preventive approach can be administered to humans, researchers must conduct experiments under controlled circumstances in a laboratory, using test tubes and animals. Scientists analyze a treatment's physical and chemical properties in the lab and study its pharmacologic and toxic effects in animals to determine its possible effectiveness and harm. This type of evaluation, which can take several years, is called preclinical research.

If the preclinical research shows promising results, investigators may request permission to begin clinical trials by filing an application with the Food and Drug Administration. If the application is approved, researchers can begin to investigate the new therapy in people. A new treatment is normally studied in three phases of clinical trials.

Phase I
Phase I trials are the first tests of a new treatment in humans. The goal is to gather

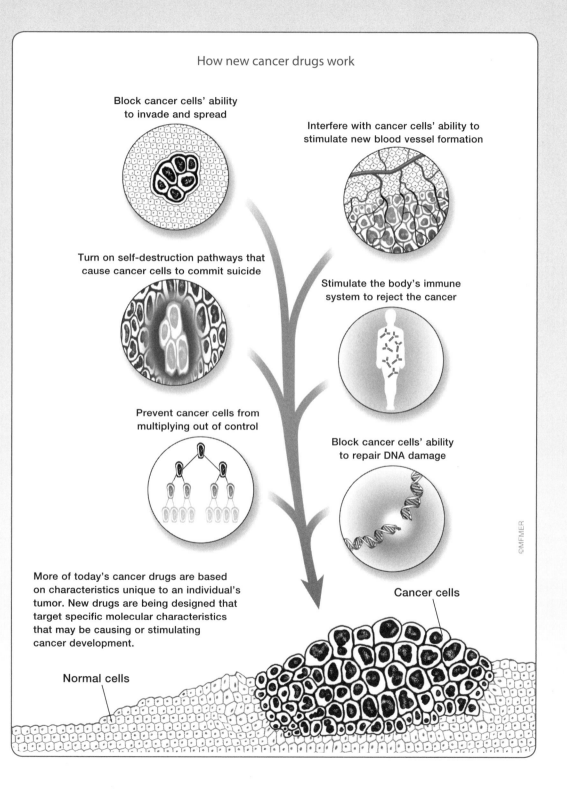

How new cancer drugs work

Block cancer cells' ability
to invade and spread

Interfere with cancer cells' ability to
stimulate new blood vessel formation

Turn on self-destruction pathways that
cause cancer cells to commit suicide

Stimulate the body's immune
system to reject the cancer

Prevent cancer cells from
multiplying out of control

Block cancer cells' ability
to repair DNA damage

More of today's cancer drugs are based
on characteristics unique to an individual's
tumor. New drugs are being designed that
target specific molecular characteristics
that may be causing or stimulating
cancer development.

Cancer cells

Normal cells

©MFMER

Enrolling in a Clinical Trial

By taking part in a clinical trial, you may have the first chance to benefit from new approaches to cancer prevention and treatment. And you'll be making a contribution to medical science while taking an active role in your own health care.

Depending on the type of trial, you may receive a current, accepted treatment, a new treatment being evaluated or a combination of the two.

In a clinical trial, no one involved in the study knows in advance if the new treatment will work or exactly what side effects or adverse reactions might occur. In addition, the trial may require some extra time for trips to the study site, treatments, hospital stays, or complex dosage requirements. Participants may be required to keep detailed records of any symptoms they may experience and to follow certain schedules and guidelines.

The best place to start in finding a clinical trial is to talk with your doctor. Doctors are usually aware of investigational drugs that might benefit their patients and clinical trials involving these drugs. You can also get a list of current clinical trials by contacting the National Cancer Institute's Cancer Information Service. For more information on clinical trials resources, see page 413.

information on the safest and most effective dose and the schedule for giving it. Doctors monitor participants carefully for any harmful side effects. These trials generally last several months to a year and involve a small number of patients, usually no more than 20 to 40.

Phase II
Once the appropriate dose and schedule are known, a phase II trial of the new therapy is done. Phase II trials are designed to see if a therapy has a biological effect in treating a specific cancer. In addition to testing for effectiveness, researchers also gather more detailed information about safety. Phase II trials take about two years and usually include 20 to 40 participants. At times, multiple phase II trials are done for a promising new agent.

Phase III
The goal of phase III trials is to compare a promising new approach with the most accepted current treatment. Researchers want to learn if the new treatment is more effective, less toxic, less expensive or can be given over a shorter period of time. Phase III trials involve large numbers of individuals, sometimes thousands of people from hundreds of research centers around the country or the world.

Participants in phase III trials are randomly assigned (randomized) into one of two or more groups. One group, the control group, receives the standard treatment. The other, the investigational group, receives the new treatment.

In double-blind trials neither the participant nor the doctor knows which treatment the person is receiving, to avoid bias. In other clinical trials, both the par-

RESEARCH UPDATE

Genomics and proteomics

Two important areas of ongoing cancer research are genomics and proteomics.

Genomics is the study of the human genome — the complete set of approximately 25,000 genes in a human being. The completion of the Human Genome Project was an enormous advance in genomics. It resulted in a map that details the sequence of chemical base pairs (nucleotides) that make up the 6 feet of tightly coiled DNA contained in each human cell. The map shows genetic landmarks along each of the chromosomes, including the locations of genes that are altered in various cancers. Information about particular genes can help identify key molecular targets for cancer diagnosis and treatment.

As work continues on refining the map of the human genome, the next frontier is proteomics, the study of human proteins. The word stems from the term *proteome*, which refers to the complete array of human proteins.

Although genes carry the instructions for making proteins, proteins are the actual players that carry out the cell's activities. Proteomics aims to evaluate the structure, function and expression of proteins. This is a huge task. The approximate 25,000 genes can be expressed in cells in different ways to produce millions of different proteins. Only a minority of them have been identified.

A major goal of proteomics is to diagram the "protein wiring" (signaling) pathways that control cell growth and activity.

ticipant and the doctor know which treatment the participant is receiving.

Researchers try to ensure that individuals in the investigational and control groups are as similar as possible in characteristics that could affect treatment outcomes. For instance, in most studies, patients in both groups should have the same type and stage of cancer.

Once a new approach has been proved successful in phase III trials, the approach becomes part of the standard treatment.

Patient safety

Patient safety is of utmost priority in clinical trials. Investigators must follow strict guidelines. Clinical trials are subject to a rigorous review, and there are oversight processes designed to protect the rights and safety of people who enroll.

Several groups have to approve the treatment procedure used in a clinical trial. These groups of experts and laypeople also review the ongoing research.

In addition, all participants in clinical trials must provide informed consent. When an individual becomes interested in a clinical trial, he or she is provided key facts about the study, including the possible risks and benefits of the treatment, or treatments, being evaluated. Before that individual can enroll in the study, he or she needs to indicate, in written form, awareness of the possible risks and benefits involved. Participants are free to leave a clinical trial at any time.

How research is paying off

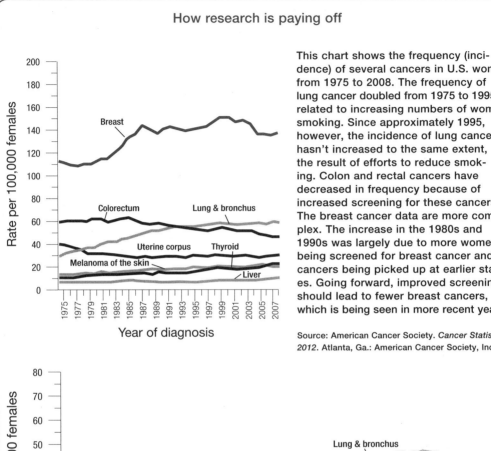

This chart shows the frequency (incidence) of several cancers in U.S. women from 1975 to 2008. The frequency of lung cancer doubled from 1975 to 1995, related to increasing numbers of women smoking. Since approximately 1995, however, the incidence of lung cancer hasn't increased to the same extent, the result of efforts to reduce smoking. Colon and rectal cancers have decreased in frequency because of increased screening for these cancers. The breast cancer data are more complex. The increase in the 1980s and 1990s was largely due to more women being screened for breast cancer and cancers being picked up at earlier stages. Going forward, improved screening should lead to fewer breast cancers, which is being seen in more recent years.

Source: American Cancer Society. *Cancer Statistics, 2012*. Atlanta, Ga.: American Cancer Society, Inc.

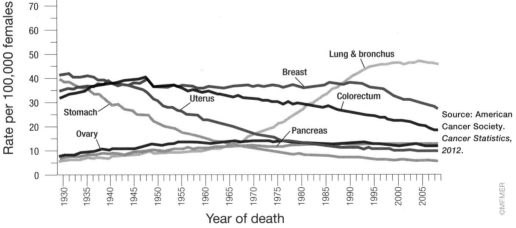

Source: American Cancer Society. *Cancer Statistics, 2012*.

This chart shows the number of deaths from several cancers in U.S. women from 1930 to 2008. The most dramatic curve is that for lung cancer, indicating how increased tobacco use changed a once-uncommon cancer (lung and bronchus) to the most deadly cancer in American women. Fortunately, research efforts in smoking cessation and the prevention of tobacco use have halted the dramatic increase in women's deaths from this disease. The deaths from breast cancer have been on the decline since the late 1980s. This decline is due to two major factors: increased screening to find cancers before they become deadly and improved treatments.

Visual Guide

Cancer biology

The normal functioning of a cell is
controlled at many levels, including
its surface (cell membrane), interior
(cytoplasm) and growth control center
(nucleus). Changes that may lead to
cancer development and growth can
occur at any of these levels.

Cell membrane
At the cell surface, chemical messengers that signal a cell to divide (growth
factors) and nutrients bind to receptors on the cell surface. Cancer cells
overexpress receptors that capture
growth factors and nutrients.

Cytoplasm
Signals from growth factors are sent
to the cell nucleus by way of a cas-
cading series of so-called secondary
messengers. Cancer cells can cause
numerous growth-promoting changes
in these signaling pathways.

Nucleus
Within the tightly coiled DNA of each
cell are the genetic instructions to make
all of the proteins a cell needs to carry
out its work. Which genes are turned on
depends on the signals received from the
cytoplasm, conveyed by transcription factors. Transcription factors bind to the DNA
of targeted genes.
  Cell division is controlled within the nucleus,
too. Before a cell can divide, it must pass through a
tightly governed cycle with several checkpoints. This is
to ensure that an injured cell doesn't divide until damaged
DNA has been repaired. Cancer cells lack these checkpoint
mechanisms, allowing altered cells to grow and proliferate.

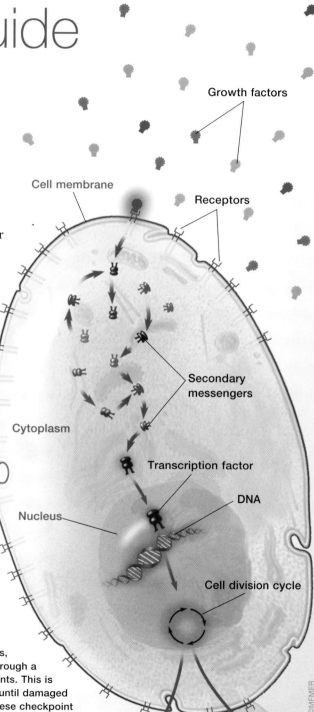

Growth factors

Cell membrane

Receptors

Secondary messengers

Cytoplasm

Transcription factor

DNA

Nucleus

Cell division cycle

©MFMER

Cancer development

Cancer is characterized by the overgrowth of abnormal cells, a multistep process called carcinogenesis. Over time, the abnormal cells accumulate into a mass, called a growth or tumor, that can invade nearby normal tissue and spread.

Atypical hyperplasia
As the excess cells stack upon one another, some start taking on an abnormal appearance.

Hyperplasia
The intricate system of cell development and growth is disrupted, causing an overproduction of normal-appearing cells.

Normal cell
Normal cells grow and divide in an orderly fashion.

Abnormal cells

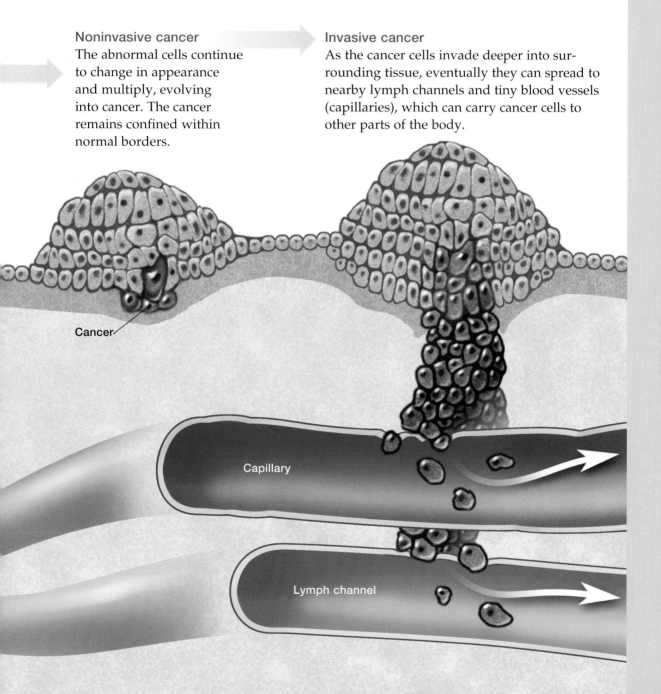

Noninvasive cancer
The abnormal cells continue to change in appearance and multiply, evolving into cancer. The cancer remains confined within normal borders.

Invasive cancer
As the cancer cells invade deeper into surrounding tissue, eventually they can spread to nearby lymph channels and tiny blood vessels (capillaries), which can carry cancer cells to other parts of the body.

Cancer

Capillary

Lymph channel

Breast cancer stages

Stage I

Stage II

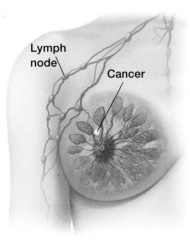
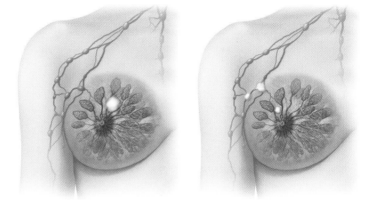

Cancer is 2 centimeters (cm) in size or less with no spread to the lymph nodes.*

Cancer is 2.1 cm to 5 cm in size, or has spread to up to three lymph nodes under the arm or to lymph nodes under the sternum, or both. Cancer greater than 5 cm with no spread to the lymph nodes is also stage II.

Stage III

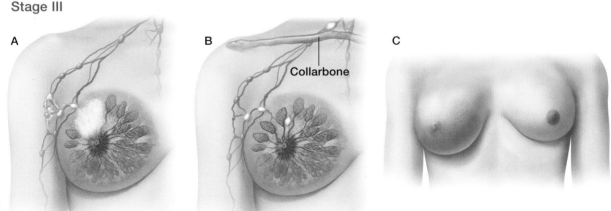

Stage III cancers include a number of criteria that make it a broad category. Here are three examples: tumor greater than 5 cm in size with involvement of at least one lymph node under the arm (A); spread to lymph nodes above the collarbone (B); spread to breast skin causing swelling and redness, known as inflammatory breast cancer (C).

*Lymph nodes containing cells that look like they came from the breast but are less than 0.2 mm are considered negative lymph nodes because there's no good evidence these are established cancers.

©MFMER

Stage IV
Cancer has spread to
distant sites, such as the
lungs, liver or bone.

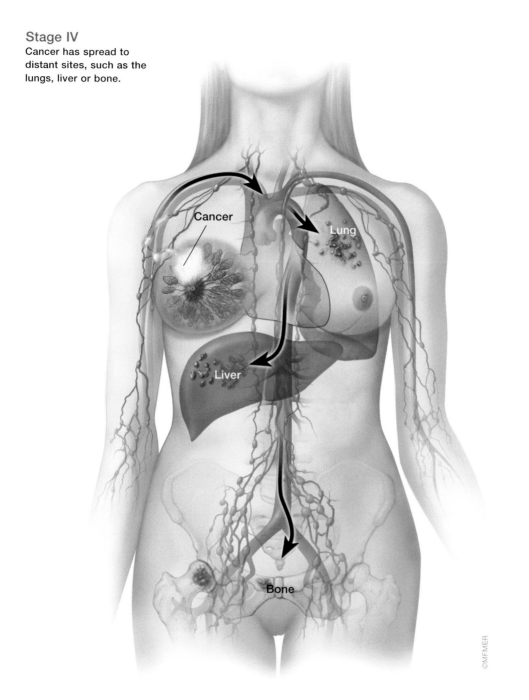

Cancer cells from a breast tumor can spread throughout the body by way of the tiny blood vessels (capillaries), which empty into veins, and by way of lymph channels, which drain into lymph nodes. Fluid and cancer cells from the lymphatic system eventually empty into large veins, which in turn empty into the heart. From the heart, cancer cells can spread to the rest of the body by way of the arteries.

Sentinel node biopsy

In this procedure, a dye is injected into the area of the tumor. The dye is absorbed into nearby lymph channels. The first lymph nodes to collect the dye, called the sentinel nodes, likely are the first to receive drainage from the breast tumor. The sentinel nodes are removed and examined for cancer cells. A small amount of radioactive material may be used instead of a dye, or a combination of the two.

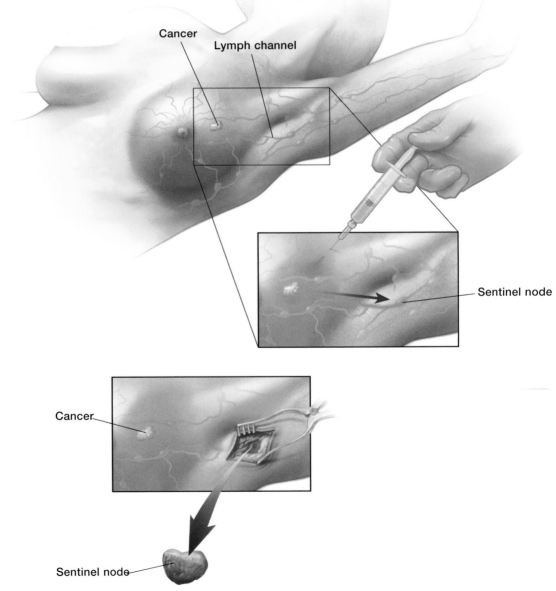

Cancer

Lymph channel

Sentinel node

Cancer

Sentinel node

Surgery

The two main types of surgery to treat breast cancer are a lumpectomy (left), in which only the tumor is removed, and a mastectomy (right), in which the entire breast is removed.

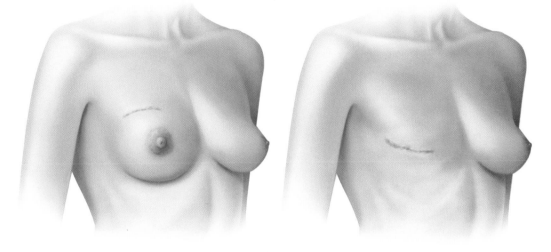

Radiation therapy

Radiation therapy uses a high-energy radiation source to kill cancer cells or interfere with their ability to grow and divide.

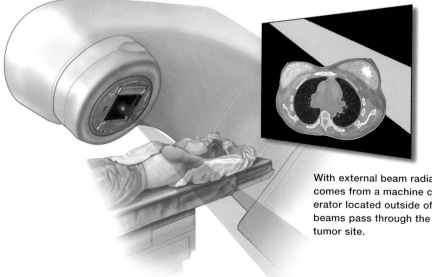

With external beam radiation, the radiation comes from a machine called a linear accelerator located outside of the body. Radiation beams pass through the skin to reach the tumor site.

Drug therapy

Medications (therapeutic agents) that kill or slow down cancer cells work at many sites within the cell. They can interfere with processes at the cell membrane. They can block the signaling cascades occurring within the cytoplasm that stimulate cell growth and division. And they can interfere with the normal functioning of DNA so that new proteins can't be made and new cells can't be formed.

Cell membrane

Medications that act at the outer layer of a cell (cell membrane) block the binding of growth factors to their receptors. Or they bind to the receptors but inhibit their activation. This prevents the transmission of growth signals to the interior of the cancer cell. The drug trastuzumab (Herceptin) is an example. It's a monoclonal antibody that binds to HER2 (also called erbB2), a growth factor receptor on the cell membrane, shutting down the receptor. Other medications being tested inhibit the erbB1 receptor, or both erbB1 and erbB2.

Cytoplasm

Several new cancer therapies target the secondary messengers within a cell that transmit growth signals from the cell membrane to the nucleus.

Nucleus

Many medications work directly at the nucleus, the control center of the cell. Most chemotherapy medications, for example, interfere with the function of DNA. Some drugs bind directly to DNA, preventing it from unfolding to manufacture proteins or to be duplicated to produce new cancer cells. Other chemotherapy drugs cause breaks in the DNA structure and inhibit the enzymes needed to repair the damage. Still other medications block the protein scaffolding that oversees cell division. The drug tamoxifen interferes with the ability of the receptor for the hormone estrogen to act as a transcription factor and turn on relevant downstream genes. Other agents work within the nucleus to induce cancer cells to undergo cell death.

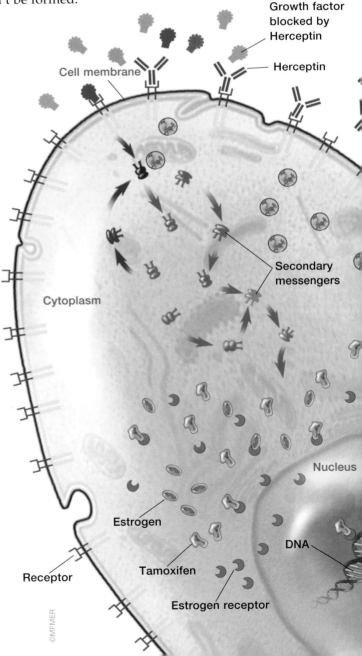

Growth factor blocked by Herceptin

Herceptin

Cell membrane

Secondary messengers

Cytoplasm

Nucleus

Estrogen

DNA

Receptor

Tamoxifen

Estrogen receptor

©MFMER

PART 2

Breast Cancer

Chapter 3: Breast Cancer

An Overview

Your Breasts	45
Breast Cancer	45
Types of breast cancer	47
Cancer growth and spread	49
What Causes Breast Cancer?	49
Genetic factors	50
Hormonal and reproductive factors	52
Environmental factors	53
Aging	54
How Common Is Breast Cancer?	54
Advancing Science	57
DNA	58
Proteins	58
Angiogenesis	60

If you've been diagnosed with breast cancer, take heart that what used to be a dismal diagnosis often no longer is. Yes, breast cancer is a serious illness, and, yes, it can be fatal. But in larger numbers than ever before, women are surviving the disease and living productive lives.

Perhaps no other disease has a greater hold on a woman's fears than does breast cancer. It's not the deadliest cancer women can get — lung cancer is. And it's not the most common life-threatening illness to affect women — that's heart disease. But ask a group of women what disease they worry about most, and the majority will likely say breast cancer.

This fear isn't unfounded. Breast cancer is the most common life-threatening cancer among women in the United States. It's the second most common cause of cancer death in women and the main cause of cancer death in women ages 40 to 55. Most women know someone who has had breast cancer — a friend, sister, mother, other relative or an acquaintance.

The disease strikes close to home in other ways as well. It can affect how a woman looks and feels about her femininity and sexuality. Many women who have breast cancer are afraid that changes in their bodies will affect not only their appearance but also the way other people perceive them.

Yet there's more cause for optimism with regard to breast cancer today than ever before. In the last 40 years, scientists have learned much more about how and why breast cancer develops and have made tremendous strides in diagnosis and treatment. Research has led to better treatments, a lower chance of death from the disease and an improved quality of life for the millions of breast cancer survivors, including women living with recurrent breast cancer.

In 1970, breast cancer was more likely to be diagnosed at a late stage, and treatment usually involved a radical mastectomy — removal of the entire breast along with underarm lymph nodes and muscles underneath the breast. Chemotherapy after surgery typically lasted a whole year.

Today, breast cancer is often detected in its early stages with a mammogram, and a radical mastectomy is rarely done anymore. Many women choose breast-sparing treatments, such as lumpectomy and radiation, and, when needed, they go through a shorter course of chemotherapy. In addition, a growing network of organizations and other supportive resources exists to help women and their loved ones who are grappling with this disease.

This chapter provides an overview of what's known about breast cancer, its causes and the women who develop it. Subsequent chapters look at risk factors, prevention, diagnosis, treatment and survivorship.

Benign Breast Conditions

A lump or thickening in the breast is the most common sign of breast cancer. That's why feeling a lump or a change in your breasts can be a scary experience. However, most breast lumps (masses) are benign, meaning that they're not cancerous. A variety of conditions other than breast cancer can produce lumps in your breasts and cause your breasts to change in size or how they feel.

Following are some common benign breast conditions. Remember, though, if you're concerned about a lump or a change in how a breast feels, make an appointment to see your doctor. It's best to have the lump evaluated, even if it turns out to be a benign problem.

- **Fibrocystic breast changes.** Fibrocystic breast changes are common, occurring in at least half the women in the U.S. *Fibro* refers to the presence of fibrous connective tissue, and *cystic* refers to cysts, which are fluid-filled sacs. You may feel a bumpy texture or lumpiness in your breasts, along with swelling, tenderness or pain, most likely just before your menstrual period. You may also experience fibrocystic changes if you're postmenopausal and taking hormones.

- **Cysts.** These are fluid-filled sacs that feel like a soft lump or tender spot. They're found most often in women ages 35 to 50. Cysts can range from tiny to about the size of an egg. They may change in size with your period.

- **Fibroadenomas.** Fibroadenomas are solid, noncancerous tumors that most often occur in women during their reproductive years. The tumors are generally painless. They may feel

Your Breasts

Breasts are composed mainly of connective and fatty tissues. Suspended within the tissues of each breast is a network of milk-forming lobes. Within each lobe are many smaller lobules, each of which ends in dozens of tiny bulbs that can produce milk. Thin tubes called ducts connect the bulbs, lobules and lobes to the nipple, which is surrounded by an area of dark skin, called the areola. No muscles are in the breasts themselves, but muscles covering your ribs lie underneath each breast.

Blood vessels and lymph vessels run throughout your breasts. Blood nourishes breast cells. Lymph vessels carry a clear fluid called lymph, which contains immune system cells and drains waste products from tissues. Lymph vessels lead to pea-sized collections of tissue called lymph nodes. Most of the lymph vessels in the breast lead to lymph nodes under the arm, called axillary nodes.

Breast Cancer

Breast cancer is the common term for a cancerous (malignant) tumor that starts in cells that line the ducts and lobes of the breast. If the cancerous cells are smooth or rubbery and may move easily under your skin when touched.

- **Benign breast disease.** This term is generally used in reference to women who have had a breast biopsy that resulted in benign findings. The majority of these findings are not worrisome. For women with hyperplasia or atypical hyperplasia, however, there is some increased risk of later breast cancer (see Chapters 4 and 9).
- **Infections.** Infection of the breast (mastitis) typically affects women who are breast-feeding or who recently stopped breast-feeding, although it's also possible to develop mastitis that's not related to breast-feeding. Your breast will likely be red, warm, tender and lumpy, and the lymph nodes under your arms may swell. You may also feel slightly ill and may have a low-grade fever.
- **Trauma.** Sometimes, a blow to the breast or a bruise can produce a lump. This doesn't mean you're more likely to get breast cancer.
- **Calcium deposits (microcalcifications).** Tiny deposits of calcium can appear anywhere within your breast. They often appear as white spots or flecks on a mammogram and are usually so small that you can't feel them. Most women have one or more areas of calcium deposits. Cellular secretions and debris or inflammation may cause them. The majority of calcium deposits are harmless, but a small percentage may be associated with cancer. Calcium deposits don't result from calcium in your diet or taking calcium supplements.

Breast anatomy

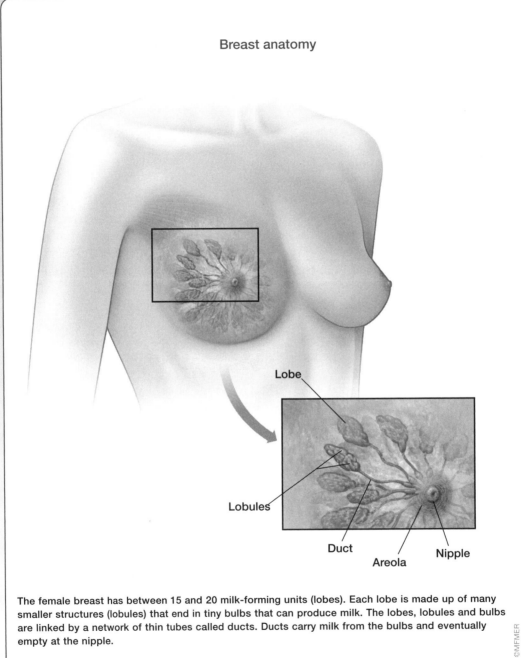

The female breast has between 15 and 20 milk-forming units (lobes). Each lobe is made up of many smaller structures (lobules) that end in tiny bulbs that can produce milk. The lobes, lobules and bulbs are linked by a network of thin tubes called ducts. Ducts carry milk from the bulbs and eventually empty at the nipple.

©MFMER

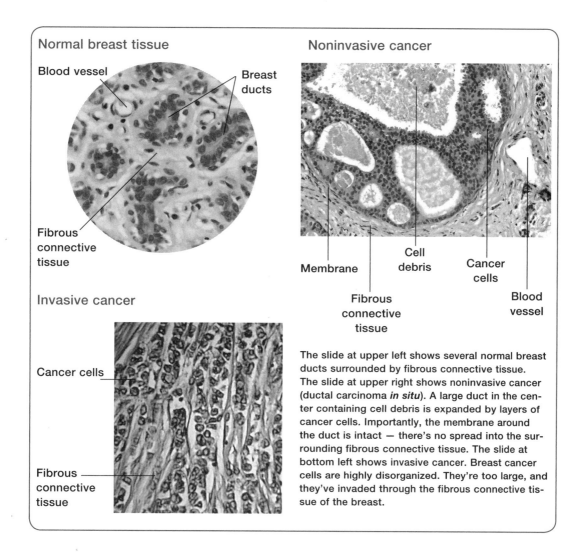

Normal breast tissue

Blood vessel

Breast ducts

Fibrous connective tissue

Noninvasive cancer

Membrane

Fibrous connective tissue

Cell debris

Cancer cells

Blood vessel

Invasive cancer

Cancer cells

Fibrous connective tissue

The slide at upper left shows several normal breast ducts surrounded by fibrous connective tissue. The slide at upper right shows noninvasive cancer (ductal carcinoma *in situ*). A large duct in the center containing cell debris is expanded by layers of cancer cells. Importantly, the membrane around the duct is intact — there's no spread into the surrounding fibrous connective tissue. The slide at bottom left shows invasive cancer. Breast cancer cells are highly disorganized. They're too large, and they've invaded through the fibrous connective tissue of the breast.

confined to the ducts or lobules and haven't invaded surrounding breast tissue, the cancer is called noninvasive, or *in situ*. Cancer that has spread through the walls of the ducts or lobules into connective or fatty tissue is referred to as invasive, or infiltrating.

Types of breast cancer

Breast cancer is categorized by the microscopic appearance of the cancer cells and by whether the cancer has invaded surrounding tissue. Following is a list of the most common types of breast cancer:

- **Invasive ductal carcinoma (IDC).** This type of cancer begins in a breast duct, breaks through the duct wall and then invades the connective or fatty tissue of the breast. There, it can gain access to blood vessels, allowing it to spread to other locations in the body. Invasive ductal carcinoma is the most common type of breast cancer. It

Breast Cancer at the Molecular Level

Genomic research has given us insights into the makeup of breast cancer cells, down to the molecules — their genes and proteins — that are driving them. There are at least four major molecular subtypes, including:

- **Luminal A.** This category accounts for 45 to 60 percent of breast cancers. They are estrogen receptor (ER) positive and progesterone receptor (PR) positive. (See page 142 for more on hormone receptor status.) They tend to be slow growing.
- **Luminal B.** These account for 10 to 15 percent of breast cancers. They are ER positive, PR positive or negative, and human epidermal growth factor receptor 2 (HER2) positive (see page 142). They tend to be faster growing.
- **HER2.** This category makes up about 10 percent of breast cancers. They are ER and PR negative and HER2 positive.
- **Triple negative/basal-like.** This category includes 10 to 15 percent of breast cancers. They are ER, PR and HER2 negative.

  In addition to differences in ER, PR and HER2, these cancer subtypes differ in their expression of many other genes and proteins. Researchers are working to define how best to use molecular subtyping in deciding which treatment to recommend for a particular individual.

represents about 75 percent of all invasive breast cancers.
- **Invasive lobular carcinoma (ILC).** This cancer starts in the lobules, breaks through to the connective or fatty tissue of the breast and can spread to other parts of the body as well. ILC accounts for about 15 percent of invasive breast cancers.
- **Other invasive cancers.** In addition to IDC and ILC, there are several less common types of breast cancer, including medullary, mucinous, tubular and papillary. These cancers account for the last 10 percent of invasive cancers.
- **Ductal carcinoma *in situ* (DCIS).** This is the most common type of noninvasive breast cancer. The abnormal cells have not spread through the walls of the ducts into the connective and fatty tissues of the breast. But if these cells aren't removed, they may develop into an invasive cancer that can spread.
- **Lobular carcinoma *in situ* (LCIS).** In this condition, the abnormal cells haven't spread beyond the lobules, and they usually don't develop into invasive cancer. For this reason, LCIS isn't considered a true cancer. However, women with LCIS are at increased risk of developing invasive breast cancer later on, in either breast. Therefore, LCIS is seen as an important marker for breast cancer risk.
- **Paget's disease.** Paget's disease is a type of breast cancer that's associated with nipple changes. The underlying cancer can be invasive or noninvasive.

  More detailed information regarding breast cancer types can be found in Chapter 8.

Cancer spread

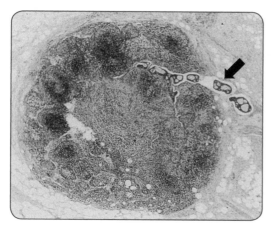

Metastatic breast cancer occurs when breast cancer cells spread to other parts of the body. The cells use lymphatic vessels and blood vessels as a means of travel to other areas. This microscopic image shows cancer cells (see arrow) entering a lymph node through a lymphatic channel.

Source: *New England Journal of Medicine.* Reprinted with permission.

Cancer growth and spread

When cancer develops in breast tissue and spreads outside the breast, cancer cells are often found in the underarm (axillary) lymph nodes. The ability of cancer cells to spread to these nodes means that the cancer has the capacity to spread to other parts of the body as well. That's why axillary nodes are examined as part of the process of determining the extent of the disease (staging).

If breast cancer spreads to other parts of the body, it's called metastatic breast cancer. Common sites for breast cancer cells to spread include the lymph nodes, skin on the chest wall, bones, liver and lungs. If, for example, breast cancer spreads to the lungs, the tumor there has the same kind of abnormal cells as the primary breast tumor. Therefore, the disease is called metastatic breast cancer, not lung cancer. It may also be referred to as distant disease.

Breast cancers grow at different rates, but some researchers estimate that the average tumor doubles in size every 100 days. Most tumors aren't large enough to feel or notice for years. In fact, it's estimated that it takes an average of at least five years for most tumors to reach a size where they can be felt. Some tumors have an even longer period in which they're undetectable (latency period).

Mammography is useful in finding tumors that are too small to be felt, but even so, most tumors have probably been growing for years before they're large enough to be visible on a mammogram. However, more aggressive breast cancers grow at a more rapid rate and can even appear in the time between a woman's yearly mammograms. By the time most breast tumors are detected — at approximately 1 centimeter in size — they have about 1 billion cells.

For more information about how cancer develops, see Chapter 2.

What Causes Breast Cancer?

It's often impossible to explain why one woman gets breast cancer and another doesn't. Breast cancer results from a series of events that transform a normal cell to an abnormal one. Multiple factors — known and unknown — contribute to the disease. There's no single cause.

Hallmarks of Hereditary Breast Cancer

What if there are two or three women in your family with breast cancer? Does that mean the cancer is hereditary?

Because breast cancer is a common disease, two or more cases of breast cancer may occur in a family simply by chance. Also, family members share many things in addition to their genes, such as similar diets and environments, weight and height, patterns of childbearing, and occupations.

All of these factors can influence a woman's risk of developing breast cancer, without the presence of an inherited alteration in a specific gene.

Breast cancer that's inherited has certain hallmarks. Some indications that breast cancer in a family may be hereditary include the following:

- Women in each generation are affected.
- Multiple relatives are affected.
- The cancer is diagnosed at an early age — before menopause.
- Some family members also have developed ovarian cancer.
- There's a family history of cancer in both breasts (bilateral breast cancer) or of male breast cancer.
- The same woman has had both breast cancer and ovarian cancer.
- The family is of Ashkenazi Jewish descent.

For more information on hereditary breast cancer, see Chapter 5.

Researchers have identified a number of factors associated with an increased risk of breast cancer. These include genetic, hormonal and environmental factors, as well as aging. These factors are interrelated and can all work together to contribute to cancer development.

Genetic factors

Most cancers, including breast cancer, acquire many genetic abnormalities — alterations to genes or chromosomes — as the cancer develops. In this sense, breast cancer is considered a genetic disease.

But most of the genetic problems seen in breast cancer aren't inherited. Genetic alterations may be either inherited or acquired (spontaneous). Inherited mutations are those you were born with — a defective gene passed on to you through one of your parents. Acquired alterations occur within your body's cells during your lifetime and aren't passed on. They're much more common than are inherited changes.

An acquired genetic error can develop in many ways, and the causes of most of these alterations remain unknown. Most breast cancers appear to result from a variety of spontaneous changes in breast cells that ultimately lead to the development of cancer cells.

Alterations in two types of genes important to cell growth can turn normal cells into cancerous ones.

- **Tumor suppressor genes.** These very important regulatory genes turn off cell growth, stopping cell division and replication. Errors in these genes allow cells to grow out of control. Inherited defects in certain tumor suppressor genes, such as the breast cancer genes BRCA1 and BRCA2, result in a marked predisposition to develop breast cancer.

- **Oncogenes.** These genes turn on (promote) cell division and growth. If this type of gene is damaged or defective, cell growth runs out of control. Several oncogenes have been associated with the development of breast cancer. They include the HER2, EGFR and ras genes. Although abnormalities in these oncogenes can contribute to breast cancer, they're not inherited.

Hereditary breast cancer

An estimated 5 to 10 percent of breast cancers are hereditary — that is, they're caused by inherited alterations in the chemical order of a gene. Individuals from some families inherit and pass on altered genetic material that significantly increases the risk of breast cancer. If your father or mother has an altered gene, you have a 50 percent chance of inheriting that gene from him or her.

For example, inherited mutations in two tumor suppressor genes have been linked to an increased risk of breast cancer. The two most common genes associated with hereditary breast cancer are breast cancer gene 1 (BRCA1) and breast cancer gene 2 (BRCA2). People with defects in these genes have a high risk of developing breast cancer over their lifetimes. Women with an alteration in one of these genes have a 45 to 80 percent lifetime chance of developing breast cancer. Men also can carry a defect in BRCA1 or BRCA2, and when they do, they're at an increased risk of breast cancer. This is especially true for men who inherit a BRCA2 mutation.

The BRCA1 and BRCA2 genes are large, and many different alterations in them have been associated with an increased risk of breast cancer. Defective BRCA1 and BRCA2 genes account for about 40 percent of hereditary forms of breast cancer. Abnormalities in these genes also result in an increased risk of other cancers, especially ovarian cancer.

Miscarriage, Abortion and Fertility Treatments

Because hormonal and reproductive factors are known to influence breast cancer risk, a great deal of research has been conducted to determine whether having a miscarriage or abortion affects a woman's chances of developing breast cancer later. Early studies produced inconsistent results, and most of those studies were small and had scientific flaws. Since then, larger, better designed studies have found no consistent link between miscarriage or abortion and breast cancer.

Researchers have also questioned whether treatments to boost fertility, such as those used during assistive reproductive technology procedures, can contribute to breast cancer development. Women undergoing treatment for infertility are exposed to high concentrations of estrogen and progesterone. Studies indicate that this type of ovarian stimulation doesn't appear to increase a woman's risk of breast cancer.

Several other inherited syndromes also significantly increase risk of breast cancer. These include Li-Fraumeni syndrome, Cowden syndrome and Peutz-Jeghers syndrome. These conditions account for less than 1 percent of all breast cancers. Alterations in other tumor suppressor genes, including p53, PTEN and ATM, are also linked to increased breast cancer risk.

See Chapter 5 for more information on hereditary breast cancer.

Hormonal and reproductive factors

Researchers have long observed that many of the risk factors for breast cancer relate to a woman's lifetime exposure to estrogen and other reproductive hormones. From a woman's first menstrual cycle to the birth of a child to the onset of menopause, the hormones estrogen and progesterone are stimulating breast cells. These hormones are essential for normal breast development and function, but they can also promote breast cancer.

Breast cancer risk is affected to some extent by several reproductive factors that increase the amount of time a woman's body produces or is exposed to estrogen. These include:
• An early age at first menstruation
• A late age at menopause
• Postmenopausal hormone therapy

Women who carry a pregnancy to term at a young age and those who breast-feed have a slightly decreased risk of getting breast cancer. On the other hand, women who don't become pregnant or who become pregnant at a later age have increased breast cancer risks.

Breast Cancer and Stress

Can stress cause breast cancer? The short answer is no, probably not. Most research hasn't found evidence of a direct link between stress and breast cancer. But the belief that emotional or psychological factors can cause cancer is widespread — and it's not a new idea.

Almost 2,000 years ago, the Greek doctor Galen noted that melancholic women were much more susceptible to cancer than were other women. Interest in the mind-body connection and cancer has been renewed in recent decades as scientists gain a better understanding of the complex relationships among the immune system, hormones and the nervous system. Evidence suggests that stress can disturb many components of the immune system and that an impaired immune system may increase a person's risk of cancer. Stress also impacts an individual's endocrine (hormonal) system, increasing or decreasing the secretion of various hormones.

Other researchers have theorized that cancer is more likely to occur in people with certain personality traits — those who suppress their emotions, especially anger, who put others' needs ahead of their own or who have an attitude of helplessness or hopelessness, the so-called cancer-prone (type C) personality.

Environmental factors

Environmental factors also play a role in the development of breast cancer. When used in reference to cancer risk, the word *environment* means more than just the surrounding air, water and land. Environmental factors include anything that isn't inherited or innate, including a woman's diet and lifestyle, where she lives and works, and any exposure to cancer-causing agents (carcinogens).

Research on the rates of breast cancer in different areas of the world suggests that environmental factors do affect cancer risk. For example, breast cancer rates in Asia and Africa are much lower than are those in North America. Yet, when Asians immigrate to the United States, within a couple of generations, the breast cancer rate among their descendants approaches the American rate. In addition, the rate of breast cancer in Japan has gradually increased as the Japanese lifestyle has become more westernized.

Unfortunately, determining which environmental factors contribute to breast cancer and to what extent is neither easy nor straightforward. So far, scientists haven't found many links between specific environmental factors and the risk of breast cancer.

In addition, it can be difficult or impossible to sort out environmental factors and a woman's susceptibility to such factors. For example, breast cancer rates are higher among some professional workers, but this may be because they have later pregnancies or no pregnancies, rather than because of something related to their jobs.

Over the years, researchers have put these theories to the test in a large number of studies investigating whether stressful life events or psychosocial factors play a role in the onset and progression of breast cancer. Results have been inconclusive and contradictory.

A few studies have shown an association between stressful life events, such as divorce, separation or the death of a spouse, close friend or relative, and the development, progression or recurrence of breast cancer. But other studies have shown just the opposite — that stressful life events are *not* associated with breast cancer risk. Similarly, most studies haven't found personality factors to be related to breast cancer risk.

In general, the evidence for a relationship involving psychological and social factors and breast cancer is weak. But because of the small number of high-quality studies on the topic, some researchers say it's not possible to definitively rule out stress as a contributing factor to breast cancer.

The bottom line? If you have breast cancer, don't think that your cancer resulted or recurred because you were unable to deal with life's stresses.

But at the same time, understand that a diagnosis of cancer is bound to create stress. To help you deal with stress, be sure to seek out the help and support you need.

Nonetheless, researchers have identified some lifestyle and environmental factors that appear to affect a woman's chance of developing breast cancer. They include:

- **A sedentary lifestyle.** Some data suggest that women who are physically inactive may have a mildly increased risk of breast cancer.
- **Excessive alcohol use.** Studies show that women who drink more than one alcoholic drink a day have a greater risk of developing breast cancer than do nondrinkers or those who drink less than one drink a day.
- **Excess body weight.** Being overweight or obese has been shown to increase the risk of postmenopausal breast cancer.
- **Radiation exposure.** Women whose breasts have been exposed to significant X-ray (ionizing) radiation — such as women who received radiation to their chest lymph nodes to treat Hodgkin disease — have an increased risk of breast cancer. The amount of radiation necessary to increase risk is much greater than that which accompanies yearly mammograms.

Researchers have also conducted studies to determine whether pesticides, pollution or on-the-job exposure to hazardous agents may contribute to breast cancer. Most of the evidence is inconclusive. For more information on breast cancer risk factors, see Chapter 4.

Aging

Increasing age is a major risk factor for breast cancer. One reason the disease is more common now than it was 100 years ago is that women are living almost twice as long (see Chapter 2). Breast cancer is uncommon among women under age 30, but your risk of getting it increases as you get older. Seventy-five percent of breast cancers occur in women older than age 50.

The National Cancer Institute estimates that about 1 in 8 women in the United States will develop breast cancer at some point during her lifetime. But this figure is somewhat misleading because it refers to the risk a woman has during her entire life if she lived to be more than 89 years old. For a woman who lives to age 80, the chance of getting breast cancer is 1 in 10.

How Common Is Breast Cancer?

Breast cancer is the most common life-threatening cancer to affect women worldwide, with approximately 1.5 million new cases of breast cancer occurring each year.

Breast cancer rates are highest in developed, affluent regions, such as the United States, the United Kingdom, Northern and Western Europe, and Australia. But even in these regions, the death rate from breast cancer has begun to decline, thanks to improved detection and treatment.

Low incidence and death rates for breast cancer are found in most Asian and African countries, and intermediate rates are found in Southern European and South American countries.

In the United States, more than 200,000 women are diagnosed with invasive breast cancer each year, and another 50,000 women receive a diagnosis of

A woman's chance of developing breast cancer increases with age

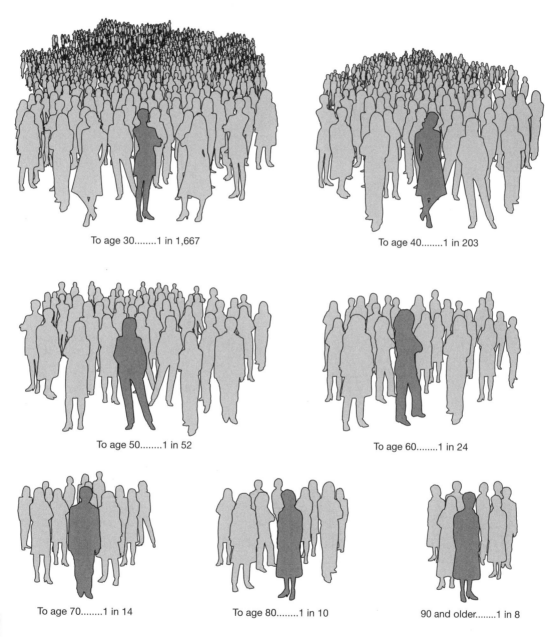

To age 30........1 in 1,667

To age 40........1 in 203

To age 50........1 in 52

To age 60........1 in 24

To age 70........1 in 14

To age 80........1 in 10

90 and older........1 in 8

©MFMER

Modified from Surveillance, Epidemiology, and End Results (SEER) data, National Cancer Institute, 2011.

Incidence of breast cancer worldwide

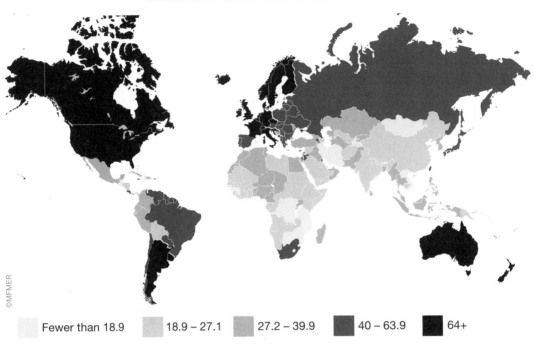

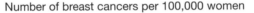

Fewer than 18.9	18.9 – 27.1	27.2 – 39.9	40 – 63.9	64+

Number of breast cancers per 100,000 women

Developed regions such as the United States, the United Kingdom, Northern and Western Europe, and Australia have the highest rates of breast cancer. Lifestyle is thought to be a key factor in breast cancer incidence.

Source: Ferlay J, Shin HR, Bray F, Forman D, Mathers C and Parkin DM. GLOBOCAN 2008 v1.2, Cancer Incidence and Mortality Worldwide: IARC CancerBase No. 10. Lyon, France: International Agency for Research on Cancer, 2010; accessed 4/18/2012.

ductal carcinoma *in situ* (DCIS). Estimated deaths from breast cancer annually number around 39,000.

The number of women diagnosed with breast cancer has generally increased in the last 30 years. A major increase occurred from 1975 to 1985. This was the result of more women being screened with mammograms, which identified many cancers that had previously gone undetected. Eventually, the number of new cancer cases began to level off and then decline. Researchers believe an important factor in the reduction of new breast cancers is less use of hormone replacement therapy after menopause.

The frequency of breast cancer also varies according to a woman's race and ethnicity. In the United States, white and black women have the highest levels of breast cancer risk, while Hispanic and American Indian women and women of Asian and Pacific Islander groups have lower levels of risk. Some of the lowest levels of risk occur among Korean and Vietnamese women. Breast cancer is more frequent in Jewish women than in non-Jewish women.

Racial and ethnic differences in survival rates

There are racial and ethnic disparities in survival rates among American women with breast cancer. Black, Native American, Hispanic, Indian and Pakistani women are more likely to receive a diagnosis of advanced breast cancer than are white women, according to a study of nearly 125,000 U.S. women from 17 different races and ethnic groups.

The study also found that black, Native American, Hawaiian, Hispanic and Vietnamese women face a greater risk of dying of breast cancer, once they develop it, than do white women, even though breast cancer isn't as common among these racial and ethnic groups as it is among white women.

Researchers speculate that some of these disparities are due to delays in diagnosis and to differences in the treatment received by women of various ethnic and racial groups. Other possible explanations include socio-economic, cultural and lifestyle factors, such as reduced access to health care and lack of health insurance, as well as underuse of mammography screening.

Advancing Science

As is true of any type of cancer, the biology of breast cancer is extraordinarily complex. Still, in the last two decades, scientists have made remarkable strides in understanding the differences between normal cells and cancer cells, and in developing new treatments to take advantage of this expanding wealth of knowledge.

Advances in technology and the completion of the Human Genome Project — an effort to identify all of the genes in humans — have further increased the pace of scientific discovery. Researchers are now better able to determine breast cancer risk and to tailor therapies to target specific molecular characteristics that can cause or stimulate cancer development.

Frequency of invasive breast cancer among U.S. women

Race/ethnicity	Rate per 100,000 women (2004-2008)
All races	124.0
White	127.3
Black	119.9
Asian and Pacific Islander	93.7
Hispanic	92.1
Native American and Native Alaskan	77.9

Source: *SEER Cancer Statistics Review, 1975-2008*. National Cancer Institute, 2011.

DNA

New technologies now allow scientists to probe the molecular machinery of breast cancer cells in greater detail.

For a cancerous tumor to grow, its cells must gain the ability to divide uncontrollably. When a cell divides, its DNA is replicated so that the newly formed cells have a copy of the person's genetic material. As cells reproduce, the DNA can be damaged. Damaged DNA can lead to uncontrolled cell division and the development of cancer.

Researchers can now study the activity of many genes simultaneously, using a process called microarray technology. This technology allows scientists to compare microscopic amounts of gene products from 25,000 genes at one time. Scientists can compare genetic patterns in breast cancers with those in normal tissue, or patterns in aggressive breast cancers with those in cancers that aren't aggressive.

Proteins

Scientists are learning more about the role proteins play in the development of breast cancer. Proteins are the products of genes.

Proteomic techniques, as described in Chapter 2, allow scientists to study circulating protein patterns that occur when breast cancer begins. Identification of these protein patterns could potentially be used as a new screening tool. At the same time, the proteins provide clues regarding

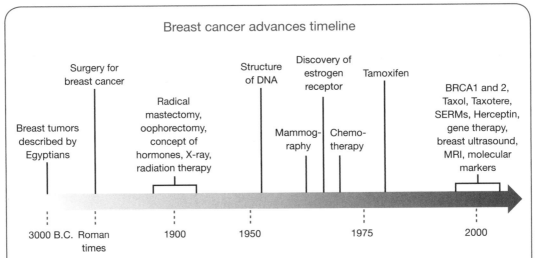

Breast cancer advances timeline

For centuries, surgery has been used to treat breast cancer. After discovery of the X-ray in 1895, radiation therapy came into use. The first use of hormone therapy was in 1896 when a young woman's ovaries were removed to treat metastatic breast cancer. But it wasn't until after discovery of the estrogen receptor and development of the drug tamoxifen that hormone therapy became a common form of treatment. Chemotherapy emerged as a standard treatment in the early 1970s. In just the last decade, the pace of discovery has accelerated dramatically.

Data from *The History of Cancer*, American Cancer Society, 2011, and other sources.

The Story of Herceptin

A major success story in the development of cancer drugs is trastuzumab (Herceptin), a drug used to treat breast cancer. The story begins with the discovery of the HER2 oncogene in 1987. Oncogenes — genes that can drive tumor growth — were first identified by molecular biologists in the early 1970s. Ten years later, researchers at the University of California Los Angeles (UCLA) began studying tumors to look for genetic alterations in known oncogenes.

The researchers discovered that about 20 to 25 percent of breast cancers had extra copies of the HER2 oncogene, causing the genes to produce too much of the growth-promoting HER2 protein. This protein sends strong growth-promoting signals to cell nuclei.

The UCLA team found that the more copies of the HER2 oncogene there were in a tumor, the more aggressive was the disease.

Researchers began looking for ways to block the activities of the HER2 protein. They became interested in a genetically engineered antibody called trastuzumab (Herceptin). Antibodies are part of the body's immune-system defense against foreign invaders. Genetically engineered antibodies target specific invaders that would normally escape notice by the immune system.

In the lab, trastuzumab inhibited the growth of breast cancer cells that depended on excess HER2.

By 1991, the researchers began clinical trials to test trastuzumab in humans.

The first (phase I) trial showed it was well absorbed and produced few side effects. Phase II trials found that trastuzumab was safe and effective in women with metastatic breast cancer in which HER2 was overexpressed. A phase III trial was then conducted. In this trial, women received either trastuzumab and standard chemotherapy or chemotherapy alone. The women who received trastuzumab and chemotherapy had slower tumor growth, greater reductions in tumor size and longer survivals, on average, than did those who received chemotherapy alone. In another study, women received trastuzumab alone. In about 25 percent of these women, the tumor got smaller or disappeared.

In 1998, trastuzumab was approved by the Food and Drug Administration (FDA) for the treatment of metastatic breast cancer in which HER2 was overexpressed. The drug was considered a triumph because it was the first approved cancer drug directed against a specific molecular alteration. Subsequent studies in earlier stage HER2-positive breast cancers showed a substantial reduction in disease recurrence when trastuzumab was combined with usual chemotherapy.

Trastuzumab is the first in an emerging wave of more tailored therapies designed to fight cancer at its roots — treatments akin to a bullet rather than a sledgehammer. It's noteworthy that this whole process took over a decade of work, from the early identification of the HER2 oncogene in 1987 to FDA approval in 1998.

early changes within cells that allow for the development of breast cancer.

One protein being studied is called p53, produced by the p53 gene. This gene is an important tumor suppressor that's activated when a cell is damaged. Its job is to stop or slow further cell growth until the damage has been repaired. If the damage is too extensive to be repaired, it sends the cell into a suicide pathway.

Breast cancer, along with other cancers, often inactivates the p53 gene so that it can't perform its job. Breast cancers associated with changes to p53 tend to be highly invasive and aggressive.

Another protein important to cell growth is HER2. This protein is over-expressed — that is, too much of it is produced — in about 20 to 25 percent of breast cancers. Scientists have developed a test to detect the presence of both the HER2 protein and its gene, a type that normally promotes cell division.

Tumors that test positive for HER2 generally grow faster and are more likely to spread than are other tumors. These tumors often respond to treatments designed to block HER2, such as the drugs trastuzumab (Herceptin) and lapatinib (Tykerb).

Angiogenesis

To continue growing, a cancer needs nourishment. It gets the nutrients it needs by promoting the growth of new blood vessels in a process called angiogenesis. The word *angio* refers to blood or lymph vessels, and *genesis* means birth or generation. The new network of blood vessels supplies the tumor with nutrients and oxygen and takes waste products from it.

Normally, angiogenesis is a tightly regulated process that's controlled by the production of molecular chemicals (some that promote and some that inhibit angiogenesis). An imbalance of these factors is seen in several conditions in which abnormal new blood vessels are formed, including cancer. Breast cancer, like many cancers, is very angiogenic.

Much research is being done in the area of angiogenesis. In particular, researchers are looking into ways to block the cellular signals that trigger angiogenesis, including drugs that inhibit the process. The drug bevacizumab (Avastin) has been studied in numerous clinical trials in breast cancer, and researchers are still working to identify a subgroup of women that most likely will benefit from this treatment.

Chapter 4: Breast Cancer

Making Sense of Risk Statistics

What Is Risk and How Is It Measured?	62
Absolute risk	62
Relative risk	63
Putting risk into perspective	65

Quantifying Risk	66
Gail model	66
Other models	67

Risk Factors	68
Family history	68
Hormonal and reproductive factors	68
Environmental factors	70
Prior breast cancer	72
Benign breast disease	73
Breast density	74

Most women want to know what their chances are of developing breast cancer and whether there's anything they can do to reduce their risk. Among women who've had breast cancer, one of the most common questions is, "What's my daughter's risk?" Being able to estimate a woman's risk of breast cancer is essential for making decisions about medical care.

But statistics about breast cancer risk can be confusing. It seems that practically every week headlines highlight some new medical finding on cancer risk — followed the next week or month by a study producing contradictory results. Sorting through this information and figuring out what's valid and what's not can be tricky.

The way risk statistics are presented only adds to the confusion. Maybe you read that eating a certain food increases your risk of breast cancer by 20 percent, or that a particular drug causes a threefold increase in breast cancers. Risk estimates are calculated in different ways and may be shown as percentages, ratios or plain numbers. How the information is presented can sway how you react to a finding and whether you consider changing your behaviors.

This chapter will help you make sense of information on breast cancer risk, including how risk is assessed. A risk factor is anything associated with a greater chance of getting a disease. Different cancers have different risk factors. The main risk factor for breast cancer is simply being a woman. Age also is an important risk factor. Your likelihood of getting breast cancer increases as you get older.

Understanding your risk of getting breast cancer can help you make informed decisions about your medical care and lifestyle. It can help you avoid overestimating or underestimating your risk. Having realistic information allows you to take appropriate steps and may ease your anxieties about breast cancer. Accurate risk assessment is especially important for women at high risk of getting breast cancer. For these women, aggressive surveillance or risk-reducing (preventive) measures may be considered.

At the same time, it's important to realize that while medical professionals know some of the risk factors that increase a woman's chance of developing breast cancer, it's uncertain exactly how, or in some cases if, all of these risk factors will cause normal cells to become cancerous.

While we understand more about the disease than ever before, breast cancer development is still often unpredictable. Having a risk factor, or even several risk factors, doesn't guarantee that you'll get the disease. Some women with several risk factors never get breast cancer. And some women with no known major risk factors do.

What Is Risk and How Is It Measured?

Cancer researchers use the word *risk* in different ways. For example, you may hear the terms *absolute risk, relative risk* and *lifetime risk*. When scientists talk about risk, they're referring to a probability or a ratio of probabilities — the chance that something may occur but not a guarantee that it will.

Risk estimates and risk factors for breast cancer and other diseases are determined by studying large groups of people to discover the probability that any given woman or category of women will develop the disease, and to see what characteristics or behaviors are associated with increased or decreased risk.

Absolute risk

Absolute risk refers to the actual numeric chance (probability) of developing breast cancer during a specified time — for example, in the next year, in the next five years, by age 50, by age 70 or over the course of your lifetime.

One specific type of absolute risk that you hear about is lifetime risk. Lifetime risk refers to the probability that an individual will develop cancer over the course of a lifetime.

For example, the lifetime risk for an "average" American woman to develop breast cancer from birth to age 90 is about 12 percent. Another way of saying this is that the lifetime risk is 1 in 8, meaning that 1 in 8 women who live to age 90 will develop breast cancer at some point (see page 55). The lifetime risk calculated to age 80 is 10 percent, or 1 in 10.

In studies that test the effects of a treatment or prevention strategy, absolute risk refers to the actual number of health problems that happen or are prevented because of a specific treatment, such as a drug, or a risk-lowering strategy. For example, an absolute risk might be described as "10 extra cases of breast cancer in 10,000 women who took a particular drug for five years, compared with women who didn't."

Relative risk

Relative risk expresses a comparison (ratio) rather than an absolute value. It shows the strength of the relationship between a risk factor and a particular type of cancer by comparing the number of cancers in a group of people with a particular trait — such as smoking — with the number of cancers in a similar group that lacks the same trait. Relative risk can also express the likelihood that a person who uses a certain treatment or prevention strategy will have an increased or decreased risk of breast cancer, compared with someone who used another strategy or who didn't do anything.

When the difference in risk between two groups is compared, it's often shown as a ratio. This ratio is known as the relative risk. Another way to describe relative risk is to show it as a percentage increase or decrease in risk. For example, women who go through menopause after age 55

FASTFACT

Relative risk at a glance

Relative risk	% increase	Risk factor	Type of cancer
25	2,400%	Smoking	Lung
20	1,900%	BRCA1 gene mutation	Breast
6	500%	Estrogen therapy, without progesterone	Uterine
5 or greater	400% or more	Lobular carcinoma *in situ* Chest radiation therapy for Hodgkin disease	Breast Breast
3-4	200-300%	Past history of breast cancer	Breast
3	200%	Mother, sister or daughter with premenopausal breast cancer	Breast
1.8	80%	Mother or sister with postmenopausal breast cancer	Breast
1.5	50%	Postmenopausal obesity	Breast
1.25	25%	Modest alcohol intake Hormone replacement therapy	Breast Breast
1.0	None	Normal	

have a risk of developing breast cancer that's about 1.5 times the risk in women who go through menopause when they're younger than 45. A relative risk of 1.5 means that their risk of developing breast cancer is increased by 50 percent. A relative risk of 1.0 means there's no increased risk. A relative risk of 0.5 means the risk is reduced by 50 percent.

Fifty percent sounds like a very large increase in risk because many people assume when they hear a percentage that 100 percent is the highest possible increase, but that's not the case. In fact, a relative risk of 1.5 may represent a very small increase in absolute risk. Unfortunately, there isn't an easy way to translate relative risk estimates into actual numeric risks, which are usually the most understandable.

A relative risk of 1.5 is also modest in the context of all cancer risk factors. For example, smoking increases the risk of lung cancer. What is the relative risk of lung cancer in smokers compared with nonsmokers? It's 25. This means that smokers are 25 times as likely to develop lung cancer as are nonsmokers. To translate this into a percentage, subtract 1 from the number and multiply it by 100, to result in 2,400 percent increase in risk.

The message to remember is, when you hear that a study found a risk increase of 50 percent or 100 percent, keep in mind

Relative Risk vs. Absolute Risk

Research studies may be reported in terms of relative risk or absolute risk, and you may have a very different reaction to the two numbers, or you may be confused about how the studies are interpreted.

A relative risk often sounds more alarming than an absolute risk. For example, consider the results of a well-known clinical trial called the Women's Health Initiative (WHI). One of the goals of this study was to identify the risks and benefits of using hormone replacement therapy (HRT) — combined estrogen plus progestin — after menopause. The study monitored the development of a number of diseases, including heart disease, breast cancer and osteoporosis, in its participants.

In the summer of 2002, WHI researchers stopped the estrogen plus progestin part of the study because they found that the risks of the therapy appeared to outweigh the benefits. In a widely publicized finding, the investigators reported that combined estrogen and progestin increased the risk of breast cancer by 26 percent.

That percentage increase represented a relative risk of 1.26, comparing the chance that a woman taking estrogen plus progestin would get breast cancer with the chance that a woman taking an inactive pill (placebo) would get breast cancer. It didn't mean that 26 percent of the women taking hormone therapy got breast cancer. The absolute risk translated into eight more cases of breast cancer

that 100 percent is not the upper limit of the possible increase. The chart on page 63 lists some relative risks associated with various cancer risk factors.

Putting risk into perspective

Most information about cancer risk and risk factors comes from epidemiologic studies, which are studies conducted in large, well-defined groups of people. In the last 50 years, epidemiologists have identified many of the major factors that contribute to cancer, including smoking for lung cancer and sunlight for skin cancer. But uncovering more subtle cancer risks has proved more difficult.

Randomized clinical trials, such as the Women's Health Initiative (WHI), are the gold standard of research studies. The WHI tested the combination of estrogen plus progestin (the two main female hormones) versus placebo in over 16,600 women, treated for about five years. The main results of that trial are shown in the table below. For postmenopausal women who had a hysterectomy, the WHI included the Estrogen-Alone trial, comparing about five years of estrogen use to placebo. There has been much less publicity centered on this trial, which found that the risk of invasive breast cancer was lower in women taking estrogen alone than in women taking a

each year among 10,000 women taking estrogen and progestin.

For any individual woman, the absolute risks of these serious adverse events are fairly small. However, when spread across an entire population of women, the risks become more significant. That

is why the study was stopped before its completion.

When you're evaluating information about your risk of breast cancer, the statistics can be confusing. It's helpful to know the difference between relative risk and absolute risk.

Women's Health Initiative findings: Use of estrogen plus progestin

Risk or benefit	Relative risk	% change	Absolute risk each year
Heart attacks	1.29	29% increase	7 more cases in 10,000 women
Breast cancer	1.26	26% increase	8 more cases in 10,000 women
Strokes	1.41	41% increase	8 more cases in 10,000 women
Blood clots	2.11	111% increase	18 more cases in 10,000 women
Hip fractures	0.66	33% decrease	5 fewer cases in 10,000 women
Colon cancer	0.63	37% decrease	6 fewer cases in 10,000 women

Data from Rossouw JE, et al. Risks and benefits of estrogen plus progestin in healthy menopausal women: Principal results from the Women's Health Initiative randomized controlled trial. *JAMA*, 2002;288:321.

placebo. The relative risk of breast cancer was about 0.77 (meaning a 23 percent reduction). Further research is ongoing to understand the differences in risk of breast cancer between the two trials, with a focus on the role of progestin.

But large, randomized clinical trials aren't always practical for studying cancer risk factors. These types of studies can take years or decades to complete, require the participation of thousands of people, and are very costly. In addition, for some risk factors, it would be unethical to subject healthy participants to possible cancer-causing agents (carcinogens).

Instead, most studies of cancer risk factors rely on observational approaches. In these studies, researchers keep track of a group of people for several years without trying to change their lives or provide special treatment. This can help scientists find out who develops a disease, what those people have in common and how they differ from the group that didn't get sick. But observational studies are more prone to bias and are considered less reliable. Sometimes, differences between the groups are caused by something the investigators aren't aware of.

Because of these limitations, most epidemiologists agree that one observational study by itself isn't authoritative — conclusions can't be made based on one study. Further research is needed to better determine if the finding is true. The media, though, often report each new study in isolation, rather than as part of an evolving picture.

When looking at information about risk and risk factors, keep a critical perspective about the source of the information and the strength of the research.

Quantifying Risk

Estimating breast cancer risk for any individual woman is difficult, in part because most breast cancers occur in women who don't have major risk factors for the disease other than being a woman and their age. In addition, each risk factor by itself is an isolated piece of information. In reality, many factors work together to cause breast cancer, and some risk factors may interact, working in a combined fashion to further increase risk.

To quantify a woman's risk of breast cancer using a combination of risk factors that may have an additive effect, researchers have developed computer-generated risk models based on data collected from many women. The information these models provide can help doctors determine which women should be tested for possible inherited genetic abnormalities. The models also help women and their doctors make decisions about screening and options to reduce risk. Women who are at very high risk of getting breast cancer may consider risk-lowering medications or surgery.

Several different risk models are available that are based on data from large epidemiologic or clinical studies.

Gail model

One commonly used tool for general breast cancer risk assessment is the Gail model, which is based on data gathered from more than 280,000 women over a period of seven years. The Gail model was originally designed to screen women and find those at higher risk of breast cancer, who could then be enrolled in chemoprevention clinical trials. The model estimates the likelihood that a woman with certain risk factors will develop invasive breast cancer in the next five years or during her lifetime.

Risk factors used in the Gail model include:

- Current age
- Age at first period (menses)
- Age at first live birth
- Number of first-degree relatives (mother, sister or daughter) with breast cancer
- Number of previous breast biopsies
- Presence of atypical hyperplasia on a breast biopsy (see page 150)
- Race

The results from the Gail model assessment can be printed off, and they're shown as an absolute risk percentage.

While this assessment performs well across a group of women (where risk can be averaged), it's not very accurate for individual women. In fact, several studies have shown that the Gail model performs only slightly better than does chance when predicting risk for individuals.

The Gail model isn't alone in this regard. Predicting an individual's cancer risk is very difficult because many factors — some inherited, others based on a woman's lifestyle and environment — interact to affect risk. At this point, it isn't known what all of these factors are, how much weight to assign them, and whether or not they're age dependent.

Other models

The Gail model doesn't place much emphasis on family history features, such as breast cancer on the father's side of the family, breast cancer in second-degree relatives (aunts, cousins, grandmothers), the age at which relatives developed breast cancer and a family history of ovarian cancer. Thus, for women with a family history of breast cancer or ovarian cancer, the Claus model is often used.

The Claus model calculates risk either as a lifetime probability or for a 10-year period. This model is appropriate only for women with at least one female relative with breast cancer. But the model doesn't take into account some other risk factors associated with breast cancer, such as age at first menstruation or first live birth.

Other risk-prediction models have been developed for use in women suspected of having an inherited susceptibility to breast cancer. These models — including BRCAPRO, Tyrer-Cuzick (IBIS) and BOADICEA — estimate breast cancer risk based on the probability of detecting mutations in breast cancer genes BRCA1 and BRCA2 in a woman or family. These models help doctors determine if a woman is likely to benefit from genetic testing.

Another risk-prediction approach that's sometimes used in high-risk women is to use data from studies that apply to a specific group or population. For example, regardless of family history, up to 30 percent of Jewish women of Ashkenazi (Eastern European) descent diagnosed with breast cancer before age 40 have one of the BRCA1 or BRCA2 mutations common to this population. Information such as this is summarized in prevalence tables, which give estimates of the prevalence of a BRCA1 or BRCA2 mutation in particular population groups.

Risk Factors

Women who've been diagnosed with breast cancer often wonder, "What did I do? How did I let my body down?"

Let yourself off the hook because it's highly unlikely that anything you did caused your breast cancer. Very few strong risk factors for breast cancer have been identified. Therefore it's often impossible to say why one woman gets the disease and another doesn't. And most of the known risk factors, such as your sex, age, menstrual history and family history, aren't things you can control.

As mentioned earlier, simply being a woman is the main risk factor for developing breast cancer. Although men have breast tissue and can get breast cancer, the disease is 100 times more common in women. That's because women have more breast cells than men do, and these cells are constantly exposed to the growth-promoting effects of female hormones.

Age also is a major risk factor. Three-fourths of women diagnosed with breast cancer are older than age 50 when they receive their diagnosis.

Family history

After sex and age, a family history of breast cancer is the strongest known risk factor for the disease. About 15 to 20 percent of breast cancers occur in women with some family history of the breast cancer, on either side of the family.

If you have one first-degree relative — a mother, sister or daughter — with breast cancer, your relative risk of getting the disease is approximately doubled, compared with that of women who have no first-degree relatives with the disease. More specifically, the risk varies depending on the age of your relative at diagnosis. It's 1.8 if she had breast cancer after menopause and closer to 3 if she was premenopausal at diagnosis (see page 63). The relative risk is 1.5 if you have one second-degree relative, such as a grandmother, aunt or cousin with breast cancer.

In general, the more first-degree relatives you have with breast cancer, the greater your risk. In addition, the younger your relatives were when they were diagnosed, the greater your risk. These key factors signal the possibility of an inherited predisposition to the disease. Hereditary breast cancer is discussed in greater detail in Chapter 5.

Hormonal and reproductive factors

More than a century ago, the first effective treatment for metastatic breast cancer in premenopausal women was reported — removal of the ovaries. It wasn't until years later, though, that the underlying link between the ovaries and production of the female sex hormones estrogen and progesterone was established. In the 1960s, estrogen receptors were discovered. Estrogen receptors are proteins in breast tissue cells that interact with estrogen and, together, bind to DNA, which turns on gene and protein production. Estrogen receptors are also found in other tissues, such as the uterus, bones, brain and heart, which are "targets" for estrogen. When estrogen binds with an estrogen receptor, the hormone influences the cell's activities.

Experimental evidence suggests that estrogen plays a key role in the development of breast cancer. In animals, the hormones estrogen and progesterone stimulate the growth of breast tumors. Although a precise cause-and-effect relationship hasn't been established, it's known that the greater a woman's lifetime exposure to female hormones, the higher her risk of breast cancer. If a premenopausal woman has her ovaries removed — reducing her exposure to sex hormones — her risk of breast cancer drops by about 50 percent.

Several risk factors for breast cancer are related to a woman's hormonal and reproductive history.

Menstrual history

Women who start menstruating before age 12 or who go through menopause after age 50 have a slightly higher risk of breast cancer. Compared with someone who begins menstruating after age 15, a girl who has her first period before age 12 has a 30 percent greater risk (relative risk 1.3) of developing breast cancer.

At the other end of the reproductive spectrum, women who don't reach menopause until age 55 or older have a 30 to 50 percent greater chance of getting breast cancer than do women who experience menopause earlier. (The average age at menopause in the U.S. is 51.)

Earlier menstruation and later menopause translate into more years of breast tissue exposure to sex hormones.

Pregnancy and breast-feeding

Women who never become pregnant or who give birth to their first child after age 30 have approximately double the risk of breast cancer, compared with women who give birth when they're younger than age 20. Giving birth at a young age significantly reduces breast cancer risk, though if an early pregnancy isn't carried to completion, the protective effect isn't seen.

Some studies have shown that breast-feeding can lower breast cancer risk, but other studies haven't. One study of 100,000 women concluded that for every 12 months of breast-feeding, a woman's risk is lowered by 4.3 percent. The study also reported that every birth reduced a woman's breast cancer risk by 7 percent.

One reason early pregnancy and breast-feeding may reduce breast cancer risk is that these circumstances push breast cells into their final phase of maturation. Breast cells that are fully mature may be less vulnerable to the influence of carcinogens.

Use of oral contraceptives

Some studies suggest that women using birth control pills have a slightly increased risk of developing breast cancer. The increased risk appears to return to normal 10 years after a woman stops using oral contraceptives. A few studies have also shown that women with a strong family history of breast cancer — who are at increased risk of getting the disease — have an even higher risk if they use birth control pills.

It's important to note, though, that some of the studies that suggested an elevated risk of breast cancer involved early formulations of birth control pills, which contained higher concentrations of estrogen and progestin. Since their introduction in the early 1960s, the dose of hormones used in birth control pills has continued to decrease and today's pills contain much lower doses. Many other studies of oral contraceptive use and breast cancer risk haven't found evidence of increased risk.

Although the relationship between oral contraceptives and breast cancer risk remains somewhat controversial, most experts think that current versions of the pill don't increase breast cancer risk.

Hormone replacement therapy

Use of the female hormones estrogen and progesterone (progestin) to help ease menopausal symptoms came about in the early 1970s. Twenty years later, nearly 40 percent of postmenopausal women in the U.S. were using hormone replacement therapy (HRT). By this time, though, reports were beginning to appear linking hormone use with a slightly increased risk of breast cancer.

Note: The term *hormone therapy* has become the more commonly accepted term to *hormone replacement therapy* (HRT). However, because this book also covers hormone therapies used to treat breast cancer, we have chosen to use HRT to refer to hormones given after menopause.

The most conclusive evidence about HRT and breast cancer risk stems from the Women's Health Initiative (WHI), a clinical trial involving thousands of postmenopausal women. Participants in the study were selected at random to receive either an inactive pill (placebo) or HRT. If a woman had had a hysterectomy, she received estrogen alone. If she still had her uterus, she received estrogen plus progestin. (Use of estrogen alone in a woman who still has her uterus has been linked to increased risk of uterine cancer.) The WHI was designed to gather information on ways to prevent and reduce heart disease, osteoporosis and colorectal cancer, while monitoring the effect of hormones on breast cancer.

However, researchers had to prematurely stop the part of the study evaluating the use of combined estrogen and progestin because they found that the risks of the therapy appeared to exceed safety limits. There was a 26 percent increase in the risk of invasive breast cancer over a five-year period. When the relative risk estimate is translated into an actual number, it equals eight additional breast cancers among 10,000 women who take estrogen and progestin for one year.

The WHI also found that women taking combined hormones — both estrogen and progestin — were more likely to have abnormal mammograms, perhaps related to increased breast density from the hormones, requiring additional follow-up and evaluation.

What about use of estrogen alone after menopause? In women who haven't had a hysterectomy, estrogen taken alone can increase their risk of endometrial cancer. However, before concluding that estrogen has only negative effects, keep in mind that higher estrogen levels have been linked to beneficial effects on bone health and some studies have shown a reduced risk of Alzheimer's disease.

The WHI also studied estrogen-alone hormone replacement therapy versus placebo and found a slightly reduced risk of breast cancer in the estrogen-alone group.

Environmental factors

Over the years, much attention has been given to environmental and lifestyle risk factors — from a high-fat diet, to alcohol use, to the presence of pesticides and power lines — as possible risks for breast cancer. But unlike the clear connection between cigarette smoking and lung cancer, there's little strong evidence to link environmental factors and breast cancer development.

Diet
Several aspects of diet have been studied in relation to breast cancer risk. Researchers have long observed that breast cancer rates are much lower in most Asian and developing countries than they are in affluent Western countries — and dietary factors have been suggested as one reason for the variation. What's more, women who migrate from a country with a lower frequency of breast cancer to a country with a higher frequency over time acquire the same level of risk as women in the new country. Despite these intriguing hints, there isn't a clear-cut relationship between diet and breast cancer risk. Research has produced conflicting results and uncertainty.

One aspect of diet that has received a lot of hype is fat intake. Common thinking used to be that high-fat diets increased breast cancer risk. This belief was largely based on observations that breast cancer rates are highest in countries where consumption of dietary fat is highest. But well-controlled studies comparing intake of dietary fat and development of breast cancer have not been able to establish a clear link between the two. Some scientists, though, believe that the range of fat intake being studied isn't large enough to detect possible differences in breast cancer risk.

Weight
Being overweight or obese increases the risk of breast cancer in postmenopausal women by about 50 percent. Obesity in premenopausal women is actually associated with a modest reduction in breast cancer risk, but since obesity before menopause usually leads to obesity after menopause, excess weight at any age is seen as a risk factor for breast cancer.

Although your ovaries produce most of your estrogen, fat tissue can convert other hormones, such as those made by your adrenal glands, into estrogen. Thus, having more fat tissue increases your estrogen levels and it may increase your breast cancer risk. Obesity also contributes to increased levels of insulin and insulin-like growth factors, which are associated with a higher breast cancer risk.

Exercise
How exercise may affect breast cancer is a fairly new area of research. Many studies indicate that low levels of physical exercise — a sedentary lifestyle — may increase breast cancer risk. Some evidence indicates that strenuous exercise in youth might provide lifelong protection against breast cancer and that moderate to vigorous physical activity as an adult is associated with a lower risk.

Exercise may influence levels of the hormones estrogen and progesterone. It may also reduce breast cancer risk by promoting a healthy weight and healthy lifestyle habits. In postmenopausal women, less body fat translates to lower estrogen levels. Exercise is also thought to boost your body's natural immune function, which could help protect against cancer.

Alcohol consumption

Dozens of studies have consistently and clearly shown that drinking alcoholic beverages increases a woman's risk of developing breast cancer and that the more a woman drinks, the higher her risk.

Compared with nondrinkers, women who consume one alcoholic drink a day have a very small increase in risk, while women who consume more than three drinks a day have about 1.5 times the risk. Compared with women who don't consume alcohol, the relative risk of breast cancer increases 7 to 9 percent with each extra drink of alcohol consumed daily. The risk is the same whether you drink wine, beer or hard liquor.

Light consumption of alcoholic beverages — one drink a day or less — is unlikely to significantly affect breast cancer risk. If you do drink, do so in moderation.

Radiation exposure

Women who've had radiation therapy to the chest wall area, especially as a child or young adult, have an increased risk of breast cancer later in life. For example, for a woman who had radiation to lymph nodes in the chest to treat Hodgkin disease, especially if she was treated before age 30, her risk of breast cancer is five times more than that of a woman who didn't receive the treatment. Radiation exposure can damage cells. However, the small amount of radiation exposure you receive from occasional diagnostic exams, such as mammograms and chest X-rays, doesn't appear to pose a significant risk.

Pesticides and environmental pollution

Many people are concerned about the potential cancer-causing effects of pesticides, hazardous chemicals and pollutants in food, drinking water and the air.

Like the general public, cancer scientists also have been very interested in uncovering possible environmental factors that may influence breast cancer development. A great deal of research has been done — and more is being conducted — in this area. However, no environmental agents aside from radiation exposure have been consistently linked to breast cancer development in humans.

Occupational exposures

Exposure to hazardous materials may contribute to a small percentage of all cancers. Direct, frequent and high-level exposure to materials such as benzene, styrene, solvents, dyes, radioisotopes, fertilizers and pesticides may increase cancer risk.

Most of the evidence related to occupational exposures and breast cancer risk, though, is inconclusive. Although breast cancer rates are higher among some workers, the increase may be related to reproductive factors such as later pregnancies or no pregnancies rather than to something associated with their jobs.

Prior breast cancer

Having had breast cancer means that a woman is at increased risk of developing a second breast cancer. Women who have had breast cancer have a threefold to fourfold increased risk of developing a new cancer in the other breast. This is a second cancer, not a recurrence of the first cancer.

This increased risk is higher for women with a family history of breast cancer and for women who were young — less than age 40 — when first diagnosed.

MYTH vs. FACT

Myth: Smoking doesn't affect your risk of breast cancer.

Fact: There was a time when researchers didn't think that smoking played a role in a woman's risk of breast cancer. Oddly enough, they thought it might even lower breast cancer risk. But recent research involving larger and more carefully conducted studies shows just the opposite — smoking does increase breast cancer risk. For now, the increase appears to be slight, about a 25 percent increase in risk.

Research also suggests the younger a woman's age when she begins smoking, the longer she smokes and the more she smokes, the higher her risk. In addition, a woman's risk of breast cancer may remain elevated for up to 20 years after she stops smoking. Recent studies also suggest that extensive exposure to secondhand smoke is associated with an increased risk of breast cancer.

Benign breast disease

Approximately 1.5 million American women have a breast biopsy each year to evaluate an area of concern. More than 75 percent of these biopsies are benign. These women are said to have benign breast disease.

However, certain changes seen on a benign breast biopsy are associated with an increased risk of later breast cancer. Your risk is increased if a biopsy shows an overgrowth of cells that line the breast ducts or lobules (epithelial hyperplasia), especially if the cells appear abnormal (atypical).

Hyperplasia

Epithelial hyperplasia may involve an overgrowth of cells that line the breast ducts (ductal hyperplasia) or lobules (lobular hyperplasia). Based on how the cells appear under a microscope, hyperplasia is classified as usual (typical) or atypical. In usual hyperplasia, there's an increased number of normal cells in a nor-

mal arrangement. In atypical hyperplasia, the cells have not only increased in number, but have also taken on some abnormal characteristics (see page 151).

Women with usual hyperplasia have some increased risk of breast cancer — up to two times greater than that of women without the condition. Among those with atypical hyperplasia, the increase in risk is more significant — four to five times as great. See Chapter 9 for more information.

Lobular carcinoma *in situ*

Lobular carcinoma *in situ* (LCIS) refers to the presence of abnormal-appearing cells in the lobules of the breast. These cells are still confined to the membranes of the lobules and haven't spread to other breast tissue. LCIS is uncommon and is often discovered unexpectedly in tissue that's taken from the breast for another reason.

Studies indicate that women with LCIS are more than five times as likely to develop invasive breast cancer later on. The invasive cancer can occur in either breast.

5 Things That *Don't* Increase Your Risk

Many misconceptions, rumors and unproven theories about breast cancer risk factors have made the rounds. The following factors have not been demonstrated to have any significant effect on breast cancer risk:

1. Antiperspirants
People have suggested that chemicals in underarm antiperspirants interfere with lymph circulation and cause toxins to build up in the breast, leading to breast cancer. Several thorough studies haven't found antiperspirant use to increase the risk of breast cancer.

2. Underwire bras
Similar to the claim that antiperspirants cause breast cancer, individuals have suggested that some bras cause cancer by blocking lymph flow. There's no scientific basis for such a claim.

3. Coffee
Following a report that women with benign breast disease experienced relief from symptoms after eliminating caffeine from their diet, researchers speculated that caffeine may be a risk factor for breast cancer. But studies have shown no increase in breast cancer risk associated with drinking coffee or tea.

4. Large breasts
Large-breasted women have the same risk of developing breast cancer as small-breasted women do. They're not more or less likely to get the disease.

5. Breast implants
Several studies have concluded that breast implants don't increase breast cancer risk.

Increased breast cancer risk associated with LCIS is higher for women who are diagnosed with the condition at a younger age. See Chapter 9 for more information on LCIS.

Breast density

Breasts appear dense on a mammogram if they contain more glands and connective tissue (dense tissue) and less fat. Breast density is an established risk factor for breast cancer. The risk of breast cancer increases progressively with increasing levels of density. Women whose breasts are more than 75 percent dense have an approximate five-times increased risk. Besides the increased risk, dense breast tissue is more difficult to evaluate on a mammogram.

Chapter 5: Breast Cancer

Hereditary Breast Cancer

Is it Hereditary?	76
Nonhereditary disease	76
Hereditary disease	77
Inheriting a Genetic Mutation	79
Genetic Counseling and Testing	81
Who should be tested?	82
What's involved?	83
How much does testing cost?	86
Making a Decision	87
Positive test results	87
Negative test results	90

Breast cancer was recognized in families as far back as Roman times. In the mid-1800s, a famous French surgeon described multiple cases of breast cancer occurring in his own family.

In the modern era, there were two main factors that unlocked the centuries-old puzzle of breast cancer occurring in families. First — in the latter half of the 20th century — was the careful collection of family histories and blood samples from family members with a recognized breast cancer link. Second has been the development of genomic technology that can be used to study these breast cancer families. This has occurred in the past 25 years, with many more developments expected in the future.

As we begin this chapter, it's important to understand there's a difference between having some family history of breast cancer (such as one or two relatives) versus a clear hereditary cancer pattern. In the pages that follow, we describe these differences in greater detail. Once you better understand the genetics of breast cancer and how genetic testing works, you can read about the options for reducing breast cancer risk, explained in Chapter 6.

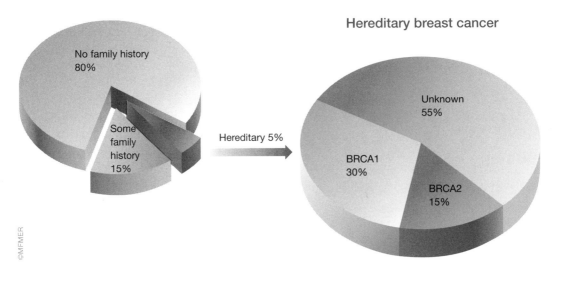

All breast cancer cases

No family history 80%

Some family history 15%

Hereditary 5%

Hereditary breast cancer

Unknown 55%

BRCA1 30%

BRCA2 15%

©MFMER

Is it Hereditary?

When a woman is diagnosed with breast cancer, one of the first things her doctor wants to determine is if she has a hereditary form of the disease. That is, is her cancer the result of an abnormal gene that's being passed on in the family?

Gathering a detailed family health history is an important first step in identifying a potential hereditary cancer. Clues that point to inherited breast cancer include:

- A history of breast cancer on either your mother's or your father's side of the family
- Multiple women on one side of the family diagnosed with the disease (rarely both parents can come from breast cancer families)
- Women diagnosed at a young age — younger than age 50
- Ovarian cancer in the family
- Male breast cancer in the family
- Breast cancer and ovarian cancer in the same woman
- Ashkenazi Jewish heritage

Nonhereditary disease

Just because a woman has one or two relatives with breast cancer doesn't mean there's a strong inherited abnormality in the family. In most women with a family history of breast cancer, there isn't one specific inherited gene that's responsible for the cancer. Instead, multiple factors that increase breast cancer risk are likely at play.

Breast cancer may occur more often in some families because of shared reproductive or lifestyle risk factors. In these women, their risk of breast cancer is much lower than that of women with an inherited mutation. For a woman who has a mother or sister with breast cancer and no other affected relatives and no identified genetic alteration, the probability that she will develop breast cancer by age 70 is between 7 and 18 percent. The risk increases as the number of relatives with breast cancer goes up, but it is still less than the risk for women who carry a known genetic mutation.

Hereditary disease

About 5 to 10 percent of all breast cancers are thought to be hereditary — caused by an inherited alteration (mutation) in a single gene. Several of these genes, known as cancer susceptibility genes, have been identified.

The first genes to be discovered were breast cancer gene 1 (BRCA1) and breast cancer gene 2 (BRCA2). Together, defects in these genes account for about 45 percent of hereditary breast cancer cases, or about 1.5 to 3 percent of all breast cancers.

BRCA1
Defects in the BRCA1 gene, located on chromosome 17, appear to be responsible for breast cancer in about 30 percent of families with multiple cases of the disease. They're also responsible for breast cancer in the large majority of families who have both breast and ovarian cancers. By age 70, a woman who carries a mutation in this gene has about a 54 percent chance of developing breast cancer and a 39 percent chance of getting ovarian cancer.

BRCA1 and BRCA2 carriers who've been diagnosed with breast cancer also have a higher risk of developing a second cancer in the opposite breast. The level of risk depends on a woman's age when receiving her first breast cancer diagnosis — as her age increases her risk decreases.

A woman who was younger than age 40 when she developed her first breast cancer has about a 60 percent chance of developing breast cancer in the opposite breast over the next 25 years.

Defects in the BRCA1 gene may also be associated with an increased risk of fallopian tube and primary peritoneal cancer (See Chapter 17 for more information about this risk and what you can do.) Men with a BRCA1 mutation have a threefold increased risk of prostate cancer.

BRCA2
Mutations in the BRCA2 gene, located on chromosome 13, account for about 15 percent of hereditary breast cancers. By age 70, carriers of a BRCA2 mutation have about a 45 percent chance of developing breast cancer and a 16 percent chance of developing ovarian cancer.

BRCA2 mutations may also be associated with an increased risk of several other cancers, including cancers of the prostate, pancreas, gallbladder and stomach, as well as the skin cancer melanoma. BRCA2 families also have an increased risk of male breast cancer.

The role of BRCA genes
BRCA1 and BRCA2 are tumor suppressor genes found in all humans. Normally, they regulate activity within a cell that helps to suppress the chance of cancer development. The BRCA genes produce proteins that help detect and repair DNA damage that can occur during normal cell division. When a BRCA gene is altered (mutated), the DNA repair process can go awry, and genetic defects can accumulate. This allows abnormal cells to multiply and cancer to develop.

Gene Search

For years, researchers had known that women with a strong family history of breast cancer were at higher risk of getting the disease than were other women. In 1994, they identified the first gene with a clear association to hereditary breast cancer — BRCA1.

The search for a gene responsible for breast cancer began with studies of families with multiple cases of breast cancer. By studying these families, researchers were able to identify a pattern (autosomal dominant inheritance pattern) for how the disease was passed on to family members (see page 80).

With the advent of technology that made it possible to analyze DNA, researchers were able to begin searching for the actual gene that was altered in people with a family history of breast cancer. In 1990, a team of scientists narrowed the search by discovering a link between early-onset breast cancer in families and a region of chromosome 17. The researchers called the region BRCA1. Four years later, the region was narrowed to the specific gene where mutations were found to occur. This discovery enabled the development of genetic testing for mutations in BRCA1. The first commercial testing for BRCA1 mutations was performed in 1996.

BRCA2 was identified on chromosome 13 in 1995.

Discovery of BRCA1

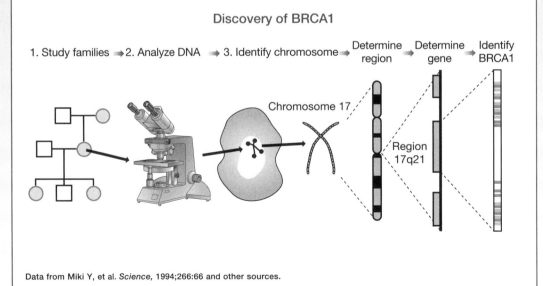

1. Study families ➡ 2. Analyze DNA ➡ 3. Identify chromosome ➡ Determine region ➡ Determine gene ➡ Identify BRCA1

Chromosome 17

Region 17q21

Data from Miki Y, et al. *Science*, 1994;266:66 and other sources.

BRCA1 and BRCA2 are both very large genes that contain codes for large proteins. More than 1,500 distinct mutations in BRCA1 and BRCA2 have been described. For example, in one mutation seen in women of Ashkenazi Jewish ancestry, just two pieces of the genetic code are missing out of a sequence of 6,000 — this one small deletion can result in an increased susceptibility to breast cancer. The mutations associated with an increased risk of cancer cause either missing or nonfunctional protein products.

Breast tumors that arise as a result of an inherited BRCA1 defect have some features of more aggressive cancers — their cells appear more abnormal (higher grade), and they usually are estrogen receptor negative. These traits are explained in Chapter 8. BRCA2-related breast cancers are more likely to be estrogen receptor positive, similar to nonhereditary breast cancers. Estrogen receptor status is one of many factors used to determine the best course of treatment.

BRCA in a nutshell

Before BRCA1 and BRCA2 were found, women with a strong family history of breast cancer were usually assumed to be carriers of a gene mutation, but no tool was available for testing these women. Thanks to advances in gene mapping and genetic testing, many women can now be tested for genetic mutations to help guide them in making decisions.

It's important to note that in families where an altered BRCA1 or BRCA2 gene is present, not all family members will inherit the gene mutation. That's why genetic testing may be especially helpful. Only family members who test positive for a known genetic mutation are at increased risk. In family members who aren't carriers, their risk isn't any greater than is the average woman's, and they won't pass the gene on to their children.

It's also important to understand that BRCA1 and BRCA2 account for only a portion of hereditary breast cancers (see the figure on page 76). Researchers continue to work to identify other breast cancer susceptibility genes. More specifics on genetic testing can be found later in this chapter.

Inheriting a Genetic Mutation

Mutations in BRCA1 or BRCA2 are inherited in what's called an autosomal dominant pattern. What this means is that one parent, either the father or the mother, has one normal copy of the gene and one abnormal copy. Either gene can be passed on. That means, each child has a 50 percent chance of inheriting the mutation.

Because both men and women have chromosomes 17 and 13, a mutation in one of these genes can come from either your father or your mother. Women may not realize they have a family history of breast cancer if the cancer is on their father's side of the family. Inheriting a genetic mutation associated with the development of breast cancer greatly increases the likelihood of getting the disease, but it's not a given. Some women with a BRCA1 or BRCA2 mutation develop early and multiple cancers, while others develop cancer later in life or not at all.

Passing on a defective gene

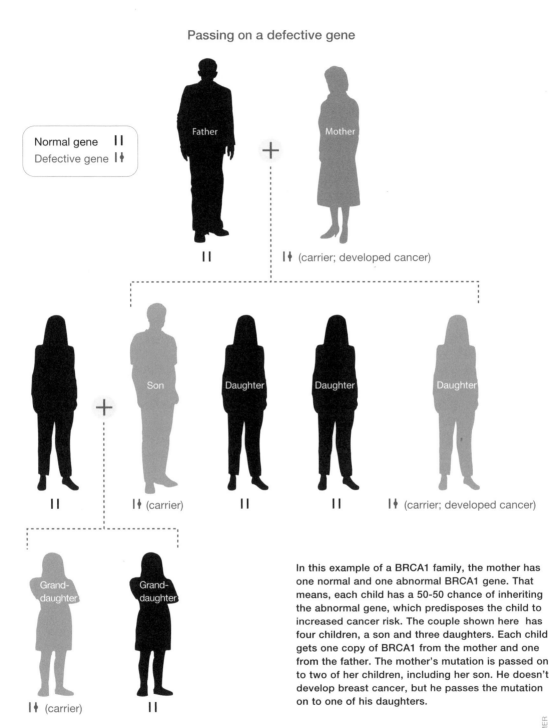

Normal gene   II
Defective gene   I⫯

Father

Mother

II

I⫯ (carrier; developed cancer)

Son

Daughter

Daughter

Daughter

II

I⫯ (carrier)

II

II

I⫯ (carrier; developed cancer)

Grand-daughter

Grand-daughter

I⫯ (carrier)

II

In this example of a BRCA1 family, the mother has one normal and one abnormal BRCA1 gene. That means, each child has a 50-50 chance of inheriting the abnormal gene, which predisposes the child to increased cancer risk. The couple shown here has four children, a son and three daughters. Each child gets one copy of BRCA1 from the mother and one from the father. The mother's mutation is passed on to two of her children, including her son. He doesn't develop breast cancer, but he passes the mutation on to one of his daughters.

©MFMER

There are several possible reasons for the individual variation in cancer susceptibility among carriers of BRCA1 or BRCA2 alterations. First, genetic mutations located at different places in these genes may lead to different levels of risk. Second, other risk factors, such as a woman's reproductive history, may influence breast cancer risk associated with these mutations. Lifestyle factors may also interact with the genetic susceptibility, and other genes may interact with the BRCA genes to modify an individual's risk.

Genetic Counseling and Testing

Women thought to be at high risk of carrying an inherited genetic mutation for breast cancer are often referred to a geneticist for a cancer risk assessment. A geneticist is a medical professional who specializes in genes and heredity. A genetic assessment may include genetic counseling and testing.

For breast cancer and other women's cancers, such as ovarian cancer, genetic testing analyzes one or more specific genes — usually BRCA1 and BRCA2. Genetic testing can help determine whether you carry a specific genetic mutation that puts you at increased risk of cancer. And it can let you know what is the probability that you'll develop the disease in your lifetime.

Genetic testing is a valuable tool that can be used to help doctors gauge a woman's breast cancer risk. But remember that it's just one component of a comprehensive cancer risk assessment plan.

Estimated breast cancer risk in BRCA mutation carriers

Age	BRCA1 carriers	BRCA2 carriers
30	1.8%	1%
40	12%	7.5%
50	29%	21%
60	44%	35%
70	54%	45%

This chart indicates the likelihood, by age, that a 20-year-old carrier of a mutant BRCA gene will develop breast cancer. For example, by age 70, 54 out of 100 BRCA1 carriers are expected to develop breast cancer.

Estimated ovarian cancer risk in BRCA mutation carriers

Age	BRCA1 carriers	BRCA2 carriers
30	1%	0.2%
40	3.2%	0.7%
50	9.5%	2.6%
60	23%	7.5%
70	39%	16%

This chart indicates the likelihood, by age, that a 20-year-old carrier of a mutant BRCA gene will develop ovarian cancer. For example, by age 70, 39 out of 100 BRCA1 carriers are expected to develop ovarian cancer.

Data from Sining Chen and Giovanni Parmigiani, Meta-Analysis of BRCA1 and BRCA2 Penetrance. *Journal of Clinical Oncology*, 2007;25:1329.

Who should be tested?

Doctors generally recommend genetic testing only for individuals with a family history that suggests they may be carriers of a BRCA1 or BRCA2 mutation.

The preferred approach is to begin the testing in a family member who has developed breast or ovarian cancer, since that person is the most likely to have a gene mutation. If a mutation is found in

this person, then other relatives can be tested for the same mutation.

Family members who are found to have the same mutation are gene carriers with increased cancer risks. An individual who tests negative for the mutation has the same risk level as women in the general population.

If it's not possible to begin testing in a family member who has had breast or ovarian cancer, then a person without

Mapping Your Family Health History

To help determine if you have an inherited risk of breast cancer, your doctor may construct your pedigree. A pedigree is a chart that shows your family tree and indicates which family members developed cancer, what kind of cancer they had and at what age they developed it. A pedigree, like the one illustrated below, can reveal a strong inheritance pattern for breast, ovarian and other cancers.

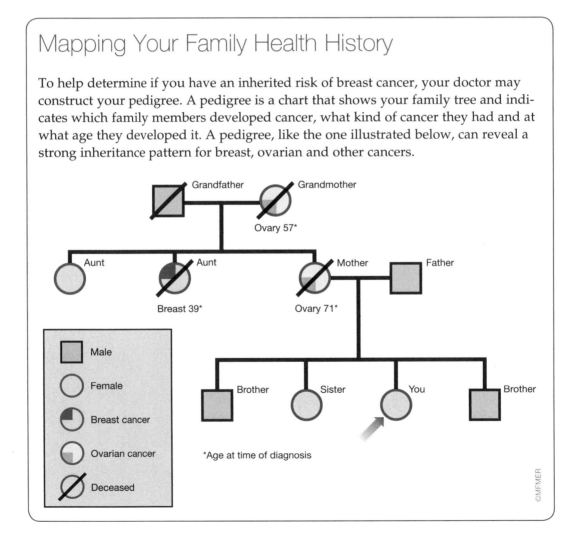

*Age at time of diagnosis

©MFMER

Questions to Ask

If you are referred for genetic counseling, you may have many questions. Feel free to ask about any concerns you may have. They may include:
• Where can I be tested?
• How much will the test cost?
• Does insurance cover it?
• When will I get my results?

• Who else will know my results, and will it affect my ability to get insurance?
• Should all my family, including my children, be tested?
• How might this information affect my relationship with my family?
• If I test positive, what are my options?

cancer can be tested. If the test reveals a mutation that's known to increase breast cancer risk in other families, then the person is a gene carrier with an elevated cancer risk.

If no mutation is found, there are a couple of possible explanations. It may be that there is a BRCA1 or BRCA2 mutation present in this family, but it happens that the individual tested is negative for it — she or he is not a carrier. Another possibility is that BRCA1 or BRCA2 mutations are not present in this family, but another mutation in some other gene is present — one that we cannot test for at this time (a so-called BRCA-negative family). In this case, the person may or may not be a carrier.

Obviously, the risk associated with these different scenarios is very different, underscoring the need to work with a genetic counselor as testing is done.

BRCA-negative families

In many families with a hereditary pattern for breast cancer, BRCA1 and BRCA2 testing is done and the results come back negative. In these families, there's likely a gene at work responsible for the cancer,

but we don't yet know the identity of that particular gene. In these situations, women who develop breast cancer are thought to be carriers of the gene mutation. Family members who don't develop breast cancer may or may not be carriers.

In more than half of inherited breast cancers, the specific genes involved are unknown (see figure on page 76). An example of a BRCA-negative family is highlighted in this chapter, beginning on page 88.

Even when BRCA1 and BRCA2 test results come back negative, genetic counseling is helpful. As new genes that predispose women to breast cancer are identified, tests for the genes are developed. A genetic counselor can also help with options for reducing cancer risk.

What's involved?

Genetic counseling is typically recommended to make sure you fully understand the risks, benefits and psychological effect of learning that you may carry a gene that puts you at increased risk of developing cancer. The counseling team may include a genetic counselor, nurse, doctor, psychologist and social worker.

A major topic covered during a genetic consultation is the likelihood that you have inherited a BRCA1 or BRCA2 mutation. The tables below show the likelihood of a person inheriting a mutation

in BRCA1 or BRCA2. The estimate is based on the individual's family history of cancer (shown across the top) and the individual's own cancer history (shown down the far left column).

For example, in the table on this page, Beth has been diagnosed with ovar-

Estimated likelihood of having a BRCA1 or BRCA2 mutation (Non-Ashkenazi population)

Family History

Personal History	No breast cancer younger than age 50 (<50) or ovarian cancer in any relative	Breast cancer <50 in one relative; no ovarian cancer in any relative	Breast cancer <50 in more than one relative; no ovarian cancer in any relative	Ovarian cancer at any age in one relative; no breast cancer <50 in any relative	Ovarian cancer in more than one relative; no breast cancer <50 in any relative	Breast cancer <50 and ovarian cancer at any age
No breast cancer or ovarian cancer at any age	1.5%	2.6% (Carol)	5.6%	3.0%	5.3%	7.2%
Breast cancer age 50 or older (≥50)	2.2%	3.8%	8.0%	4.9%	9.5%	10.6%
Breast cancer younger than age 50 (<50)	4.7%	10.4%	21.2%	10.3%	21.9%	26.6%
Male breast cancer	6.9%	17.4%	36.6%	15.9%	33.3%	28.3%
Ovarian cancer at any age, no breast cancer	7.7%	14.3% (Beth)	27.4%	14.7%	22.7%	34.4%
Breast cancer ≥50 and ovarian cancer at any age	12.1%	23.6%	50.0%	23.6%	44.2%	39.4%
Breast cancer <50 and ovarian cancer at any age	26.3%	40.0%	64.5%	41.2%	45.5%	57.4%

Adapted from BRCA1 and BRCA2 Prevalence Tables. Myriad Genetic Laboratories, Inc.

ian cancer. She has no family history of ovarian cancer, but her cousin was diagnosed with breast cancer at age 45. These combined factors, as is shown in the table, put Beth's chance of having a BRCA1 or BRCA2 mutation at 14.3 percent. Meanwhile, Beth's sister Carol has not had cancer. The chance that Carol has inherited a mutation is only 2.6 percent.

As you look at these tables, you see the features that significantly increase a person's chance of having a mutation, such as ovarian cancer in the family. The table on page 84 applies to non-Ashkenazi

Estimated likelihood of having a BRCA1 or BRCA2 mutation (Individuals of Ashkenazi ancestry)

Personal History	Family History					
	No breast cancer younger than age 50 (<50) or ovarian cancer in any relative	Breast cancer <50 in one relative; no ovarian cancer in any relative	Breast cancer <50 in more than one relative; no ovarian cancer in any relative	Ovarian cancer at any age in one relative; no breast cancer <50 in any relative	Ovarian cancer in more than one relative; no breast cancer <50 in any relative	Breast cancer <50 and ovarian cancer at any age
No breast cancer or ovarian cancer at any age	8.2%	13.0%	16.4%	12.7%	22.3%	22.9%
Breast cancer age 50 or older (≥50)	3.3%	7.1%	10.8%	13.2%	13.6%	16.7%
Breast cancer younger than age (<50)	7.9%	17.5%	26.9%	18.1%	20.0%	33.0%
Male breast cancer	13.5%	26.8%	46.2%	21.1%	66.7%	55.6%
Ovarian cancer at any age, no breast cancer	16.2%	26.4%	47.4%	26.2%	57.1%	57.8%
Breast cancer ≥50 and ovarian cancer at any age	20.5%	18.2%	30.0%	31.3%	100.0%	55.6%
Breast cancer <50 and ovarian cancer at any age	42.1%	63.2%	85.7%	62.5%	100.0%	36.4%

Adapted from BRCA1 and BRCA2 Prevalence Tables. Myriad Genetic Laboratories, Inc.

86 Part 2: Breast Cancer

Chapter 5: Hereditary Breast Cancer **86**

When the Results Are Unclear

When genetic testing for BRCA1 and BRCA2 is done, you don't always get a clear-cut answer. Sometimes, there's an alteration in a gene but scientists don't know if the alteration leads to a defective protein.

To understand this, it's important to know that the molecular spelling of all of our genes differs slightly from one person to another. However, these minor changes don't affect the function of the protein that's produced from the gene — the protein still does what it's supposed to.

In between these minor changes, which aren't harmful, and over 1,500 genetic mutations that are known to be harmful, lies a gray area of genetic changes called variants of uncertain significance (VUS). About 5 to 20 percent of the time, genetic testing of BRCA1 and BRCA2 will produce a VUS result. This means that the laboratory cannot determine if the gene change is a harmless one or harmful one.

This is a complex area where genetic counseling can be very helpful, partly because the individual who was tested may be confused or frustrated with the results. People who receive VUS results should stay in contact with their genetics specialist. As further research is done, these variants may be reclassified as harmful or harmless.

individuals. Because BRCA1 and BRCA2 mutations are more common in individuals of Ashkenazi Jewish descent, a separate table is necessary for them (see page 85). Again, the table shows the likelihood that a person has inherited a mutation, based on that person's family history and personal cancer history. Please keep in mind that the figures in these tables are only estimates and should not be taken as guarantees.

Other topics covered during a genetic consultation may include:
- Limitations, risks and benefits of testing
- Your perceptions of risk and motivation for testing
- Education about genetics, inheritance and risk
- Genetic testing procedures
- Screening and prevention options
- Privacy and confidentiality issues
- Emotional and psychological consequences of testing

How much does testing cost?

For many women, the cost of genetic testing is a major concern. The price varies, depending on the situation. For a woman who's the first person in her family to be tested, the test currently costs about $3,500. This is because BRCA1 and BRCA2 are very large genes and a mutation could be present along their entire lengths. If the woman tests positive for a specific genetic mutation, then another relative in her family can be tested for that specific mutation at a lesser cost, generally about $500. The testing is less costly for other family members because the geneticists know exactly where to look for the mutation.

For women of Ashkenazi Jewish descent, the initial test screens for the three most common genetic alterations in the Ashkenazi population, which account for 80 to 90 percent of hereditary cases of breast and ovarian cancer in Ashkenazi Jewish women. The cost for this initial test is approximately $600. If the result is negative, a woman may choose to have more extensive testing done.

Many insurance plans cover the cost of genetic testing or part of it. But some health plans don't, and some women aren't comfortable having their insurer know they're being tested. While many women are concerned that genetic testing could lead to insurance discrimination, there are few known instances in which this has occurred. To learn what your options are, talk to your doctor or insurer.

Making a Decision

Whether to undergo genetic testing is a personal decision. Many women proceed and feel relieved to know their risk status, even if they have a mutation, because this knowledge makes them feel empowered. They believe that the information they've gained will help them make the right decisions. Others worry about discrimination from health insurers or employers or about the cost of testing. For most women, the issue of genetic testing is emotionally charged, which is why counseling is critical.

Following are some factors to consider as to how you may react to either a positive or negative test result. If you decide

to be tested, the appropriate test will be selected and ordered, and your blood will be drawn. The test is a simple blood test. It generally takes about three to four weeks to get the results. The counseling team will likely discuss your results with you in person.

Positive test results

If genetic testing reveals a BRCA gene mutation, you might experience a range of responses to learning your test results:

- **Relief of knowing your risk status.** Now that you know what you're up against, you can step up your surveillance efforts or take risk-reducing steps, such as preventive surgery or medications.
- **Anxiety about developing cancer.** In this chapter, we've provided estimates as to the risk of a person with a BRCA1 or BRCA2 mutation developing breast or ovarian cancer. These are only estimates, but knowing that you're at increased risk may cause you anxiety. A genetics counselor or your doctor can help review the numbers, and your options.
- **Strained family relationships.** Some of your relatives may not want to know there's been a gene mutation detected within the family. But it may be hard to keep the truth from close family members. Give thought to how — or even if — you'll share test results with your family members.
- **Guilt about passing a gene mutation on to your child.** Learning your genetic status may stir fears that your child or children have also inherited the gene mutation.

One Family's Story

Here is one story of a family with hereditary cancer that was revealed over a several-month period.

When Janet noticed a dimpling under her left breast while doing her monthly breast self-exam, she knew it was cancer, though she had no reason to suspect it. Janet was only 38 years old, a runner and in good health. She didn't smoke, didn't drink and wasn't aware of any family history of breast cancer — because Janet's mother was adopted, the health history on that side of the family was unknown.

Being a physician, Janet was only too aware that dimpling is a common sign of breast cancer. Then there was also the mild pain she had been experiencing while breast-feeding her youngest son, something she had easily dismissed to nursing — until now. What she didn't know standing in front of a mirror that November day was how her discovery would profoundly change not only her life but also the lives of four other women.

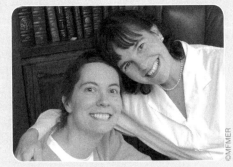

Jill, left, and Janet, right, following their cancer treatments.

Janet immediately saw her doctor. A mammogram and additional tests confirmed her fears. It was cancer. While awaiting the final test results, Janet sat in her husband's lap and cried, agonizing over how her young sons would cope without her. "In my mind, I just went right to the worst-case scenario, that I had stage IV cancer."

Fortunately, the cancer was only at stage II. Janet had her left breast removed, followed by a regimen of chemotherapy, radiation and the hormone medication tamoxifen.

Not surprisingly, Janet's diagnosis came as a shock. She grew up in a tightknit family, and her parents and three sisters were devastated when Janet called with the news. Her younger sister, Jill, drove from Michigan to Minnesota to be with Janet and help take care of the boys during Janet's first round of chemotherapy.

At Janet's insistence, her sisters each made appointments to have mammograms. The news was good; the results came back fine. A sigh of relief, but unfortunately it would be short-lived.

It was less than six months after Janet's diagnosis when her sister Jill experienced a perplexing event. A young child jumped into Jill's arms, accidentally kicking her in the breast. The incident caused intense pain, and it bothered Jill that such a minor mishap should bring about such pain. Later, while examining her breasts at home, Jill felt a lump — the same one she first noticed before her recent mammogram. Her doctor had told her then that the lump was likely a cyst and not to worry about it. And, for a while, Jill didn't, having been reassured by the "normal" finding on her mammogram that everything was OK. But Jill didn't like that the lump hadn't gone away and that it didn't seem to move. To be safe, she made another appointment to see her doctor. Still feeling it was just a cyst, Jill's doctor ordered a biopsy to comfort Jill's concerns. The results weren't comforting. It was cancer.

That summer, while Janet was beginning her radiation therapy, 31-year-old Jill underwent a mastectomy. For Jill, the diagnosis was more severe. The tumor was close to 8 centimeters, and she had several involved lymph nodes — a stage III cancer. Her treatment would be even more extensive than Janet's.

Janet made plans to travel to Michigan to be with Jill during her initial round of chemotherapy. Though tired from her radiation treatments, Janet was determined to be there for Jill, just as Jill had been there for her. Shortly before she was getting ready to leave, Janet's mother, Charlotte, called. The call didn't turn out to be the routine, "Hi, how are you doing?" Charlotte had just been in for a mammogram. She had had previous mammograms, but this was the first since her two youngest daughters had been diagnosed with breast cancer. The results showed an "axillary abnormality." She didn't know what it meant. Janet did. Her mother had an enlarged lymph node under her arm, likely due to breast cancer. For Janet, the news was almost too much to bear. "I was talking to her on the phone and I said, 'I cannot take another diagnosis of cancer right now.' This was literally weeks after Jill's diagnosis." Within a few days, 71-year-old Charlotte underwent surgery to remove a small cancerous mass in her breast that had spread to lymph nodes under her arm.

For the two oldest sisters, Julann and Jean, it suddenly felt as if their breasts had turned into ticking time bombs. Julann made an appointment with a surgeon to discuss the possibility of preventive (prophylactic) mastectomy. Though genetic tests showed that the family didn't carry the BRCA1 or BRCA2 breast cancer gene, it was apparent that some inherited genetic abnormality was at play, which current technology can't yet identify. After a battle with her insurance company, 46-year-old Julann finally received approval for surgeons to remove and reconstruct both of her breasts. As Janet sat in the waiting room and received updates from the operating room nurse, she became worried. The general surgeon was still in the room. "He should be done by now," Janet thought. "This isn't good." The surgeon would later tell Janet what she already suspected. During the surgery, the surgical team found cancer. Fortunately, it was still in its early stages.

For the fourth time in just over a year, cancer had raised its ugly head in this family. For these women, their once-normal routines became vague recollections. Janet recalls a single week in January. Her mother was in the hospital, Jill was just completing radiation treatments, Julann was starting chemotherapy, and Jean was going in for a breast biopsy because a mammogram had revealed an abnormal mass.

Finally, for Jean, there would come a break. Her biopsy results came back negative. But she decided there would be no more waiting, no more gambling with time. She decided to have prophylactic surgery.

As they did during those long and often grueling months, faith, family and a sense of humor continue to keep the women going today. "As hard as it was, sometimes you just had to step back and laugh," says Jill. "If you didn't laugh about it, you would cry all the time."

The women remain cancer-free. They credit their good fortune to the fact that they were proactive. They performed self-exams, had regular mammograms and took preventive action.

- **Concerns over health insurance discrimination.** Keep in mind that in the United States, the federal Genetic Information Nondiscrimination Act of 2008 protects individuals undergoing genetic testing. It prohibits insurers from denying insurance or raising premium or contribution rates on the basis of genetic information. The law also covers protection from employment discrimination.

Negative test results

For women in families with a BRCA1 or BRCA2 mutation who test negative for the mutation, there can be various reactions:

- **Relief that you don't have an increased cancer risk.** If there's a known mutation in your family, and your test result is negative, you may feel relieved knowing that your breast cancer risk is not any greater than that of the general population.
- **'Survivor' guilt.** Testing negative for a BRCA mutation may produce feelings of guilt — especially if other family members test positive.

Chapter 6: Breast Cancer

Preventing Breast Cancer

Lifestyle Factors	92
Diet	92
Alcohol	97
Physical activity	97

Women at High Risk	99
Prophylactic mastectomy	100
Prophylactic oophorectomy	102
Prevention medications	106

Future Directions	109

What can you do to make sure you don't get breast cancer? Unfortunately, there are no clear answers to that question. Research holds promise for developing better risk-reduction strategies, but there's no guaranteed way to prevent the disease.

What is possible? For all women, it's important to follow screening guidelines. Although screening won't prevent breast cancer, it can lead to early detection, which increases the likelihood of successful treatment. For more information about screening and detection, see Chapter 7.

It's also important that you understand your risk of getting the disease, as discussed in Chapters 4 and 5, so that you can decide what steps to take, if any, to reduce your risk. For women at average risk, a change in certain lifestyle habits, such as limiting alcohol use and maintaining a healthy weight, may lower their risk to some degree. For women at high risk, options to prevent breast cancer include prevention medications or surgery to remove the breasts or ovaries. Because these are major, difficult decisions, high-risk women are urged to learn all they can about their specific risks and the strategies for reducing those risks.

This chapter looks at lifestyle factors that can be changed (modified) to reduce your risk of breast cancer, and it discusses prevention options if you're at high risk of getting the disease.

Lifestyle Factors

If you're like most women hoping to avoid breast cancer, you're looking for something you can do — some change you can make in your life — that will lower your risk of the disease. It's great to want to do everything you can. Despite a great deal of research, though, few lifestyle factors have been strongly linked with breast cancer.

Most lifestyle changes result in only a modest reduction in cancer risk, if any. Among those that have received the most attention are factors related to diet, alcohol consumption and physical activity.

Diet

Researchers began investigating the role of diet in the development of breast cancer after noticing striking variations in breast cancer rates in different populations. For example, breast cancer is less common in countries of the Far East where people eat less fat and a lot of soy foods. However, there are many differences between present-day American women and these populations, only one of which is diet.

Researchers are also exploring the interactions between diet and genetic factors. For example, nutrients in the diet can protect deoxyribonucleic acid (DNA) from being damaged and thus may help prevent the development of abnormal (mutated) genes related to cancer. Some believe that dietary factors combined with physical activity and weight control might delay or prevent the development of breast cancer in people with an increased genetic susceptibility to the disease.

Research on diet and breast cancer risk is often widely publicized, but despite a great deal of research, there's a lack of consensus on the topic. Although several dietary factors could influence cancer risk, most studies haven't found a clear-cut relationship between reduced consumption of particular foods or beverages and breast cancer prevention.

Fats

Probably no aspect of diet has received more attention with regard to cancer than has fat. Early studies suggested that high intake of dietary fat was associated with a higher incidence of breast cancer. And in the 1980s, public health organizations recommended that people eat less fat to reduce their risk of cancer. Since then, however, most studies have found no correlation between higher dietary fat consumption and an increased risk of breast cancer.

One group of researchers looked at the combined results of seven different studies that examined dietary fat and breast cancer risk. The seven studies collected information on the dietary habits of more than 350,000 women. The investigators found no association between fat in the diet and breast cancer — the risk of breast

The Skinny on Fat

Fats are classified according to the type of fatty acids — the molecular building blocks of fats — they contain. Saturated fatty acids are found in higher concentrations in animal foods such as meats and dairy products. Saturated fats, such as butter, whole milk, lard and shortening, are solid at room temperature. Polyunsaturated fatty acids are found in foods of plant origin. They include safflower, corn and sunflower oils. Polyunsaturated fats are liquid at room temperature. Monounsaturated fatty acids are found in highest concentrations in olive oil, canola oil, peanut oil, avocados and most nuts. These fats are liquid at room temperature but begin to solidify when chilled.

cancer was the same for women who had a high intake of fat and for those who ate a low-fat diet. The study concluded that even diets very low in fat don't protect against breast cancer. The Women's Health Initiative also studied a low-fat diet and found no reduction in breast cancer risk.

The (mostly) negative results in studies of breast cancer and dietary fat may be due to several factors:

- Studies that show different breast cancer rates in different countries can't easily separate diet from other risk factors.
- It's difficult to study the effects of an individual nutrient, such as fat, because foods contain multiple nutrients.
- Diets high in fat are also high in calories and can contribute to obesity, which is a risk factor for breast cancer among postmenopausal women. Obesity is also known to increase levels of estrogen and other hormones that may influence breast cancer development.
- It's possible that the effect of diet on breast cancer risk is time-dependent — that aspects of diet during childhood and adolescence, when breasts

are developing, affect breast cancer risk decades later.

- The effect of dietary fats on breast cancer may depend on the type of fat that's consumed. Several studies have tried to determine if saturated, monounsaturated and polyunsaturated fats have different effects on the development of breast cancer. Some preliminary studies have shown a modest protective benefit from olive oil, which is high in monounsaturated fat. But studies of other types of monounsaturated fat haven't found the same association, suggesting that the benefits of olive oil may come from other nutrients in the oil besides its fat.
- At this time, experts recommend replacing saturated fats with olive oil or other monounsaturated fats to reduce the risk of heart disease. Doing so may also have a slight effect on breast cancer risk.

Omega-3 and omega-6 fatty acids

Two types of polyunsaturated fat that have been studied in relation to breast cancer are omega-3 and omega-6 fatty acids. Omega-3 fatty acids are found in

Weight Control and Breast Cancer Prevention

There's little debate when it comes to the association between weight and breast cancer risk. Obesity is associated with an increased risk of breast cancer in postmenopausal women. And 75 percent of breast cancers occur in women older than age 50, an age when women tend to be particularly vulnerable to weight gain.

Excess body fat can lead to higher levels of estrogen, other hormones and growth factors, which are associated with increased breast cancer risk.

Excess weight is also reported to increase your risk of developing cancers of the colon, uterine lining (endometrium), gallbladder, esophagus, pancreas and kidney. For this reason, the American Cancer Society recommends that all people maintain a healthy weight throughout life.

If you're a woman who is past menopause and who's overweight and not very active, health experts recommend you lose weight and become more physically active. Doing so can not only help prevent cancer but also improve your overall health.

A good weight-loss program generally includes dietary changes, exercise, behavior modification and ongoing medical supervision. Contact your doctor if you need help losing weight.

fatty, cold-water fish, such as salmon, mackerel, sardines, herring, bass, shark, swordfish and tuna, and in flaxseed, walnuts and canola oil. In animal studies, a high intake of omega-3 fatty acids from fish oils has been shown to slow the development and growth of breast tumors. But most human studies have found little evidence to support the idea that high consumption of fish reduces breast cancer risk.

Omega-6 fatty acids are plentiful in vegetable oils. Some studies suggest that the ratio of omega-3 to omega-6 fatty acids in the diet is important in reducing breast cancer risk. In animal studies, a high omega-3 to omega-6 ratio has been shown to decrease the number, size and growth of breast tumors. A few preliminary human studies have found that a high omega-3 to omega-6 ratio is associated with a lower breast cancer risk in premenopausal women.

A study in breast cancer survivors
An important study, called the Women's Healthy Eating and Living (WHEL) trial, examined if a diet particularly low in fat and high in vegetables, fruit and fiber could lower the risk of breast cancer recurrence in women who had already had the disease. The trial compared a group of women following this enhanced diet and another group who ate a usual diet that followed standard nutritional recommendations.

After more than seven years of follow-up, there was no difference in the likelihood of recurrence in the women eating the healthier diet versus the usual diet. While these results were disappointing for survivors who are working hard to

Q: Will eating fruits and vegetables help prevent breast cancer?

A: Although eating a diet rich in fruits and vegetables provides a host of health benefits, these foods don't appear to offer particular protection against breast cancer.

Studies that have looked at consumption of fruits and vegetables and breast cancer risk have produced inconsistent results. One analysis of 26 studies did report a reduction in breast cancer risk with high vegetable consumption, and a modest reduction with high fruit intake.

However, another analysis of eight previously published studies including more than 350,000 women did not find an association between fruit and vegetable consumption and breast cancer risk.

But eating fruits and vegetables brings many other health benefits, including a reduced risk of diabetes, obesity and heart disease. And it may reduce your risk of other cancers, such as lung and colon cancers. The American Cancer Society recommends eating five or more servings of vegetables and fruit each day.

improve their health, it doesn't mean that a healthier diet — especially if it leads to a healthier weight — would not reduce the risk of developing breast cancer in the first place.

Vitamins and minerals
Several vitamins and minerals have been studied for their possible role in preventing breast cancer. These include vitamins A, C, D and E, folate (a B vitamin), isoflavones (phytoestrogens most commonly found in soy), and the mineral selenium.

Vitamin D is essential to bone health and other vital functions. It's obtained primarily by exposing your skin to sunshine, but it can also be obtained from some foods and dietary supplements. Some studies have suggested that low vitamin D levels increase the risk of breast cancer. It's important for your overall health to maintain normal vitamin D levels either through diet or supplements.

Studies also suggest that an adequate intake of folate may be important in preventing breast cancer, particularly among women who drink alcohol regularly. Folate occurs naturally in food, and folic acid is the synthetic form of the vitamin that's found in supplements and fortified foods, such as breakfast cereals. The recommended daily intake of folate is 400 micrograms a day. Alcohol interferes with the body's absorption of folate and increases the excretion of the vitamin by the kidneys.

Soy and phytoestrogens
Reports of the potential health benefits from soy have made soy foods increasingly popular. You may have heard that eating soy foods helps prevent breast cancer. Some studies, though, have suggested just the opposite — that soy is harmful for women with a high risk or history of breast cancer.

Soybeans are a source of isoflavones, a type of phytoestrogen. Phytoestrogens are plant chemicals that behave like estrogen in your body but are less potent than your natural estrogen.

Much of the basis for the suggestion that soy foods protect against breast cancer comes from studies that show lower breast cancer rates in many Asian countries, where soybean products are a food staple. Studies also show that when Asian women move to the United States and adopt a Western lifestyle, their risk of breast cancer rises. Clearly, many changes in lifestyle could explain these patterns. Soy consumption is just one factor.

Hundreds of studies have attempted to determine if eating soy does indeed help prevent breast cancer. Most studies haven't found that high soy intake cuts breast cancer risk. Nor have good studies found an increased risk of breast cancer in women eating soy products. Similarly, in breast cancer survivors, eating soy products has not been linked to the disease.

The bottom line? As with most things, moderation is key. If you enjoy soy foods, it's reasonable to use soy products in your diet in moderation, whether or not you're at risk of breast cancer or have had the disease. But experts don't recommend taking soy for the sole purpose of trying to lower your breast cancer risk. Common sources of soy protein in the American diet are tofu, soy milk, energy bars, soy protein powder and soy nuts.

Lignans

Lignans are another naturally occurring compound found in plants. Like isoflavones, several lignans are phytoestrogens.

Antioxidants and Cancer Prevention

Carotenoids, selenium, vitamin C and vitamin E are all antioxidants — substances that bind to and protect the body's cells from the damaging effects of free radicals. Free radicals are highly reactive and potentially toxic oxygen metabolites located within cells.

Free radicals are created as a byproduct of normal metabolism, the biochemical process in which your body uses oxygen and nutrients to produce energy. The natural aging process and chronic diseases also produce free radicals in the body. When produced in small amounts, these oxygen metabolites help the immune system do its job, but as production of free radicals increases, they can damage cells.

The effects of free radicals are neutralized by antioxidants. Antioxidants are substances found in food. They're derived from vitamins, minerals and plant chemicals in fruits and vegetables. Antioxidants also are available as supplements.

Because damage from free radicals is associated with increased risk of cancer, antioxidants are thought to possibly protect against cancer by decreasing the adverse effects of free radicals.

The richest source of lignans is flaxseed, sometimes called linseed. Flaxseed oil, however, doesn't contain a significant amount of lignans. Other sources of lignans include whole grains, soybeans, cranberries, some vegetables — broccoli, carrots, cauliflower and spinach — and black and green teas.

Like isoflavones, lignans are being studied for possible use in breast cancer prevention. But, as with isoflavones, the evidence isn't consistent enough to make the case for their preventive benefits. Some studies have shown a lower incidence of breast cancer among people who eat more lignan-containing foods, and in animal studies, lignans inhibited the growth of breast tumors.

More studies are needed about the potential benefits of flaxseed and other lignan-containing foods.

Alcohol

Drinking alcohol is associated with a higher risk of developing breast cancer. Having two drinks a day of beer, wine or liquor increases your risk of breast cancer by about 20 percent. The risk goes up with each drink consumed in a day.

Excessive use of alcohol is also associated with a number of other health problems. Moderation, again, is key. Moderate drinking is defined as no more than one drink a day for women. One drink is defined as 12 ounces of beer, 5 ounces of wine or 1.5 ounces of 80-proof distilled spirits.

Physical activity

Physical activity, ranging from yardwork to intensive exercise sessions, pays off

However, studies haven't found a specific benefit of antioxidants — whether from food sources or supplements — in protecting against breast cancer.

An important note for women with breast cancer who are receiving chemotherapy or radiation: Those treatments work, at least in part, by causing damage to DNA and other large molecules, especially in rapidly growing cells like cancer cells. If taken at the same time, antioxidants could help clean up this damage, something you wouldn't want. This is why taking antioxidants during cancer treatment isn't recommended.

In one study of 90 women with breast cancer, those who took high-dose combinations of vitamins and minerals in addition to standard cancer treatments fared worse in terms of survival time than did women who didn't take the supplements. In another large study involving smokers, participants who took supplemental vitamins developed more lung cancers than did participants who took inactive pills (placebos).

Because of the uncertainty surrounding so many supplements, the best advice is to get your antioxidants by way of food you eat — in other words, from a healthy diet — rather than in the form of a pill.

Diet and breast cancer

Many questions still remain regarding the relationship between food, alcohol and breast cancer prevention. Here's a summary of what's currently known about various foods and alcohol:

Dietary factor	Effect on breast cancer	Recommendation
High-fat diet	Doesn't directly increase risk, but contributes to obesity, which is associated with increased risk	Aim for a total fat intake of no more than 30 percent of calories, with 10 percent or less from saturated fat. Minimize animal sources of fat, such as meats and high-fat dairy products.
Olive oil	May have protective effect; further research is needed	Replace saturated fat with olive oil or other monounsaturated fats.
Fruits and vegetables	Limited	To reap other health benefits, eat five or more servings daily.
Vitamin D	Low levels may increase risk	Maintain normal levels — from sunshine or from milk and juices fortified with vitamin D, or from supplements.
Soy products	No clear increase or decrease in risk	Eat dietary soy in moderation. Soy supplements aren't recommended.
Folate or folic acid	Decreases risk, especially in women who drink alcohol	Consume the recommended daily intake of 400 micrograms.
Fish and fish oils	Reduce breast cancer development in animals; no strong effect shown in humans	Consume fish and fish oils as part of a healthy diet.
Flaxseed	Unknown	Eat in moderation.
Alcohol	Increases risk	If you drink, do so in moderation.

with a number of health benefits. Among them are cardiovascular fitness, which can help protect against heart disease, and a reduced risk of diabetes. Exercise may also decrease the risk of certain cancers, such as colon and breast cancers.

There is good evidence that regular physical activity lowers the risk of breast cancer. Over 60 studies have investigated the association between breast cancer and physical activity, and most show a reduced breast cancer risk in women who were most physically active.

The relationship between exercise and breast cancer risk is complex, and several underlying biological factors may account for the reduction in risk that comes with physical activity. Regular exercise helps

FASTFACT

Too much weight
and too little exercise

The International Agency for
Research on Cancer estimates that
between one-fourth and one-third of
cancers of all types could be attributed to the combined effects of being
overweight and physically inactive.

prevent obesity and weight gain, which
are associated with breast cancer risk.
Both physical inactivity and obesity affect
the normal metabolism of insulin. Regular
exercise may reduce levels of insulin and
insulin-like growth factors — high levels
of which have been associated with an
increased risk of breast cancer. Exercise
may also lower levels of sex hormones,
including estrogen. Estrogen is thought to
act as the fuel that promotes the growth
of some breast cancers.

Experts such as the American Cancer
Society recommend engaging in at least
150 minutes a week of moderate aerobic
activity (think brisk walking or swimming) or 75 minutes of vigorous aerobic
activity (such as running), preferably
spread out throughout the week. Any
physical activity that raises your heart
rate or causes you to sweat is beneficial,
from recreational sports to heavy house-
work or yardwork, even if done in short
sessions.

If you're already living an active lifestyle, consider doing a bit more. Evidence
suggests that higher amounts of physical
activity may provide even greater reductions in cancer risk. Although the optimal
length, frequency and intensity of exercise
for cancer prevention aren't known, 300
minutes or more a week (the equivalent of
one hour, five days a week) of moderate
or greater intensity physical activity may
be a goal to strive for.

Women at High Risk

If you're a woman identified as having
a high risk of breast cancer, prevention
becomes even more critical. Women at
high risk include those who test positive
for a BRCA1 or BRCA2 mutation, women
from BRCA1 or BRCA2 families who do
not wish to be tested themselves, women
with strong family histories, and women
whose families are tested and found to be
negative for a BRCA1 or BRCA2 mutation
(BRCA negative families).

A woman may also be at high risk if
she is from a family where genetic testing isn't feasible (such as when relatives
with cancer are deceased) or when no one
in the family wants to pursue testing. A
personal history of atypical hyperplasia or
lobular carcinoma *in situ* (LCIS) may place
a woman at high risk. (See Chapters 4 or 9
for more information on these conditions).
A woman may also be considered at high
risk if her lifetime risk of breast cancer is
20 percent or more.

Women at high risk face a number of
difficult issues:

• Understanding and coming to terms
  with the meaning of their risk status
• Dealing with fear of harm, disfigure-
  ment, pain or death
• Coping with guilt about passing on a
  hereditary risk
• Managing stress and worries

• Making decisions about preventive therapy

Before pursuing any type of treatment aimed at reducing your risk, it's essential that you have an accurate estimate of your breast cancer risk. Make an appointment with your doctor or a breast specialist to determine your risk status. For many women, genetic counseling can be helpful. You can read more about this process in Chapter 5.

Doctors don't always agree on the most effective way to manage the care of high-risk women. Some focus on close surveillance and early detection of the disease, while others focus on risk reduction.

The goal of screening and surveillance, sometimes referred to as secondary prevention, is early detection of breast cancer — since early diagnosis usually means more successful treatment. Screening in high-risk women typically involves breast examinations by your doctor twice a year, monthly breast self-examinations, and annual mammograms beginning five to 10 years before the age of the earliest breast cancer diagnosed in the family. In addition, annual screening using magnetic resonance imaging (MRI) is now recommended for many high-risk women.

Some women at high risk of breast cancer prefer to take more proactive steps to reduce their risk. They may consider surgery to remove their breasts (preventive, or prophylactic, mastectomy) or surgery to remove their ovaries (preventive, or prophylactic, oophorectomy). In women who haven't yet reached menopause, removing the ovaries significantly reduces the amount of estrogen that their bodies produce. This can halt or slow the growth of breast cancer. Another option is the use of medications to reduce cancer risk. These strategies are sometimes referred to as primary prevention.

Each of these options has benefits and risks. Deciding what course to take is a highly personal decision. There's no one right answer for all high-risk women. Risk-reduction counseling can help you evaluate your options and make the decision that's right for you. With any primary preventive strategy, there's always the chance that some women who pursue it would not have developed breast cancer at all. For this reason, it's important to have a thorough understanding of your individual risk and your options for reducing that risk.

Prophylactic mastectomy

Risk-reducing mastectomy, also known as prophylactic mastectomy, is the surgical removal of one or both breasts to reduce the risk of breast cancer. For example, a high-risk woman with breast cancer may have a mastectomy to treat the cancer and choose to have her remaining breast removed prophylactically. Although prophylactic mastectomy was discussed as early as the 1920s, the operation wasn't commonly performed until the 1960s and 1970s, when breast implants became available for breast reconstruction and the medical community gained a greater awareness of increased breast cancer risk in some families.

Studies have shown that removal of both breasts (bilateral mastectomy) is very effective in reducing the risk of breast cancer. However, the surgery doesn't prevent all cases of breast cancer. That's because breast tissue is widely distributed on the chest wall, extending into the armpit, and even to the collarbone, in most women. Therefore, it's impossible for a surgeon to remove all breast tissue. It's possible that breast cancer could still develop in the small amount of remaining breast tissue.

Researchers at Mayo Clinic compared women with a family history of breast cancer who had bilateral prophylactic mastectomies between 1960 and 1993 to their sisters who didn't have the surgery. In 214 high-risk women who had a bilateral prophylactic mastectomy, just three breast cancers occurred during 14 years of follow-up. Based on their sisters' experiences, 30 breast cancers should have occurred in that time frame in the high-risk women. Thus, prophylactic mastectomy reduced the risk of their getting breast cancer by about 90 percent, and the surgery also resulted in a significant reduction in the number of deaths from breast cancer. Instead of an expected 19 deaths, there were two.

Subsequent research has consistently confirmed that prophylactic mastectomy decreases the risk of breast cancer by 90 percent or more, even in BRCA carriers.

Other studies have found that an opposite-breast (contralateral) prophylactic mastectomy significantly reduces the risk of a second breast cancer in women who've had cancer in one breast and are at high risk of developing it in the other.

Who's a candidate?
Prophylactic mastectomy is an elective procedure, and there aren't precise guidelines defining who should have the surgery. A number of factors are taken into

consideration. The surgery may be appropriate for women who:
- Carry a BRCA mutation
- Have a strong family history of breast cancer without a known genetic mutation
- Have already had one breast removed due to cancer and have a family history of the disease
- Have had lobular carcinoma *in situ*

To make the best individual decision about whether prophylactic mastectomy is appropriate, it's crucial that you understand your true risk of breast cancer. Many women overestimate their individual risk.

It's highly recommended that women considering prophylactic mastectomy talk with a genetic counselor before making this decision. Meeting with a breast surgeon beforehand to discuss the potential risks and benefits of the surgery is also essential. Women interested in breast reconstruction — plastic surgery to restore the shape of a breast mound — after a mastectomy should meet with a plastic surgeon to discuss options available. A woman may also want to meet with a psychologist or other mental health professional to discuss potential issues related to body image and other concerns that may follow this type of surgery.

How it's done
The recommended procedure for prophylactic mastectomy is a mastectomy that removes the entire breast and nipple. The skin over the breast may be preserved to enhance breast reconstruction. Subcutaneous mastectomy, an operation that removes breast tissue but spares the nipple, isn't the preferred procedure

because it leaves a substantial amount of breast tissue behind.

After a mastectomy, most women choose to have breast reconstruction. Mastectomy and breast reconstruction are discussed in more detail in Chapters 11 and 12.

Risks

Like any major surgery, prophylactic mastectomy may result in some physical complications, either immediately after the operation or months to years later. Problems with breast implants are among the most common concerns.

One study evaluated 592 women who had both breasts removed and implant reconstruction. Almost all these women had subcutaneous mastectomies. Over the next 14 years, about half the women required a second operation. The most common reason for this second operation was a problem with implants, often the development of a tight, firm capsule around the implant.

In addition to possible physical complications, prophylactic mastectomy can have psychological and social effects. Limited research has been done regarding the emotional and psychological effects of prophylactic mastectomy. In one study at Mayo Clinic, researchers surveyed women who had had prophylactic mastectomy, asking several questions about the psychological and social consequences of the surgery. About 15 years after the surgery, 70 percent of the women were either satisfied or very satisfied with their surgery. Almost 75 percent of the women said they had a lower level of emotional concern about developing breast cancer. The majority of women

also reported either favorable effects or no change in emotional stability, stress, self-esteem, sexual relationships and feelings of femininity. When asked whether they would choose to have the surgery again, two-thirds said they definitely or probably would.

Women who felt they had the surgery mainly on the basis of a doctor's advice were more likely to be dissatisfied. Women who had strong support from family and friends were most satisfied with their decisions.

In smaller studies, women who had had prophylactic mastectomies reported significantly lower levels of anxiety after the surgery, but some women experienced difficulties with body image, sexual interest and functioning, and self-esteem.

Because of the potential physical and psychological effects, the decision to have prophylactic mastectomy must be made on an individual basis after carefully weighing the risks and benefits. It's important to fully consider all of your options before making a decision. You need to understand the procedure and the effect it will have on body image and, potentially, your sexuality. Some women find it helpful to talk with others who have had the surgery.

Prophylactic oophorectomy

Another surgical option available to women at high risk of breast cancer is prophylactic salpingo-oophorectomy — removal of the fallopian tubes and ovaries. Removing the ovaries in premenopausal women greatly decreases the amount of estrogen a woman's body

Lisa's Story

After watching her mother die of breast cancer at the age of 49, Lisa, a nurse, developed cancerphobia.

Lisa's fear of cancer grew as she took stock of her family history and learned that many of her relatives had been diagnosed with either breast or ovarian cancer: her maternal grandmother, four of seven maternal aunts and two paternal aunts. "I always thought that I would die of breast cancer. So many of my family members did. I vowed to try to detect it early."

Lisa's insurance company wouldn't pay for a mammogram before age 40, so she and her husband decided to bear the cost. Doctors detected a lump when Lisa had her first mammogram. After a biopsy revealed that the lump was benign, Lisa's surgeon ordered yearly mammograms and checkups every six months, and the insurance company began to pay for the screenings.

Over the course of five years, mammography identified four lumps in Lisa's breasts. She underwent a biopsy each time — all of the lumps were benign.

But Lisa, her husband, Todd, and their two daughters began to dread the routine screenings — and the possibility that results would reveal an aggressive cancer. Noting her family history and her level of distress, Lisa's surgeon asked Lisa if she had ever considered prophylactic mastectomy.

After thinking about it, Lisa decided that she was interested in learning more about the surgery. She conducted extensive Internet research on prophylactic mastectomy and weighed its pros and cons.

In addition, Lisa decided to have a complete genetic evaluation and risk assessment. After three days of undergoing diagnostic tests, genetic tests and genetic counseling, as well as consulting with a breast surgeon, Lisa and Todd had all of the information they needed to make a decision. Her family history and history of previous breast biopsies all added up to a very high risk.

"The decision to proceed with prophylactic mastectomy became a no-brainer after we saw all those black circles indicating breast cancer on Lisa's family history pedigree," says Todd. "I was going to love her whether she had breasts or not. It didn't matter."

The procedure took about two hours. Immediately following that surgery, a plastic surgeon began an intricate reconstruction procedure that took about 14 hours to complete.

Lisa required 16 weeks of rest to fully recover, but says that she's pleased with the results.

"Never once did we doubt our decision," Lisa points out. "Never once did we have second thoughts. I've felt the world lifted off my shoulders. My life has started all over."

produces and may halt or slow breast cancers dependent on estrogen to grow.

Oophorectomy is usually motivated by the need to reduce ovarian cancer risk. However, if the procedure is performed before a woman reaches menopause, it also reduces breast cancer risk.

Prophylactic salpingo-oophorectomy reduces the risk of breast cancer by about 50 percent in premenopausal women. It reduces the risk of ovarian cancer (including tubal and peritoneal cancer) by 90 percent in both pre- and postmenopausal women. Peritoneal cancer, which behaves like ovarian cancer, can still develop in cells lining the abdominal-pelvic cavity, even after prophylactic salpingo-oophorectomy.

Oophorectomy is usually recommended for women who are at increased risk of both breast cancer and ovarian cancer due to an inherited mutation in the BRCA1 or BRCA2 gene. Even though the risk of ovarian cancer may be lower than the risk of breast cancer (see the tables on page 81), ovarian cancer is much more difficult to detect at an early stage. For this reason, it's also more likely to be deadly.

For BRCA1 carriers, oophorectomy is usually done between ages 35 and 40. For BRCA2 carriers, ovarian cancer risk is less than 1 percent until age 45, so the procedure may be delayed somewhat. Prophylactic oophorectomy may also be recommended for women with a strong family history of breast and ovarian cancers but no known genetic alteration.

Some women at high risk choose to have a prophylactic oophorectomy instead of prophylactic mastectomy because of their concerns about body image and because breast cancer is more likely to be detected at an earlier stage than is ovarian cancer.

When an oophorectomy is performed, the fallopian tubes are removed as well (this procedure is known as salpingo-oophorectomy) to avoid the possibility of tumors developing in the tubes. In addition, the fallopian tubes are no longer needed if the ovaries are removed.

Risks

Removal of the ovaries may bring some negative consequences that need consideration. In premenopausal women, oophorectomy causes premature menopause. One important consideration, especially for younger women, is that this brings about the loss of fertility. Premature menopause can also increase the risk of osteoporosis. Signs and symptoms of menopause, which include hot flashes, vaginal dryness, sexual problems, sleep disturbances and, possibly, cognitive changes, may affect quality of life. Some women who have such surgery experience emotional and sexual effects, though there's insufficient research in this area.

Using hormone replacement therapy (HRT) after prophylactic oophorectomy is an option for reducing some of the signs and symptoms of menopause, especially for women who have the procedure at a young age. The effect of such hormones on breast cancer risk isn't entirely clear, but the amount of hormone given is considerably less than what your ovaries would have made.

If you're considering prophylactic oophorectomy, make sure you fully understand the risks and benefits of the

Janice's Story

It came as such a shock to Janice when her sister was diagnosed with breast cancer at a such young age. It turns out, the cancer had gone undetected for some time and had spread beyond the breast. The diagnosis was not good, and Janice's sister died two years later at the age of 43. Five years after her sister's death, Janice's mother was diagnosed with inflammatory breast cancer that had spread to her lymph nodes. Her mother's diagnosis triggered a warning for Janice — maybe these cancers weren't unfortunate coincidences, maybe they had some sort of genetic link.

To gather more information and help her sort through the situation, Janice called a local breast clinic. From there, she was referred for genetic counseling. During genetic counseling, Janice filled out a questionnaire about her family history of cancer. The results revealed not only a few cases of breast cancer on her mother's side but also a strong history of colon cancer on her father's side. For Janice, the results of the evaluation indicated that she was at increased cancer risk.

The next step was deciding what to do about it — if anything. Janice learned that she had a number of options to reduce her risk. Because she didn't feel there was one clear-cut preventive strategy that would be best for her, Janice decided to take her time and keep her options open.

For the time being, Janice has a mammogram regularly to check for any breast changes. She also decided to have her uterus and ovaries removed. The purpose of this surgery was twofold: Removing her uterus would reduce her risk of uterine cancer, which is greater in families with a strong history of colon cancer. And removing her ovaries would decrease the amount of estrogen produced in her body, helping reduce her risk of breast cancer.

While Janice had initially been reluctant to have genetic testing, she later decided to proceed and is awaiting the results.

For Janice, one of the hardest parts is keeping the situation in perspective. "You kind of live in this worst-case scenario world," she says. At times, it's been difficult for Janice to not get wrapped up in the uncertainty of her future — to not feel like the cancer risk is a death sentence. "You need to try to separate yourself from what's going on around you." Janice's advice to others is to try not to dwell on the what-ifs.

The results of her genetic tests may also benefit more than just Janice. Janice is concerned that her daughter and niece may be at increased cancer risk, and the results of her tests may help them with their health decisions.

Janice has also decided to turn this time of struggle and uncertainty into an opportunity to pursue her dream. She has always wanted to be a writer and she loves learning, so Janice has returned to school to work toward a master's degree in health journalism. She's enjoying school, she feels well and, so far, she's happy with the decisions she's made.

procedure. Genetic counseling is recommended before oophorectomy. The timing of the procedure depends on the age at which a woman is considered at greater risk of ovarian and breast cancers. (As mentioned earlier, BRCA1 carriers are at risk of getting ovarian cancer at an earlier age than are BRCA2 carriers.) After having an oophorectomy, some women choose to undergo other preventive strategies for breast cancer, such as chemoprevention or mastectomy. Prophylactic oophorectomy is discussed in more detail in Chapter 17.

Prevention medications

Using medication to prevent the development of cancer is called chemoprevention. However, some people object to this term because *chemo* brings to mind chemotherapy, which involves much stronger medications and more dramatic side effects. For this reason, terms such as *prevention medications* or *preventive therapy* are used instead.

For breast cancer, several large, randomized clinical trials have been performed in healthy women — who had some increased risk of breast cancer — comparing an anti-estrogen drug (such as tamoxifen) with an inactive placebo. It's important to understand that the women who participated in these studies could have a wide range of risks. For example, being over age 60 was considered sufficient risk for entry into some of these trials. While many participants had some family history of breast cancer, there were very few BRCA1 or BRCA2 carriers among participants. Genetic testing was not done at the start of the study but has

been done later on stored blood samples in select women.

Tamoxifen and raloxifene (Evista) both belong to a class of drugs called selective estrogen receptor modulators (SERMs). These drugs bind to the same protein partner that the hormone estrogen needs to exert its effects — the estrogen receptor.

Estrogen is thought to act as a fuel that promotes the growth of breast cancer cells. But SERMs are different from estrogen. In some tissues they mimic the effect of estrogen, and in others — such as in breast tissue — they block or work against estrogen. The pattern of activity varies with each SERM.

In the remainder of the chapter, tamoxifen, raloxifene, aromatase inhibitors, nonsteroidal anti-inflammatory drugs and newer agents are discussed in more detail.

Tamoxifen

Tamoxifen has been used to treat breast cancer for decades. Four large clinical trials — one in the United States and three in Europe — studied the drug's ability to prevent breast cancer.

In more than 28,000 women in the studies, tamoxifen was compared to an inactive substance (placebo). By pooling the results of these four studies, researchers showed that tamoxifen reduced the risk of a woman developing invasive breast cancer by 43 percent. Only estrogen receptor positive breast cancers were reduced. There was no effect on estrogen receptor negative cancers. The risk of ductal carcinoma *in situ* (DCIS) was also reduced by 37 percent.

The 43 percent risk reduction refers to relative risk. What does this mean in real

Options for women at high risk of breast cancer

Option	Advantages	Disadvantages
Surveillance	• Preserves breasts • Allows for other options • Requires no treatment for women who don't develop breast cancer • MRI screening adds sensitivity.	• Doesn't prevent disease • Mammography has a high rate of false-negatives in younger women. • MRI screening can lead to false-positives. • Lacks good research on its effectiveness
Prevention medications	• Anti-estrogens reduce breast cancer risk by about 50 percent. • Preserves breasts • Allows for other options	• Effective only for estrogen receptor positive breast cancer • Effectiveness for BRCA1 and BRCA2 carriers uncertain • Several side effects, depending on the drug • Tamoxifen can be used in either premenopausal or postmenopausal women; raloxifene and exemestane are for postmenopausal women only. • No effect on breast cancer deaths has been shown.
Prophylactic mastectomy	• Reduces risk of breast cancer by at least 90 percent • Has a long-term effect	• Requires major surgery that results in loss of breasts • Is an irreversible decision • Has potential psychological and physical effects • Has a high rate of re-operation with implant reconstruction
Prophylactic oophorectomy	• Reduces risk of breast cancer by 50 percent in premenopausal women • Reduces risk of ovarian cancer by 90 percent • Preserves breasts	• Effect on estrogen receptor negative breast cancer less certain • Results in premature menopause with associated side effects • Results in loss of fertility • Is an irreversible decision

terms? To make this easier to understand, let's say that tamoxifen cuts a woman's risk in half (so slightly more than the 43 percent reduction actually seen). Say that a particular woman has a 4 percent actual risk of developing breast cancer in the next five years if she doesn't take tamoxifen. By taking the drug, she reduces the risk to 2 percent. In other words, out of 100 women with a similar level of risk, four would develop the disease over five years if they didn't take tamoxifen. If they did take the drug, two would develop the disease.

A very important finding in these clinical trials was that deaths from breast cancer weren't reduced. This is because the treatment didn't prevent the more aggressive, estrogen receptor negative breast cancers.

Side effects and risks

The most common side effects of tamoxifen are hot flashes and vaginal discharge. Some premenopausal women also experience menstrual irregularities.

Women who take tamoxifen are at increased risk of developing blood clots, although this is uncommon, occurring in less than 1 percent of women who take the drug. Tamoxifen also increases the risk of two types of cancer that can develop in the uterus — endometrial cancer, which begins in the lining of the uterus, and uterine sarcoma, which arises in the muscular wall of the uterus.

In these trials, women who took tamoxifen had about three times the chance of developing uterine cancer, compared to women who took a placebo. The absolute risk of this is small — about three additional cases of uterine cancer among 1,000 women taking tamoxifen each year. The increased risk was seen only among women who were age 50 or older. Women under 50 who took tamoxifen had no increased risk of uterine cancer.

Raloxifene

Like tamoxifen, raloxifene binds to estrogen receptors in breast tissue and blocks estrogen's effects in the breasts. On bone tissue, on the other hand, the drug behaves like estrogen, stopping bone loss.

Raloxifene was originally developed for the treatment of breast cancer but was found to have low activity in women with metastatic disease. Because of its favorable effect on bone density, it was then tested in women with osteoporosis. In the bone trials, scientists saw that women who took raloxifene were less likely to develop breast cancer. Thus, in 1999, the National Cancer Institute launched the Study of Tamoxifen and Raloxifene (STAR) trial. This study included almost 20,000 women and compared raloxifene to tamoxifen in postmenopausal women at increased risk of breast cancer. The results: With eight years of follow-up, raloxifene was not quite as effective as tamoxifen. Raloxifene has about three-fourths the effectiveness that tamoxifen did in reducing the risk of breast cancer.

Raloxifene hasn't been studied in premenopausal women. Because its safety in younger women is unknown, the drug isn't recommended for these women.

Similar to tamoxifen, raloxifene increases the risk of blood clots slightly. Early reports suggested that raloxifene, unlike tamoxifen, didn't increase the risk of uterine cancer. However, the most recent analysis of STAR trial results show that the likelihood of uterine cancer was the same in those taking raloxifene as in those taking tamoxifen. Both tamoxifen and raloxifene have been approved by the FDA for prevention of breast cancer. For raloxifene, this approval is only in postmenopausal women.

Aromatase inhibitors

Aromatase inhibitors are drugs that reduce estrogen levels in a woman's body by blocking an enzyme called aromatase, which is involved in converting other hormones to estrogen. These medications present an alternative hormonal approach to breast cancer treatment. Three aromatase inhibitors, anastrozole (Arimidex), exemestane (Aromasin) and letrozole (Femara), are currently used to treat breast cancer in postmenopausal women. These drugs can't be used in younger women whose ovaries produce estrogen.

A large clinical trial compared exemestane to a placebo in postmenopausal women to help prevent breast cancer. The trial showed a 65 percent reduction in the risk of estrogen receptor positive breast cancer but, like tamoxifen, had no effect on estrogen receptor negative disease. Arthritis and menopausal symptoms were more common in those given exemestane.

Serious adverse effects such as blood clots and uterine cancer were not seen with aromatase inhibitors. Some aromatase inhibitors may contribute to bone loss, but the extent of this potential side effect has not yet been fully determined.

Nonsteroidal anti-inflammatory drugs

Several studies have tried to determine if aspirin and nonsteroidal anti-inflammatory drugs (NSAIDs) have an effect on breast cancer risk. NSAIDs include many common over-the-counter painkillers, such as ibuprofen (Advil, Motrin, others) and naproxen sodium (Aleve). All the studies to date have been observational studies, which don't provide the strongest level of evidence.

Some research has found that people who regularly take aspirin or NSAIDs have a slightly decreased risk of breast cancer. But other studies have not shown a significant association between breast cancer risk and the use of NSAIDs. In studies involving animals, NSAIDs have been shown to inhibit the development of breast tumors.

Of note, the benefits of NSAIDs in lowering breast cancer risk were seen only with standard doses, not in low (baby aspirin) doses. Acetaminophen (Tylenol), which isn't an NSAID and has a different mechanism of action, hasn't been associated with a lower risk of breast cancer.

It's not known for certain how aspirin and NSAIDs may help protect against breast cancer. In animals, these drugs are capable of triggering cell death in abnormal breast cells. The medications work by blocking cyclooxygenase (COX) enzymes, which are involved in many important body processes, including inflammation and cancer development.

Future Directions

Of course, it would be great if doctors knew just what to do to prevent breast cancer. But in reality few factors are known to provide strong protection against the disease.

Preventive options for women at high risk are fairly limited and far from ideal. The good news is, breast cancer prevention is the focus of a wide range of ongoing research. Advances in the understanding of cancer are providing more targets and tools to achieve the ultimate goal of preventing breast cancer.

Chapter 7: Breast Cancer

The Latest on Screening

Ongoing Controversies	112
Mammography trials	112
Screening risks	113
Making sense of it all	114
Screening Recommendations	115
Breast Self-Awareness	116
How to do a breast self-exam	116
Clinical Breast Examination	119
Mammography	120
Screening mammograms	120
Diagnostic mammograms	120
Preparing for your mammogram	121
The day of the test	122
Understanding the results	123
Limitations of mammography	123
Where to get a mammogram	124
New Approaches	126

Until scientists find a way to prevent breast cancer, the best way to fight the disease remains the same — to find it as early as possible. You've likely heard or read this many times, but it bears repeating: The earlier cancer is detected, the better the chance for successful treatment and long-term survival. That's why breast cancer screening is so important.

The purpose of screening for a particular disease is to identify the condition before it starts producing signs and symptoms and while it's the most receptive to treatment. The makeup of most cancers is such that if a mass of cancerous (malignant) cells is caught early enough, the need for aggressive treatment is reduced and the chance for a cure is increased.

Screening for breast cancer has traditionally been accomplished with three methods, described in detail in this chapter:

- Mammography, a procedure in which X-rays are taken of your breasts to detect masses too small to be felt
- Clinical breast examination (CBE), a procedure in which your doctor examines your breasts for lumps or changes
- Breast self-examination (BSE), a procedure in which you examine your own breasts for lumps or changes

Many experts believe that increased awareness and use of breast cancer screening, particularly mammography, has played an important role in the decrease in breast cancer deaths. Breast cancer death (mortality) rates have been declining every year in the U.S. since 1989.

Finding better ways to screen for breast cancer continues to be a top priority. This chapter looks at the standard methods, along with breast magnetic resonance imaging (MRI) and newer approaches.

Ongoing Controversies

Despite a steady decrease in deaths, many details regarding breast cancer screening remain controversial. Largely because of conflicting studies, not all doctors and medical organizations agree on the benefits of today's screening methods, the age at which women should begin screening and how often they should be screened (screening intervals).

As a result, there are differences of opinion on when or how often screening should be done, or even if it should be done at all. Much of the controversy centers on mammography screening, although both clinical breast examinations and breast self-examinations have come under scrutiny as well. Use of breast MRI for high risk women has its supporters as well as opponents.

Since breast cancer screening is such a hot topic, it's helpful to understand the benefits and limitations of today's screening methods, so you can make wise decisions about your personal care.

Mammography trials

It seems so simple — that screening for breast cancer should be good for everyone. But, of course, nothing is that simple, and recommendations from the medical community must be based on solid evidence. This evidence comes from randomized clinical trials, the first of which started in 1963. That trial compared screening versus usual medical care without screening. One mammography trial was performed in the U.S., the others were done in Sweden, Canada and Britain. Once it became apparent that screening with mammography was beneficial, it no longer was considered ethical to perform randomized trials that included women who didn't receive mammograms.

This is why a lot of data regarding breast cancer screening is controversial. Much of the evidence is based on older clinical trials that contained flaws and that were performed when the quality of imaging was less than optimal.

In addition, the data on the benefits of screening for women under age 50 are less convincing. There are fewer breast cancers in younger women, and younger women often have more dense breast tissue. Mammography isn't as good at identifying cancer in dense breast tissue as it is in more fatty tissue.

However, updates to these older trials indicate that screening with mammography saves lives. For women in their 40s, regular screening led to a 15 percent relative reduction in breast cancer deaths.

What does this figure mean in terms of actual women? Think of it this way: 1,900 women in their 40s need to be screened regularly to prevent one death from breast cancer. For women in their 50s, 1,340 women need to be screened to prevent one breast cancer death.

For women in their 60s the results are stronger, with a 32 percent relative reduction in breast cancer deaths. This means that only 377 women at this age need to be screened to prevent one death. Most of the mammography trials didn't include women in their 70s or older, so good data are lacking for this group.

Another advantage of mammography is that mammograms tend to pick up cancers earlier. Early detection may avoid the need for aggressive surgery and chemotherapy.

In addition to mammography, there have been questions regarding the value of clinical exams and breast self-examination. These issues are discussed later in the chapter.

Screening risks

Adding to the controversy regarding mammography, researchers point out that screening has some risks. It's possible that a tumor may be missed during screening — what's known as a false-negative result — leading to a false sense of security. If a woman notices a lump in her breast and a mammogram isn't able to detect the tumor, resulting in a negative, or "normal," finding, the woman may be inclined to think "It's nothing," when it may be cancer. On the other hand, a mammogram may detect an abnormality when no cancer is present — a false-positive result — resulting in unnecessary anxiety and testing.

In addition, some individuals believe that certain cancers that are detected with a mammogram may be a type that grows so slowly they may never pose a threat to the lives of the women who have them. These individuals are concerned that identifying such cancers can lead to unnecessary tests and procedures, as well as needless fear and anxiety. Follow-up tests and procedures to diagnose and treat the cancer may pose some risk of side effects, and they can be expensive and time-consuming. Unfortunately, it's not possible to judge which cancers might fit into this category.

Are You at High Risk?

The following groups are considered to be at high risk of developing breast cancer:
- Women with a BRCA1 or BRCA2 mutation
- Women from BRCA1 or BRCA2 families who haven't been tested themselves
- Women with a strong family history of breast cancer who have a lifetime risk of 20% or more
- Women with atypical hyperplasia or lobular carcinoma *in situ* (LCIS)
- Women who had chest wall radiation between ages 10 and 30

For more information on breast cancer risk factors, see Chapter 4.

Screening guide

The following chart offers an overview of the latest recommendations and where most organizations stand on screening:

Age	Consensus	Recommendation
Women in their 20s and 30s, average risk	General agreement	• Breast self-exam optional • Clinical breast exam every three years, as part of general physical • No mammogram
Women ages 40 to 49, average risk	Some disagreement	• Breast self-exam optional • Clinical breast exam annually, as part of general physical • Mammogram every year
Women ages 50 to 74, average risk	Some disagreement	• Breast self-exam optional • Clinical breast exam annually, as part of general physical • Mammogram every year
Women age 75 and older, average risk	Some disagreement	• Regular screening as long as an individual is in good health
Women of all ages, high risk	General agreement	• Breast self-exam recommended • Clinical breast exam every 6-12 months, as part of general physical • Mammogram every year • Talk to your doctor for an individualized program. You may benefit from starting screening earlier and using other screening tools, such as MRI.

Making sense of it all

Breast cancer is a well-publicized disease, and with the media attention given to one study and then to another, it's easy to feel lost in a sea of statistics and opinions. You may find yourself asking, "If these exams aren't that useful, then why am I doing them?"

The truth is, despite their limitations, screening methods are useful. Many women have found their cancers by doing breast self-exams. It's also a fact that doctors do detect breast changes when performing clinical breast exams as part of a general physical. And most research shows that breast cancers found in women who have regular mammograms are more likely to be smaller in size and easier to treat than those cancers found in women who don't get regular mammograms.

Screening Recommendations

So, when should you be screened and how often? Most health organizations support regular breast cancer screening with mammograms. Organizations such as the American Cancer Society, the American College of Obstetricians and Gynecologists, and the National Comprehensive Cancer Network recommend that women at average risk of breast cancer have their first screening mammogram at age 40. If you're at high risk, you and your doctor may decide to begin screening tests at an earlier age.

An alternative viewpoint put forward by the U.S. Preventive Services Task Force in a 2009 report was that women under the age of 50 should decide whether to have a mammogram based on their individual circumstances and the benefits and disadvantages of the test.

The benefit of mammography increases with age, with the strongest benefit

Fibrocystic Breasts

Fibrocystic breasts are composed of tissue that feels ropy, lumpy or bumpy in texture. Doctors refer to this as "nodular" or "glandular" breast tissue. The nodular tissue may be accompanied by fluid-filled cysts in the breasts, which adds to the lumpy feeling. This condition, called fibrocystic breasts or fibrocystic breast changes, tends to be more prominent in the upper outer region of your breasts.

Fibrocystic breasts are often associated with variations in hormone levels during your menstrual cycle, sometimes causing painful breasts. Symptoms tend to be most bothersome just before menstruation.

More than half of women experience fibrocystic breast changes at some point in life. The condition is more common in women in their 20s and 30s. Having fibrocystic breasts doesn't mean that you're more likely to develop breast cancer, but if your breasts are lumpy, performing breast self-exams can be more challenging. Try to become familiar with what's normal for your breasts. This will help make the detection of new lumps or changes easier.

For pain associated with fibrocystic breasts, talk to your doctor about options for relieving the pain.

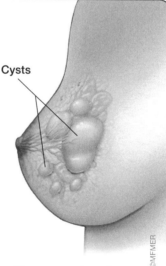

Cysts

©MFMER

Many women have lumpy (fibrocystic) breasts. The condition is most often associated with changes in hormone levels that occur with menstruation.

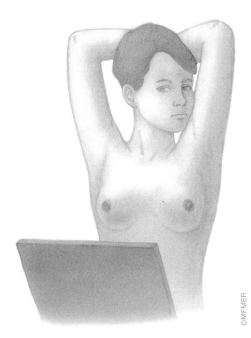

In front of a mirror, visually inspect your breasts for changes in shape and size, dimpling, and nipple and skin changes, such as discoloration or scaling.

coming after age 50. This occurs partly because your chances of developing breast cancer increase as you get older. In addition, normal breast tissue is generally less dense in postmenopausal women, making cancers easier to detect.

Breast Self-Awareness

For years, doctors and women's health advocacy groups have emphasized the need for regular breast self-examination (BSE) to promote early detection of tumors. However, because recent research has failed to show that regular breast self-examination reduces the number of deaths caused by breast cancer, there's less emphasis on this screening method. Doctors are increasingly taking the stance that if breast self-examination causes you more anxiety than it's worth, it's OK not to do it or to do it only on occasion.

This doesn't mean, though, that self-exams are never useful. Over the years, many women have detected breast tumors through self-examination or incidentally. This examination method can help identify breast cancer in its earlier stages, before signs and symptoms develop. Because of this, some organizations continue to support self-exams as part of a comprehensive screening program.

Perhaps more important than adhering to a strict monthly self-exam schedule is to increase your awareness of your breasts — what they look like and how they feel. If you make a habit of examining them every so often, you'll find it easier over time to notice what's normal for you and what's not. When a change is detected, seek prompt medical attention.

How to do a breast self-exam

A self-exam includes three basic steps:
1. Visual examination in front of a mirror
2. Examination while standing in the shower
3. Examination while lying down

The following tips can help you get the most out of a breast self-exam, but don't obsess so much with technique that you avoid doing it for fear of doing it wrong.

It's also important for premenopausal women to remember that breast tissue changes throughout the month. It responds to changes in hormone levels that occur during the menstrual cycle,

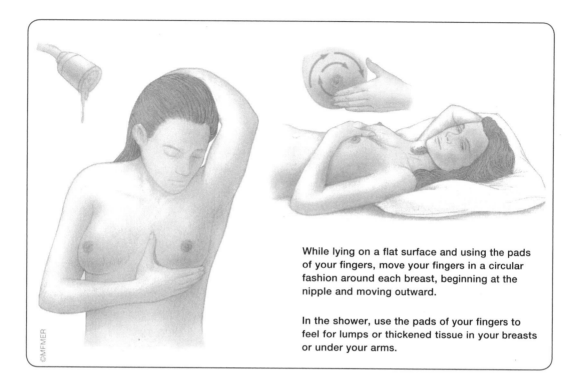

While lying on a flat surface and using the pads of your fingers, move your fingers in a circular fashion around each breast, beginning at the nipple and moving outward.

In the shower, use the pads of your fingers to feel for lumps or thickened tissue in your breasts or under your arms.

causing swelling and engorging of the breasts due to increased blood flow. With your menstrual flow (menses), your breasts return to normal size.

If you're premenopausal, the best time to examine your breasts is about one week after the start of your period. That's when breasts are less likely to be tender or swollen. Women who are pregnant or breast-feeding also should be aware that during these times their breasts are likely to feel more lumpy than normal.

Visual examination

Here are some suggestions to help you view your breasts from different angles. You might want to do a visual exam right before you get in the shower.

- Stand in front of a mirror with arms at your sides, inspecting both breasts carefully. Turn from side to side to view the outer portions of your breasts. If this is your first time, get a good look at them and try to familiarize yourself with their size and shape. During subsequent self-exams, look for changes since the last time you inspected them.
- Rest your palms on your hips. Press down firmly on your hips to flex your chest muscles and firm your breasts, and again, turn from side to side.
- Raise both arms above your head and press your palms together to flex your chest muscles and firm your breasts. Again, turn from side to side.

Standing in the shower

It's usually easier to feel (palpate) your breasts for changes when your skin is wet and soapy.

Possible signs of cancer

Some changes to watch for when examining your breasts include lumps, dimpling or thickening in a breast or under the arm; a nipple that's not pointing straight ahead (retracted); redness of breast skin, flaking or redness around a nipple; nipple discharge that's clear or bloody; and breast skin that takes on the appearance of an orange peel (*peau d'orange* changes). If you notice any changes, bring them to your doctor's attention, even if your mammograms have been normal.

Dimpling

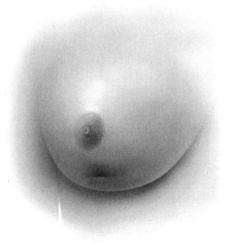

Nipple retraction

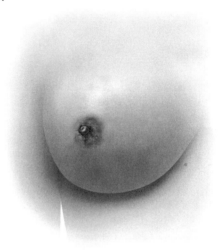

Inflammation

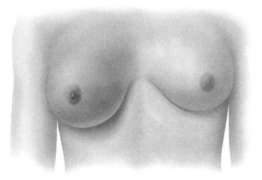

***Peau d'orange* changes**

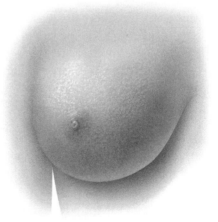

©MFMER

- Use your right hand to examine your left breast. Raise your left arm overhead to allow your breast to lie flat against your chest, or if you have larger breasts, support your breast with your left hand.
- Use the pads of your fingers instead of your fingertips to examine your breast.
- Move your fingers systematically all over your breast. This can be in a circular, up-and-down line or wedge pattern. Just be sure to feel all your breast tissue. Remember that breast tissue extends up toward the collarbone and under your arm, where lymph nodes are located. Lymph nodes are small nodules that filter foreign substances from your system. A ridge of firm tissue in the lower curve of each breast is normal.
- Check the tissue under the nipple and look for discharge from the nipple.
- Perform a similar exam of your right breast.
- Do this exam the same way every time so that you can notice any changes.

Lying down

Lie down on a flat surface and use the same procedure that you used in the shower, plus these additional steps:

- To examine your right breast, place a folded towel under your right shoulder blade. Place your right hand behind your head to distribute the breast tissue more evenly on your chest.
- Repeat the exam on your left breast with the folded towel under your left shoulder blade and your left hand behind your head.
- You may want to use lotion or powder on the pads of your fingers to make the motion easier.

Clinical Breast Examination

A clinical breast examination (CBE) is a screening test performed by your health care provider. During this exam, your doctor visually inspects your breasts for changes in shape, size and appearance. He or she also feels your breasts for lumps or other abnormalities. In addition, your doctor may examine your armpits (axillae) for enlarged lymph nodes, another indication of possible breast cancer.

A clinical breast exam is often performed in conjunction with mammography or as part of your annual physical examination.

Research involving large populations of women has not found that clinical breast exams reduce breast cancer deaths. Nevertheless, numerous health organizations, including the U.S. Preventive Services Task Force and the American Cancer Society, recommend clinical breast exams as part of breast cancer screening.

If a clinical breast exam is done shortly before your mammogram, areas within your breasts that feel suspicious during the exam can be targeted for special attention during mammography. If you or your doctor find a suspicious lump, it should be investigated further, even if the mammogram comes back normal. At times, a clinical breast exam can find a cancer that mammography doesn't.

The presence of a lump, however, doesn't mean cancer. The lump may be noncancerous (benign). In addition, normal breast tissue can feel lumpy. Of lumps that appear to be benign, less than 1 percent actually turn out to be a cancer.

Mammography

Mammography is generally performed in two situations. It's used to screen for breast cancer and to help make a diagnosis if breast cancer is suspected.

Screening mammograms

A screening mammogram is a breast X-ray that's taken to look for suspicious masses or breast tissue changes in women who have no signs or symptoms of breast cancer. It requires two views of each breast — one from above (cranial-caudal view) and one from an inside angle of the breast (mediolateral-oblique view).

For a cranial-caudal view, the X-ray film — or detector, in case of a digital mammogram — is placed below the breast, and the X-ray beam is aimed from above the breast down through the breast (see image A on the opposite page). A mediolateral-oblique view is obtained by having the X-ray film or detector placed to the side, basically under the armpit (see image B). If a tumor or suspicious area is identified, a radiologist can put these two images together to determine its approximate location.

Rather than using X-ray film to capture breast images, some medical facilities may use digital mammography. The testing is performed in the same way, but the images are captured digitally. In research studies comparing the two approaches — standard X-rays and digital mammography — cancer detection was similar for both in women over 50. In younger women, who are more likely to have extremely dense breasts, digital mammograms may perform better.

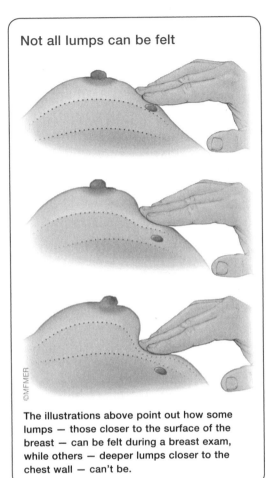

Not all lumps can be felt

The illustrations above point out how some lumps — those closer to the surface of the breast — can be felt during a breast exam, while others — deeper lumps closer to the chest wall — can't be.

Your first screening mammogram is typically called your baseline mammogram. Radiologists — doctors who specialize in interpreting images — will compare it with future mammograms to look for changes.

Diagnostic mammograms

A diagnostic mammogram is a breast X-ray used to further investigate breast changes, which may include one or more of the following: a lump, nipple thickening, nipple discharge, difference in

Two mammography views

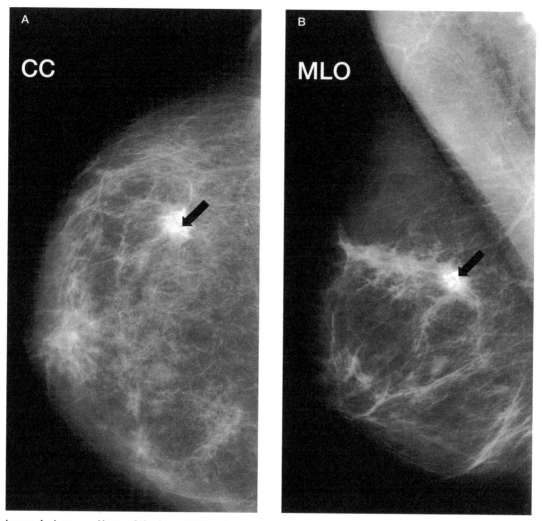

Image A shows an X-ray of the breast taken from above the breast, looking down. This is known as a cranial-caudal (CC) view. Image B shows a side-view X-ray of the breast, taken from the middle of the chest, looking toward the armpit. This is known as a mediolateral-oblique (MLO) view. By putting the two images together, radiologists can determine the location of a tumor. In this case, it's located in the upper outer portion of the breast.

breast size or shape, or a change in the overlying breast skin. A diagnostic mammogram is usually more complex, and it takes longer than does a screening mammogram. For more information on diagnostic mammograms, see Chapter 8.

Preparing for your mammogram

When scheduling your first screening mammogram, or if you're switching to a new doctor, your doctor will likely want to know about your personal and family history of breast disease. If you don't know this information, try and gather it before your appointment. In addition, be prepared to discuss the following:

- Any problems with your breasts
- Past breast biopsies or surgeries
- Whether you have breast implants
- Whether you're pregnant or nursing
- Whether you're taking hormone replacement therapy (HRT) or hormone treatments for a breast disorder
- The timing of your menstrual cycle or when you started menopause

If you've moved or changed doctors and this is the first time you're having a mammogram at a new facility, bring your prior mammograms with you for comparison. Bring the original mammogram, either the films or a disc, not copies, plus accompanying reports. This allows the radiologist to make the best possible interpretation.

Because your breasts will be compressed during mammography, avoid testing at times when your breasts may be most tender. This often includes the week before and the week of your period. Usually, your breasts are least tender the week after your period. If you have a history of breast pain (mastalgia) or tenderness, you might consider taking an over-the-counter pain medication about an hour before your mammogram.

You'll likely be given instructions before you come in for the test. Don't apply deodorants, antiperspirants, powders, lotions, creams or perfumes under your arms or on your breasts. Metallic particles in powders and deodorants could be visible on your mammogram and make interpretation difficult.

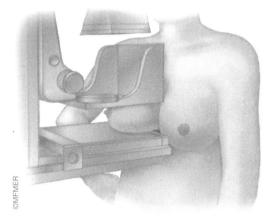

During mammography, your breast is pressed against the X-ray platform by a clear, plastic plate used to spread out the breast tissue. The breast is compressed to even out its thickness and allow X-rays to penetrate and distinguish tissues.

The day of the test

At the screening facility, you're typically given a gown and asked to remove neck jewelry and clothing from the waist up. For the mammogram itself, you stand in front of a specialized X-ray machine. This machine delivers a lower dose of radiation than do many standard X-ray devices. The technician places one of your breasts on a platform that holds the X-ray film and raises or lowers the platform to match your height. The technician also helps you position your head, arms and torso to allow an unobstructed view of your breast.

Your breast is then gradually pressed against the platform by a clear, plastic plate. Pressure is applied for a few seconds to spread out the breast tissue. The pressure isn't harmful, but it may be uncomfortable, and some women find it painful. If you experience too much discomfort, tell the technician.

Because of the low dose of radiation administered, your breast must be compressed to even out its thickness and permit X-rays to penetrate and distinguish tissues that might hide an abnormality. The pressure also holds your breast still, decreasing the chance of blurring from movement. You'll be asked to stand still and hold your breath during the X-ray exposure, which takes a few seconds.

After the technician has taken pictures of both breasts, the quality of the images will be checked. If they are inadequate for technical reasons, you may have to repeat part of the test. The entire procedure usually takes less than 30 minutes.

A radiologist interprets these images and sends a written report of the findings to your doctor.

Understanding the results

Most women who have a mammogram receive normal results. About 10 percent of women who are screened have an abnormality that requires further testing. Usually, other imaging tests can clarify the abnormality, but some women require a biopsy. In about 70 percent of women who have a biopsy, the results are negative for cancer.

So, for every 1,000 women who have a screening mammogram, approximately 100 will be called back for additional testing, about 10 will need a biopsy, and three will have cancer.

Abnormalities that may prompt additional testing include:
• Calcium deposits (calcifications) in ducts and other tissues
• Masses
• Distorted tissues

• Dense areas in only one breast
• Dense areas not seen on your last mammogram

Calcifications may be the result of cell secretions or debris, inflammation, trauma to the breast, previous radiation therapy, or foreign bodies. They're not related to dietary calcium or calcium supplements.

There are two types of calcifications. Tiny, irregular deposits called microcalcifications may be associated with cancer. Larger, coarser deposits called macrocalcifications tend to result from benign conditions such as aging, injury and common noncancerous tumors (fibroadenomas).

Breast calcifications are common. Many women have at least one breast calcification that can be seen on a mammogram. Most calcifications are benign, but if they appear worrisome, a radiologist may order a diagnostic mammogram that gives magnified views of the suspicious area. If the pattern or appearance of the calcifications remains suspicious after further testing, your doctor may recommend a biopsy.

Dense areas on a mammogram may indicate tissue with many glands that make calcifications and masses more difficult to identify, or they may represent cancer. Distorted areas on a mammogram may suggest tumors that have invaded neighboring tissues.

A mammogram alone generally can't prove that an abnormal mass is breast cancer. Additional tests usually are necessary to make that determination.

Limitations of mammography

Mammography isn't foolproof. The accuracy of the procedure depends in part on the quality of the X-rays taken and the experience and skill of the radiologist. If these are inadequate, cancerous growths may be missed. However, even with the best techniques and radiologists, some breast cancers aren't detectable with mammography. Some women have more dense breast tissue than that of other women. Dense tissue can hide tumors and make interpretation of a mammogram more difficult.

In general, younger women and women who've been through menopause and are taking estrogen have denser breasts than do older women. However, some older women not taking estrogen also have breasts that appear dense on a mammogram.

Drawbacks associated with screening mammography include:

- **False-negatives.** *False-negative* is the term for a test result that comes back normal when cancer is actually present. According to the National Cancer Institute, up to 20 percent of breast cancers are missed during mammography screening. False-negatives are more common in younger women because of higher breast density.
- **False-positives.** *False-positive* is the term for test results that indicate cancer may be present when it's not. False-positives are more common in younger women, women who've had previous breast biopsies, women with a family history of breast cancer and women who are taking the hormone estrogen.
- **Limited benefit.** Discovery of a tumor with a mammogram doesn't always mean that survival is guaranteed. Mammography can detect most tumors that are 5 to 10 millimeters (mm) — about ¼ inch — and some as small as 1 mm. But certain types of breast cancer grow very rapidly and are more aggressive in spreading to other parts of the body. Such a cancer may grow and develop into a noticeable lump in between regular mammogram visits.

In addition, some women will be diagnosed with very slow-growing, nonaggressive breast cancers that wouldn't have caused a threat to their lives. Because low aggressiveness can't be determined by today's tests, these women may end up being over-treated.

Where to get a mammogram

Mammograms may be performed at your doctor's office, in a hospital or in a clinic.

QUESTION & ANSWER

Q: Should I be worried about radiation from a mammogram?

A: Modern mammography machines use very low amounts of radiation, usually 0.1 to 0.2 rads per image. A rad is a measure of the amount of radiation. For comparison, a woman who has breast cancer and is treated with radiation therapy typically receives a dose of around 5,000 rads. A woman who is screened with a mammogram every year from age 40 to age 80 receives less than 20 rads.

Detection can be difficult

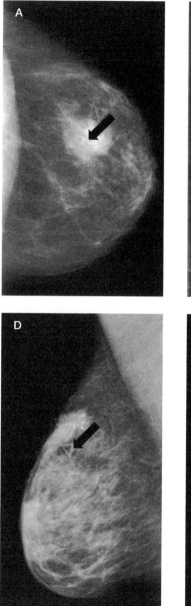

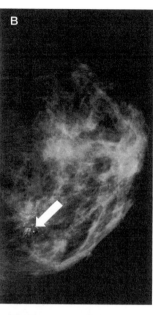

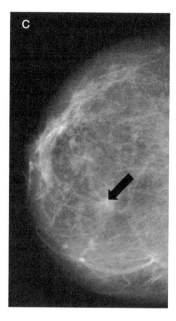

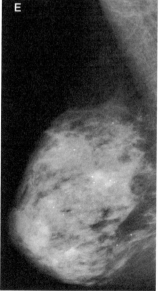

Image A shows a large tumor in a woman with less dense breasts. The tumor is clearly visible. But not all tumors or potentially cancerous lesions are that easy to identify. Image B shows tiny, irregular deposits (microcalcifications) that may be associated with cancer. Image C shows an area of more subtle tissue distortion that may be associated with cancer. Image D comes from a woman with more dense breasts. The triangle is a marker put on the woman's skin, indicating an area where a doctor felt a lump. On the mammogram, the lump isn't easily identifiable. Image E comes from a woman with very dense breasts. In women with dense breasts — typically younger women — tumors and microcalcifications may be difficult to see on mammography.

©MFMER

Or your doctor may refer you to a mammography facility or an X-ray or imaging center. Mobile units may offer screening at various locations.

All mammography facilities are required to have Food and Drug Administration (FDA) certification. To be certified, a facility must meet strict quality standards set up by the Mammography Quality Standards Act. To get the best quality mammogram, go to a medical facility that regularly performs mammograms and has a radiologist dedicated to interpreting them.

New Approaches

Although mammography is currently the best accepted tool for breast cancer screening, experts agree it's not perfect. An ideal screening tool would be accurate, reliable, inexpensive and readily available. Other approaches include:

Magnetic resonance imaging
Magnetic resonance imaging (MRI) uses a magnetic field and radio waves to create a detailed, two-dimensional (2D) image.

In breast imaging, MRI is done in conjunction with a contrast material that's injected into a vein just before or during the procedure. The contrast material enhances areas with abnormal blood vessels, such as cancers.

Breast MRI may be used to further assess suspicious areas seen on other imaging tests to determine the extent of the cancer. MRI may also be used as a screening tool, in addition to a mammogram, for some women with a significantly increased risk of breast cancer (see page 113).

Although breast MRI has powerful imaging abilities, the test has some limitations, including the possibility of false-positive results, leading to additional testing. Breast MRI is also very expensive.

Ultrasound
Ultrasound is an imaging procedure that uses high-frequency sound waves to display images of the inside of the human body on a screen. To produce the images, sound waves are bounced off body tissues, and the returning waves are measured and recorded. By analyzing a computer image of breast tissue, a doctor may be able to tell if a lump detected on a mammogram or a physical exam is a cyst or solid mass. Cysts, which are sacs of fluid, aren't cancerous, but a solid mass may be.

Ultrasound is often used to help determine if a lump or suspicious area on a mammogram or clinical exam is solid or fluid-filled, or to better visualize an area of concern in dense breast tissue.

Nuclear medicine studies
Nuclear medicine studies of the breast, also called molecular breast imaging, use tiny amounts of a radioactive tracer that's picked up mainly by tumor cells. For example, the tracer may go to cells that are dividing rapidly or that possess some specific breast cancer feature that normal cells don't have. The tracer is injected into a vein in your arm. A special camera detects the tracer in your body and produces images in areas where it has accumulated.

Side effects from the procedure are minimal. The radiation dose is very low, and the tracer usually leaves your body within a few hours.

Chapter 8: Breast Cancer

Diagnosing Breast Cancer

Signs and Symptoms	128
Medical History	128
Physical Examination	129
Imaging Tests	130
Diagnostic mammography	130
Ultrasound	130
Biopsy Procedures	132
Fine-needle aspiration biopsy	133
Core needle biopsy	134
Surgical biopsy	136
Pathology Report	139
Type of cancer	140
Tumor grade	141
Hormone receptor status	142
HER2 status	142
Staging	143
Staging tests	143
Staging classification	145
Estimating survival	147

What happens if you find a lump in your breast or if a mammogram or another test shows an abnormality? Although this may suggest the possibility of cancer, it doesn't automatically mean that you have cancer. It does indicate, though, the need for further tests to determine what the lump or abnormality is. This is called the diagnostic process.

The evaluation of a new breast lump often involves a number of steps, including asking about your signs and symptoms, if you have any; examining your breasts; reviewing the results of imaging tests; and, ultimately, the removal and examination of a sample of cells from the abnormal area (biopsy). If cancer is present, other tests are typically performed. These tests can help determine if the cancer has spread to other parts of your body, and they can identify certain characteristics of the tumor that may help you and your doctor decide on the type of treatment you should receive.

The diagnostic process may take several days. This is often a time of great uncertainty and emotional stress. Not knowing whether you have cancer can sometimes be worse than knowing that you do. Knowledge allows for action. Uncertainty hinders your ability to plan and move forward, causing anxiety.

This is precisely why diagnosis is so important. An accurate diagnosis is key to your plan of action, and getting the diagnosis right often takes more than one test. Waiting for the results can be difficult. It might help to use this time to learn more about breast cancer and how it's treated. This way, if the tests reveal cancer, you're more prepared for what comes next. At the same time, remember that noncancerous (benign) breast conditions are far more common than cancerous (malignant) ones.

Signs and Symptoms

The most common sign of breast cancer is a lump (mass) or thickening in one breast that can be felt (palpated). Often, the lump is painless, but occasionally it may be associated with pain or tenderness. A lump that's cancerous is usually firm to hard and it may have irregular borders, although some cancerous lumps are more soft and rounded. Most tumors develop in the upper outer portion of your breast, close to your armpit.

A tumor that can be felt (a palpable mass) is most often discovered by a woman herself, either by accident or through breast self-examination. Sometimes a feeling of discomfort or a bump to a breast may draw attention to a lump. Less often, a lump is discovered by a partner during lovemaking or by a doctor during a routine physical exam.

Even an experienced doctor can't reliably distinguish between a noncancerous (benign) lump and a cancerous one based on a physical exam alone. That's why all lumps and physical changes to the breast need to be evaluated with imaging tests.

In addition to a lump, other signs and symptoms may include:

- Differences in the size and shape of one breast compared with the other
- A generalized swelling of part of your breast
- A spontaneous nipple discharge from one breast that's not breast milk (bloody or clear in color)
- A recent inversion of one of your nipples that can't be turned outward again
- Thickening or irritation of a nipple that may be accompanied by an itching, burning or scaly rash (Paget's disease of the nipple)
- Dimpling, thickening or puckering of the skin of one of your breasts
- A change in the skin of the breast in which it takes on the consistency of an orange peel (*peau d'orange*)
- Enlarged lymph nodes in your armpit area, or less commonly, above your collarbone

In the earliest stages of breast cancer, and even in some of the later stages, there are no signs or symptoms. This is where screening mammography becomes helpful. A mammogram may reveal a lump or abnormality that can't otherwise be visually or palpably detected.

Medical History

If there's any suspicion of breast cancer, one of the first things your doctor likely will do is get your complete medical history, if he or she doesn't already have it. Most women who develop breast cancer don't have risk factors for the disease, but information about your health may help your doctor assess your situation.

Your doctor may wish to gather information regarding:

- Recent changes in your breast or new signs and symptoms
- Previous breast problems or biopsies
- Previous breast cancer diagnosis and the test results that led to it
- Previous hysterectomy, including why you had it done and whether your ovaries were removed
- Your family history of breast and ovarian cancer
- Use of hormone replacement therapy (HRT)
- Use of oral contraceptives
- Your reproductive history, including at what age you had your first period and at what age you experienced menopause, if that applies to you; the number of times you were pregnant and your age at your first pregnancy; and if you breast-fed your children

Your doctor may use the Gail model risk assessment described in Chapter 4 or another method for evaluating your risk. He or she may also want to see previous mammograms and ultrasound examinations of your breasts. This may help provide a frame of reference for the current evaluation.

Physical Examination

After gathering as much information as possible about your personal and family medical history, an examination of both of your breasts usually follows. This is known as a clinical breast examination. While you're seated facing your doctor, he or she may visually inspect your breasts, making note of any differences between the two, any scars, skin redness or signs of skin dimpling or nipple inversion. Some lumps aren't immediately apparent in a normal seated position, so you may be asked to place your hands on your hips and then raise your arms above your head so that your doctor can see your breasts from different angles. Your doctor may also feel your armpits and the area around your collarbone to check for enlarged lymph nodes.

Next, you may be asked to lie down while your doctor examines your breasts, using a similar technique to that used for breast self-examination (see page 117). This way, your doctor can evaluate the size, shape and firmness of any noticeable lumps or masses. Your nipples may also be examined for asymmetry, inversion, irritation and discharge.

If your signs and symptoms are suggestive of cancer — even if prior mammograms have been normal — it's likely your doctor will recommend additional tests. For women age 30 and older, this may be a diagnostic mammogram.

Further testing is often based on the results of the mammogram. If you're under age 30, your doctor may recommend an ultrasound because at a young age dense breast tissue may prevent a mass from being seen on a mammogram. An ultrasound helps determine whether a mass is solid or fluid-filled (cystic). If the mass is solid, a biopsy procedure — usually a core needle biopsy — may be performed.

If you don't have any signs or symptoms but your screening mammogram suggests a suspicious abnormality, further testing is typically recommended, usually in the form of a diagnostic mammogram, an ultrasound or a biopsy.

Imaging Tests

The benefit of imaging tests is that they may be able to locate tumors deep within breast tissue that can't be felt. They can also show whether there's more than one suspicious area. Imaging tests may also be used to guide a needle biopsy procedure.

The most common imaging tests used in the diagnosis of breast cancer are diagnostic mammography and ultrasound. Other tests, including magnetic resonance imaging (MRI) and molecular breast imaging (MBI), sometimes are used. Positron emission tomography (PET) is rarely used to diagnose breast cancer, but it may be used once a diagnosis is made.

Diagnostic mammography

Diagnostic mammography may be used for several purposes — to assess signs and symptoms of breast cancer, to precisely locate or further evaluate an abnormality visible on a screening mammogram, and to follow up on women who've had lumpectomies for previous breast cancer.

Like screening mammography, diagnostic mammography consists of X-raying your breast. Diagnostic mammograms include more views than the standard two done during routine screening. For example, during a diagnostic mammogram, a spot compression view can focus pressure on the breast at the site of the abnormal tissue area (lump). This spreads out the breast tissue and allows for a better view of the lump or area of concern. A magnification view may zoom in on an area to bring out the details of a small mass or clusters of tiny, irregular calcium deposits (microcalcifications).

Before you're scheduled for a diagnostic mammogram, your doctor may mark the site of the lesion on your breast so that the radiologist will know where to focus attention. Your radiologist may also ask you to point out where you've experienced any signs or symptoms. Often, both breasts are X-rayed so that they can be compared for symmetry. Ideally, current mammograms are compared with previous images to look for small changes in breast tissue.

Signs of cancer on a mammogram include dense masses with irregular borders, suspicious microcalcifications, tissue distortions and asymmetrical breasts. Typically, when a finding falls into Category 4 or 5 (see opposite page), a biopsy is done.

Ultrasound

Ultrasound imaging is often used to further evaluate a finding, such as a mass, and to determine its characteristics. Benign masses, such as cysts and fibroadenomas, often have a characteristic appearance with ultrasound, and therefore a biopsy may not be needed.

Ultrasound technology, also referred to as ultrasonography or sonography, uses sound waves to create images of unseen areas within the body. A breast ultrasound works by directing very high-pitched (high-frequency) sound waves at the tissues in your breast. These sound waves bounce off the curves and variations of breast tissue and are visually translated into a pattern of light and dark areas on a screen. The patterns form a visual image of the tissue inside your breast.

Interpreting mammography results

The American College of Radiology has developed a system for interpreting mammograms that standardizes the results and provides doctors with consistent terminology with which to write their reports and make uniform recommendations to women. This reduces differences in interpretation and decreases the margin of error. The system is called the Breast Imaging Reporting and Data System (BI-RADS) and is widely used. The BI-RADS system divides results into the categories listed below:

Category	Description
Category 0: Needs additional imaging evaluation	Category 0 is usually used to describe a screening mammogram in which a possible abnormality has been found. The evaluation is considered incomplete, and more testing is necessary to arrive at a definitive category (1, 2, 3, 4 or 5). Additional testing might include mammography with spot compression, magnification or special mammographic views, or ultrasound.
Category 1: Negative	There is nothing to comment on. The breasts are symmetrical, and no masses, architectural distortions or suspicious calcifications are present.
Category 2: Noncancerous (benign) finding	This also is a negative mammogram in that no cancer has been found, but the radiologist may wish to describe a benign finding present in the breast, such as a cyst; fibroadenoma, lipoma or other characteristic.
Category 3: Probably benign finding; short interval follow-up suggested	A finding in this category generally has a high probability of being benign. However, your radiologist may feel it's better to be safe than sorry and recommend a follow-up mammography exam after a specified period of time, generally about six months.
Category 4: Suspicious abnormality; biopsy should be considered	A finding in this category doesn't have the exact characteristics of cancer but it has a definite probability of being cancerous. A biopsy is often recommended.
Category 5: Highly suggestive of being cancerous (malignant); appropriate action should be taken	Findings in this category have a high probability of being cancerous, and they should be biopsied.
Category 6: Known biopsy; proven malignancy; appropriate action should be taken	This category is reserved for findings on imaging tests in which malignancy was proved by way of a biopsy before the test.

Adapted from the American College of Radiology Breast Imaging Reporting and Data System (BI-RADS), fourth edition, 2003.

During an ultrasound exam, a gel-like substance is applied to the skin over your breast. The gel acts as a conductor for sound waves, and it helps to eliminate air bubbles between your skin and the transducer. A transducer is a small hand-held probe that sends out the sound waves and records them as they bounce back. The person performing the exam (ultrasonographer) moves the transducer back and forth over your breast, directing the sound waves into the tissue and capturing the waves' echoes. The returning echoes are digitally converted into black-and-white images on a screen.

A disadvantage of ultrasound is that it can't reliably detect microcalcifications, which commonly accompany cancer. This is one of the main reasons this procedure isn't used for screening. But ultrasound has several important uses in the diagnosis of breast cancer. They include:

- **Evaluating a questionable mammographic finding.** Ultrasound may be used to further evaluate a suspicious abnormality on a mammogram.
- **Distinguishing a cyst from a solid mass.** Cysts are benign sacs filled with fluid. Sound waves pass through fluid more easily than through a solid mass. A cyst, which isn't cancerous (malignant), generally has a different appearance on an ultrasound image than does a solid mass, which may or may not be malignant. If a definitive diagnosis of a simple cyst is made using ultrasound, usually no further testing is required. If the cyst has complex features, a fine-needle aspiration may be recommended. If the mass is solid and it feels suspicious, a biopsy is generally done.

- **Evaluating dense breast tissue.** In younger women, especially women under age 30, breast tissue can be dense. Breast density can obscure masses or abnormalities on a mammogram. In such cases, an ultrasound may provide a clearer image. That's why it's often the tool of choice for evaluating a younger woman with a mass that can be felt. If the mass turns out to be a simple cyst, no further testing is needed. If the mass is solid, a mammogram may be recommended to determine the presence of any calcifications, or a biopsy may be done to determine whether the mass is benign or malignant.
- **Evaluating breasts with implants.** Ultrasound can distinguish between the materials used in implants and breast tissue, making it useful in evaluating women with breast implants who may have an implant rupture or a new lump that can be felt.
- **Guiding needle biopsy procedures.** Ultrasound may also be used by your doctor to help guide a needle biopsy procedure. It can provide an image of the needle as it's being inserted into the breast tissue. This can help your doctor direct the needle to the appropriate area.

Biopsy Procedures

A biopsy involves removal of a small sample of tissue for analysis in the laboratory. It's generally the only way of knowing for certain that a suspicious lesion is cancer. It's most often recommended after a physical examination and an imaging test have raised the possibility of cancer. Besides identifying cancerous cells, a biopsy can provide important information about the type of cancer you may have and whether it might respond to a special form of treatment, such as anti-estrogen therapy or therapy directed at HER2 receptors.

The three common types of biopsy procedures are fine-needle aspiration biopsy, core needle biopsy and surgical biopsy. Each has its own advantages and disadvantages, and in a given situation, one may be more appropriate than another.

The pages that follow describe each of the biopsy procedures. If you don't understand why you're having one type of biopsy instead of another, ask your doctor to explain his or her recommendation in greater detail.

Fine-needle aspiration biopsy

This is the simplest type of biopsy, and it's most often used for lumps that can be felt. For the procedure, you lie on a table. A local anesthetic might be used. Sometimes an anesthetic isn't used because it may cause more discomfort than the procedure. While steadying the lump with one hand, a doctor uses the other hand to direct a very fine needle — one more slender than that used to obtain a blood sample — into the lump. The needle is attached to a hollow syringe. Once in place, a sample of cells is collected in the syringe and the needle removed.

Your doctor may use this type of biopsy as a quick-and-easy method to distinguish between a cyst and a solid mass, avoiding a more invasive biopsy.

- **Cyst.** A cyst typically yields fluid, and your doctor may drain all the fluid. If

the fluid is clear and the mass disappears, this is usually a sign of a simple cyst. The possibility of cancer needs to be considered if the fluid is bloody and part of the mass remains. In this case, the fluid is typically sent to a laboratory for examination.

- **Solid mass.** If the mass is solid, your doctor may feel resistance to the needle and no fluid will be retrieved. A sample of cells is then obtained by passing the needle through the mass several times while maintaining suction. The cells collected in the syringe are spread onto one or more slides and sent to a laboratory. A pathologist — an individual who studies tissue samples for signs of disease — will inspect the specimen for the presence of cancer cells. A repeat biopsy may be performed if an inadequate sample was collected.

Image guidance

If the mass is hard to feel, your doctor may use ultrasound or mammography imaging to help guide the needle to the correct site. With ultrasound, your doctor can watch movement of the needle on the ultrasound monitor. When mammography is used, the procedure is called stereotactic biopsy.

Stereotactic methods are typically done with a larger needle (core needle biopsy), but on occasion they're done by fine-needle aspiration biopsy. Two mammograms are taken from different angles, and the mass is mapped out by a computer, which guides the needle to the precise location. This procedure is described in more detail later in this chapter.

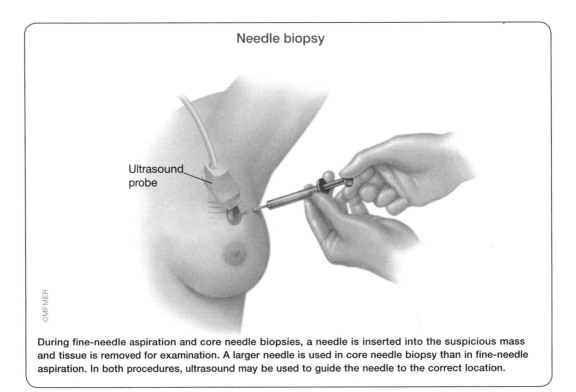

Needle biopsy

Ultrasound probe

©MFMER

During fine-needle aspiration and core needle biopsies, a needle is inserted into the suspicious mass and tissue is removed for examination. A larger needle is used in core needle biopsy than in fine-needle aspiration. In both procedures, ultrasound may be used to guide the needle to the correct location.

Pros and cons

The advantages of fine-needle aspiration biopsy are that it's quick, relatively inexpensive and fairly painless. It can be done in your doctor's office, and often the results can be determined within the same day.

The accuracy of this procedure depends on the experience of the person performing the procedure. Studies have shown that experienced staff can produce very accurate results. Fine-needle aspiration biopsies performed by inexperienced staff, though, aren't as reliable. Interpretation of the sample also requires special expertise.

A disadvantage of the procedure is that because only cells are obtained and not tissue, it may be more difficult to distinguish between noninvasive (in situ) and invasive cancer. As a result, many medi-

cal facilities in the United States prefer to use a core needle biopsy, which often can provide more definitive results.

Core needle biopsy

A core needle biopsy may be used on a mass that's visible on a mammogram or ultrasound or that can be felt by your doctor or a surgeon. A core needle biopsy uses a larger needle than does a fine-needle aspiration. With this procedure, a small cylinder of tissue (core) is withdrawn from the mass rather than just cells, giving the pathologist more tissue to examine. In most cases, the procedure is performed under the guidance of a radiologist and with imaging equipment.

A core needle biopsy can provide a definitive diagnosis in most cases. It's often the first procedure used to assess a new lump or an area of concern on a mammogram. A surgical biopsy is a more invasive procedure, so being able to perform a core biopsy may eliminate the need for a surgical biopsy. Any core needle biopsy carries a small risk of infection and bleeding.

Preparation

Before the procedure, tell your doctor if you've been taking aspirin or any blood-thinning medications. These can keep your blood from clotting properly during the procedure and may cause more bleeding. You may be asked to temporarily stop taking the medication. In addition, don't wear deodorant, talcum powder, lotion or perfume the day of the test because they may interfere with imaging used during the procedure. You may also be asked not to eat for a certain amount of time before the test. Some facilities may request that you insert an ice pack in your bra after the procedure to reduce pain and swelling.

During the procedure

With all core needle biopsies, the site of the needle puncture is usually numbed with a local anesthetic. A small incision, approximately $1/8$ inch to $1/4$ inch, may be made to allow the biopsy needle to be inserted more easily. Depending on the type of biopsy, you might hear a quick popping sound as the device removes a tissue sample. Several samples of tissue are usually taken to ensure an adequate sampling. Generally, women don't experience too much discomfort during the procedure. The tissue that's removed is then sent to a pathologist for examination.

Although it takes only about 15 minutes to remove the tissue samples, the whole biopsy process, including all of the preparation, may take up to 90 minutes.

The process will vary some depending on the procedure you have.

Stereotactic core needle biopsy
With this procedure, you generally lie facedown on a padded biopsy table with one of your breasts positioned through a hole in the table. The table is usually raised several feet, and the radiologist sits below the table. Some facilities use a standing procedure similar to a screening mammogram. Your breast is then firmly compressed between two plates while mammograms are taken to determine the exact location of the lesion for the biopsy. It's very important to keep still once your breast has been positioned so that the correct spot is biopsied.

Ultrasound-guided core needle biopsy
During this procedure, you lie on your back on an ultrasound table. You may be asked to raise your arm over your head on the side of the breast to be biopsied. This allows stretching of the soft tissue so that the radiologist can get a better image of the abnormality. The radiologist then locates the mass with an ultrasound probe. Ultrasound guidance may be used if the abnormality can be clearly seen on an ultrasound image.

MRI-guided core needle biopsy
This type of core needle biopsy is done under the guidance of magnetic resonance imaging (MRI) — an imaging technique that captures multiple cross-sectional images of your breast and combines them

using a computer, to generate detailed 2-D pictures. During this procedure you lie facedown on a padded scanning table. Your breasts fit into a hollow depression in the table. The MRI machine provides images that help determine the exact location for the biopsy.

Pros and cons

The advantages of core needle biopsy over fine-needle aspiration biopsy include obtaining a larger sample for examination, the ability to distinguish noninvasive (*in situ*) cancer from invasive cancer, greater accuracy in diagnosis and better identification of breast calcifications in the tissue removed. Occasionally, a core needle biopsy may miss a cancer (false-negative result) or, very rarely, lead to a false diagnosis of cancer when, in fact, no cancer is present (false-positive result). The procedure is more expensive than is fine-needle aspiration. Nonetheless, core needle biopsy has become relatively standard. Individuals — both women and their doctors — like to know if cancer is present before surgery because it allows for better surgical planning.

Often, a tiny, stainless steel or titanium clip is inserted in the biopsy site within the breast to mark the spot of the biopsy, in case the area needs to be checked again later. The clip can only be removed surgically and is only visible with special equipment. It can't be felt, and it doesn't set off alarms at the airport.

Surgical biopsy

In some instances, the amount of tissue obtained with a needle biopsy isn't enough, and a surgical biopsy must be performed. Or the suspicious mass is small and palpable, and your doctor may recommend both diagnosing and removing the mass in one procedure. In other situations, it may be determined that a relatively prominent lesion needs to be surgically removed, regardless of the needle biopsy results. Surgical biopsy may also be used if the location of the abnormality makes it difficult to use other procedures.

As its name implies, surgical biopsy involves minor surgery. You likely will be able to leave the hospital on the same day.

The two types of surgical biopsies are incisional and excisional:

- An incisional biopsy removes a portion of the mass for examination.
- An excisional biopsy removes the whole mass and, if all the cancer cells have been removed, may serve as treatment as well as a diagnostic procedure. This is also known as lumpectomy or wide local excision.

Preparation

The procedure is usually performed in an operating room with sedation and a local anesthetic or, in some cases, under general anesthesia. Tell your doctor if you're taking blood-thinning medications, including aspirin, nonsteroidal anti-inflammatory drugs (NSAIDs) or any other medicines or herbal products that affect blood clotting. You may also be asked to not eat for a certain amount of time before the procedure. You'll also want to arrange for someone to drive you home.

Wire localization

After a core needle biopsy, your radiologist may use a technique called wire localization to map the route to the mass for the surgeon. This is usually done immediately before surgery. For the procedure, you're positioned for a mammogram, and the mass in question is located on a grid. Then a needle with an attached wire is inserted into your breast at a depth corresponding to the coordinates on the grid. You may be given a local anesthetic before the procedure, but sometimes the anesthetic can be more uncomfortable than insertion of the needle.

The tip of the wire is positioned within the mass or just through it. Two more mammographic views are taken to check the position of the wire. If necessary, the wire can be adjusted. After the correct positioning is obtained, the needle is removed and the wire is left in place.

A hook at the tip of the wire keeps its position secure. A mammogram view of the wire is sent to the operating room.

Some medical facilities use radioactive seeds instead of wires. The surgeon is able to locate the area by using a probe that detects the radioactivity.

Sometimes, if ultrasound can provide a better view, a radiologist will use ultrasound instead of mammography to guide insertion of the wire.

The biopsy

Once all of the preliminary steps are complete, your surgeon carefully examines the diagnostic images to decide on the best surgical approach. During surgery, he or she will attempt to remove the entire mass, along with the wire. The surgeon may mark the edges (margins)

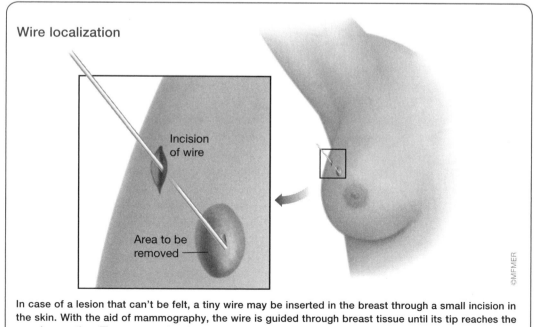

Wire localization

Incision of wire

Area to be removed

©MFMER

In case of a lesion that can't be felt, a tiny wire may be inserted in the breast through a small incision in the skin. With the aid of mammography, the wire is guided through breast tissue until its tip reaches the area in question. The surgeon then has good guidance as to where to remove tissue.

From identification to removal

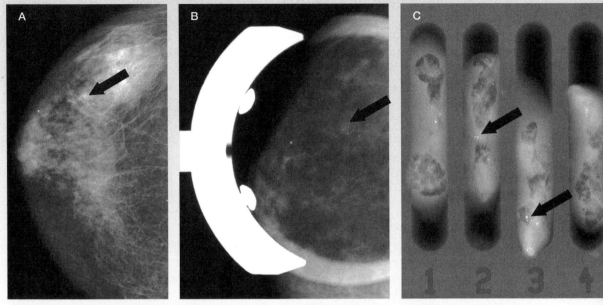

Image A is a screening mammogram indicating possible tiny, irregular deposits, called microcalcifications. Because the microcalcifications aren't easily identified, a magnification view of the area is taken, as illustrated in image B. Here the microcalcifications can be seen more easily. A needle biopsy is then performed (see the illustration on page 134). Tissue samples taken from the area in question may be X-rayed to see if

of the removed tissue (specimen) with sutures to orient the specimen for the pathologist. The specimen's margins may also be marked with ink so that when cut open, the pathologist may determine whether cancer cells are at the margins.

The surgeon may have the tissue X-rayed before it goes to the pathologist to help determine if all of the calcifications are included in the sample. If the margins have cancerous cells (positive margins), this means that some cancer may still be in the breast and more tissue needs to be removed. If the margins are clear (negative margins), it's more likely that all the cancer has been removed.

Occasionally, only by removing the breast (mastectomy) can the entire area of abnormal tissue be removed.

Risks and aftercare
The risks of surgical biopsy are similar to those of any minor surgery, including bleeding, infection and bruising around the site. You may find it best to take the rest of the day off and relax. For the next five to six days, avoid activities that may cause you discomfort.

You may shower or take a bath after the dressing is removed. The dressing is usually removed during a return appointment, or your surgeon may instruct you how to remove it a day or two after surgery. Minimal drainage is expected the

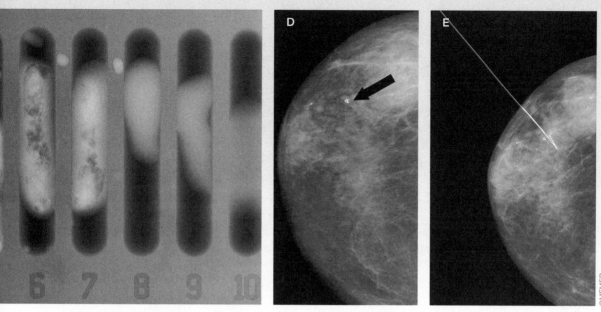

microcalcifications are present in the samples, as shown in image C. During the biopsy procedure, a small clip is placed in the location where the samples were taken, as shown in image D. Using the clip as a guide, a wire is then placed in the area to direct the surgeon where to remove additional tissue to help make sure all of the microcalcifications have been removed. This is shown in image E.

first few days. A small gauze pad inside your bra may help absorb the drainage. A bra also provides support to the incision. Call your doctor if you develop symptoms of infection, such as foul-smelling drainage, increased swelling, redness or tenderness at the incision, or a fever.

Pathology Report

After a pathologist has studied the tissue that was removed, he or she writes up a detailed pathology report describing the specimen. The report may also list relevant parts of your medical history and any special requests to medical personnel.

It explains the site from where the specimen was taken and gives a description of what the specimen looks like to the naked eye. Its size, color and consistency may be noted. The pathologist should indicate whether cancer cells were present at the edges of the specimen (positive or negative margins) and what the noncancerous tissue looks like. He or she may also detail how many tissue sections of the specimen were taken for examination.

If cancer is present, a pathologist will outline a number of details about the cancer to help you and your doctor decide on the best type of treatment. These details include the type of cancer present (invasive or noninvasive), histologic type (ductal, lobular or special type), how abnormal the cancer cells appear (tumor grade), whether the tumor cells contain certain proteins called hormone receptors (estrogen and progesterone receptor status), and whether the tumor cells have a surface protein receptor called HER2.

Type of cancer

By looking at the distribution of cancer cells in the specimen, a pathologist is able to tell if the cancer is invasive (infiltrating) or noninvasive (in situ). Invasive cancer spreads beyond the membrane that lines a breast duct or lobule, into surrounding connective tissue (see page 35). From there it's able to travel (metastasize) to other parts of the body. Noninvasive cancer usually stays in one location, although it can become invasive. Noninvasive cancer has a much better projected outcome (prognosis) than does invasive cancer.

Invasive
The most common type of invasive cancer, which accounts for about 80 percent of all invasive breast cancers, is invasive ductal carcinoma. Invasive lobular car-

cinoma makes up about 10 percent of invasive breast cancers. The remaining 10 percent of invasive cancers are rare or special types.

Invasive lobular cancers can be particularly hard to detect with mammograms, and they may not be identified until they're larger and can be felt.

Some of the special types of invasive breast cancer include medullary, tubular and mucinous breast cancers. These invasive cancers tend to have a better prognosis than does invasive ductal or lobular carcinoma and may be treated differently from the more common invasive cancers. Metaplastic cancer is a rare type of cancer, and it can behave more aggressively than does invasive ductal cancer.

Noninvasive
Noninvasive cancer (carcinoma *in situ*) is less common than is invasive breast cancer. Ductal carcinoma *in situ* (DCIS), the most common type of noninvasive breast cancer, appears to be confined to the breast's duct system, and it doesn't invade the breast's connective tissue (see Chapter 10).

Lobular carcinoma *in situ* (LCIS) begins in the lobules instead of the ducts. Most breast cancer specialists don't consider LCIS to be a true breast cancer. But women with this diagnosis have an increased risk of developing future invasive cancer in either breast, not just the breast containing the LCIS (see Chapter 9).

With appropriate treatment and follow-up, both of these noninvasive conditions carry an excellent prognosis.

Tumor grade

In addition to determining what type of cancer is present, a pathologist also assigns a grade to the cancer. The grade is based on how normal or abnormal the cells appear when examined under a microscope. The lower the grade, the better the prognosis.

Pathologists generally use a grading system called the Scarff-Bloom-Richardson system, or some variation of this system, for grading invasive breast cancers.

In medical terms, the grade refers to the appearance of the cancer. It's based on three features of the tumor: tubule formation, nuclear grade and mitotic activity. Each of these features is given a score of 1 to 3.

- **Tubule formation.** Normal breast ducts are shaped like small tubes (tubules). Cancer cells tend to become more and more distorted as the cancer progresses. A specimen that contains more than 75 percent tubular structures is given a score of 1. A tubular composition of 10 to 75 percent represents a score of 2. If less than 10 percent of cells have a tubular form, the score is 3.

- **Nuclear grade.** The nuclear grade reflects how the nucleus of each cell appears. The nucleus of a normal cell has a regular structure, and the cells are small and uniform (well-differentiated). The more aggressive a cancer is, the greater the variation in size and structure of the cancer cells' nuclei (poorly differentiated). A score of 1 for nuclear grade implies a close resemblance to a normal nucleus, 2 represents a moderate increase in size and variability, and 3 represents marked variation between normal and cancerous cells.

- **Mitotic activity.** Mitosis is the process of cell division. The score for mitotic activity indicates how many of the cancer cells are dividing. To obtain this score, a pathologist counts the number of cells undergoing mitosis compared with the total number of cells observed. A score of 1 implies slow growth, a score of 2 implies intermediate growth and a score of 3 implies fast growth.

The scores of each of the three measurements are then added together to obtain an overall tumor grade — a total score of 3 to 9 points is possible:

- A total score of 3, 4 or 5 is classified as grade 1 (low-grade or well-differentiated).
- A total score of 6 or 7 is grade 2 (intermediate-grade or moderately differentiated).
- A total score of 8 or 9 is grade 3 (high-grade or poorly differentiated).

Grade 1 implies the cells still look fairly normal, and the mass appears to be growing slowly. If the specimen is a grade 3, it means the cells have lost their proper structure and function, or they're dividing rapidly, or both. Grade 2 cancers are in the middle — they aren't as normal in appearance as grade 1, but they aren't as abnormal as grade 3.

Hormone receptor status

Scientists have discovered that two female hormones, estrogen and progesterone, affect the growth of most breast cancers. One of the tests that's often performed on a biopsy specimen is a hormone receptor test. A receptor is a cell protein that binds to specific chemicals, drugs or hormones traveling through the bloodstream.

Normal breast cells have receptors that bind with estrogen and progesterone. When bound to the receptors, the hormones interact with appropriate genes, helping to promote breast development during puberty and prepare breasts during pregnancy. Most breast cancer cells also have these hormone receptors.

If a pathologist detects estrogen receptors (ER) or progesterone receptors (PR) on the cancer cells, he or she will report the tumor cells as ER positive or PR positive, respectively, or both. If no ER or PR receptors are detected, the tumor is reported as ER negative or PR negative, respectively, or both.

In addition to determining if a cancer has estrogen or progesterone receptors, the pathologist will report on the percentage of tumor cells with receptors and the degree of receptor positivity. This information is helpful to doctors in determining which cancer medications may be most effective.

The good news about being ER positive or PR positive is that you may benefit from hormone therapy, which consists of medications designed to interfere with the hormone stimulation of these cancers. Hormone receptor positive cancers typically grow more slowly than do hormone receptor negative cancers.

HER2 status

Human epidermal growth factor receptor 2 (HER2) is a protein receptor that's produced by the HER2 gene. Normally, substances that attach to this receptor stimulate cell division. When too many of these receptors are present, they can cause increased cell growth. About 20 to 25 percent of breast cancers have an excess of the HER2 protein.

There are two ways to test for HER2 receptors: One is by a technique called immunohistochemistry (protein overexpression) and the other is by a method called fluorescent *in situ* hybridization (FISH), also known as gene amplification.

- **Immunohistochemistry tests.** These tests, which were developed first and are less expensive than FISH tests, are generally done first. They use certain easily identifiable antibodies that bind to HER2 to measure the number of receptors on a cancer cell surface. Scores range from 0 to 3+. A score of 0 or 1+ is considered negative and means the tumor cells don't have an excess of HER2 receptors. A score of 3+ indicates the tumor cells are overexpressing HER2 protein and is considered positive. A 2+ score is considered borderline.
- **FISH test.** For 2+ immunohistochemistry results, a doctor may recommend a FISH test to confirm whether the HER2 gene is overamplified (positive). FISH

uses fluorescent DNA markers to find extra copies of the HER2 gene. The results are generally reported as being either positive or negative.

Knowing that your cancer cells contain too much HER2 can be important information that can help determine the treatment you receive. The drug trastuzumab (Herceptin), for example, is a specific antibody that binds to HER2 shutting it down and, thereby, reducing the growth rate of the cancer (see Chapters 3 and 11).

Staging

Once a doctor knows that cancer is present, he or she wants to know if the cancer is confined to the breast or if it has spread to other areas. This knowledge is obtained through what's called staging. Staging is another aspect of the diagnostic process that's essential to determining the best form of treatment. It's also a very significant factor in predicting your prognosis.

Staging tests

Several additional tests may be needed as your doctor determines the stage of your cancer. These include blood tests, a chest X-ray, bone scan, magnetic resonance image (MRI), computerized tomography (CT) scan and positron emission tomography (PET) scan. It's important to note, though, that most women don't need all of these tests. This is partly because the tests have limited usefulness and partly because the chances that the cancer has spread beyond the breast and lymph nodes are low.

Blood tests

A complete blood count (CBC) can help your doctor assess your general health. A CBC measures:
• Red blood cells, which carry oxygen
• White blood cells, which help fight infections
• Platelets, which help your blood to clot when you bleed

A blood chemistry test measures the level of substances that indicate whether your organs, such as your kidneys and liver, are functioning correctly.

Abnormal levels of certain substances in your blood, called tumor markers, might suggest the presence of cancer. But unless other evidence suggests your cancer has spread to distant parts of your body — which occurs in only 5 to 10 percent of women when they're initially diagnosed — tests for these markers generally aren't used because they don't provide much useful information at this point. In addition, no one tumor marker is specific for breast cancer.

Chest X-ray

Your doctor may recommend a chest X-ray to check for any evidence that the cancer has spread to your lungs. If your tumor is very small and the cancer cells haven't spread to your lymph nodes, a chest X-ray may not be necessary.

Bone scan

A bone scan is used to check for spread of the cancer to your bones. The test usually isn't done unless other evidence indicates possible spread, such as pain in your bones or abnormal blood tests.

During the test, you receive an injection containing a tiny amount of a radioactive tracer. The tracer is drawn to cells involved in bone remodeling. Throughout a person's lifetime, bone tissue is continuously removed and replaced by new bone tissue, a process called remodeling. When cancer cells spread to bone, remodeling typically increases. A special camera scans your body and records whether the tracer has accumulated in certain areas (hot spots). A hot spot may indicate that cancer has spread to your bones, but it could also indicate infection or arthritis, another cause of increased bone remodeling.

Computerized tomography scan

Computerized tomography (CT) is an X-ray technique that produces more-detailed images of your internal organs than do conventional X-ray studies.

The procedure involves an X-ray tube that rotates around your body and a large computer to create cross-sectional, 2-D images (slices) of the inside of your body. When these images are combined, a doctor may be able to see tumors, measure them and later biopsy them if necessary. This test is generally only used if your doctor suspects the cancer has spread.

Magnetic resonance imaging

Like computerized tomography, a magnetic resonance image (MRI) also views the inside of your body in cross-sectional slices, but it uses an extremely strong magnet instead of X-rays. The magnet manipulates water molecules in your body so that they tumble, which produces a faint signal. A sensitive receiver — similar to a radio antenna — picks up those signals. A computer used to generate the pictures manipulates the resulting signal.

Diagnostic Basics

Most women with a new diagnosis of breast cancer don't need to undergo all the diagnostic tests available. The following examinations and tests — in addition to a biopsy of the tumor or suspicious area — are often all that's necessary to determine the stage of the cancer:

- Medical history
- Physical examination
- Mammogram
- Chest X-ray (not always)
- Blood tests

Depending on their chemical makeup, different tissues produce stronger or weaker signals. This allows a doctor to differentiate a tumor from normal tissue. In some cases, MRI can be a more sensitive test than can a CT scan. Typically, though, this test isn't necessary to stage breast cancer.

Positron emission tomography scan

Positron emission tomography (PET) is different from an MRI or CT scan in that it records tissue activity rather than tissue structure. As opposed to normal cells, cancer cells often exhibit increased metabolic activity. During a PET scan, you will receive a small amount of a radioactive tracer — typically a form of blood sugar (glucose) — into your body. Most tissues in your body absorb some of this tracer, but tissues that are using more energy — exhibiting increased metabolic activity — absorb greater amounts. Tumors are usually more metabolically active and tend to absorb more of the sugar tracer, which allows the tumors to light up on the scan.

PET scans are typically performed with CT scans to help localize the abnormal areas. Your doctor may recommend a PET scan if he or she suspects the cancer has spread but is uncertain of the location to which it has spread.

Staging classification

After your surgery your doctor may order additional tests. Once the surgery is complete and the results of these tests are known, your doctor will have the information needed to let you know the stage or your cancer.

Ideally, staging is done after examination of tissue specimens (pathologic material) obtained during surgery. This is called pathologic staging. Staging can be attempted before pathologic examination. This method, termed clinical staging, is less accurate.

The most commonly used method of doing this is the TNM staging system created by the American Joint Committee on Cancer. It addresses three key issues:

- **T (tumor).** How big is the tumor, and has it spread to the skin or to chest wall muscle?
- **N (node).** Have cancer cells spread to nearby lymph nodes?
- **M (metastasis).** Has the cancer spread to other, distant areas of the body?

Numbers are assigned to each of these categories, indicating the degree to which the tumor has grown or spread. *T* receives a number from 0 to 4, indicating the size of the tumor and if it has spread to the skin or chest wall. *N* receives a number from 0 to 3, indicating the degree

Summary of Staging Definitions

Primary tumor status

T0:	No evidence of primary tumor
Tis:	Carcinoma *in situ*
T1:	≤ 20 millimeter (mm) of invasive cancer
T2:	20.1-50 mm of invasive cancer
T3:	> 50 mm of invasive cancer
T4:	Direct extension to the chest wall, or skin ulceration, or skin nodules, or inflammatory breast cancer

Regional lymph node/pathologic status

N0:	None involved, or node with < 0.2 mm area of tumor cells
N1:	1-3 involved axillary nodes, or microscopically involved internal mammary node detected by sentinel node biopsy procedure
N2:	4-9 involved axillary nodes *or* clinically apparent internal mammary nodes
N3:	≥ 10 involved axillary nodes, or infraclavicular node, or supraclavicular node, or axillary nodes *and* internal mammary nodes

Metastasis

M0:	No distant metastasis
M1:	Distant metastasis

of spread to the lymph nodes and how many lymph nodes are involved. *M* is rated either 0 or 1, indicating no spread or spread, respectively, to distant parts of the body.

A higher number indicates a larger tumor or more advanced spread of the cancer. More detailed notations also may be assigned to certain categories, such as to indicate whether the cancer is *in situ* (vs. invasive), or a lowercase letter to signify a subcategory. For example, a T1, N0, M0 classification means that the tumor is less than 20 millimeters (mm), it hasn't spread to the lymph nodes, and it hasn't metastasized. These classifications may be modified after surgery when the pathologic data are complete.

Once the TNM classification is made, your doctor can determine the stage of your cancer, which usually is labeled as a Roman numeral. A lower number indicates an early stage, and a higher number means a more advanced, serious cancer. The T1, N0, M0 tumor described above would be a stage I tumor.

Stages 0 to IV

Breast cancer staging is complicated and constantly changing as doctors learn more about breast cancer, its spread and prognosis. The chart on the opposite page lists the latest stage groupings for breast cancer. Your doctor can identify for you which designation describes your cancer. Following is some general information about the stages of breast cancer.

Stage 0

This is very early *(in situ)* breast cancer that hasn't spread within the breast or to other parts of the body.

Stage I

Stage IA cancer refers to breast cancer that's 20 mm or less in size — smaller than an inch — with no lymph node involvement. Lymph nodes containing cells that look like they came from the breast but are less than 0.2 mm are considered negative lymph nodes because there's no good evidence these are established cancers. This is a stage IB cancer.

Stage II

Stage II is subdivided into IIA and IIB. Stage II cancer is more extensive than stage I, but not as extensive as stage III. A tumor is stage IIA if it is 20.1 to 50 mm in size, has spread to up to three lymph nodes under the arm or to lymph nodes under the sternum, or both. A tumor greater than 50 mm in size with no spread to the lymph nodes is stage IIB.

Stage III

Stage III breast cancers are subdivided into three classifications: IIIA, IIIB and IIIC. Stage III cancers include a number of criteria that make this a broad category. Stage III cancers are sometimes referred to as local-regionally advanced cancers. One of the main criteria with stage III cancers is there's no evidence the cancer has spread (metastasized) to distant sites.

Some examples of stage III cancers are as follows:
- A tumor greater than 50 mm in size with involvement of at least one lymph node under the arm (IIIA)
- Cancer that has spread to lymph nodes above the collarbone (IIIB)
- Cancer that has spread to breast skin causing swelling and redness, known as inflammatory breast cancer (IIIC)

Stage IV

In stage IV, the cancer has spread beyond the breast and adjacent lymph nodes to distant parts of the body, such as the lungs, liver, bones or brain.

Estimating survival

Based on statistics assembled from women diagnosed with breast cancer in the past, scientists are able to estimate how many women with varying tumor features might survive for at least five years after a breast cancer diagnosis. This is commonly known as the five-year survival rate. Specifically, it refers to the percentage of women who are still alive five years after their cancers were diagnosed.

This doesn't mean that survivors live for only five years after being diagnosed with cancer. In fact, most cancer survivors live much longer. It also doesn't mean that a woman still living five years after her initial treatment is cured. Of all women who experience a breast cancer recurrence, less than half of the time it's

Breast cancer stage grouping

Stage	T	N	M
Stage 0	Tis	N0	M0
Stage IA	T1	N0	M0
Stage IB	T0	N1mi	M0
	T1	N1mi	M0
Stage IIA	T0	N1	M0
	T1	N1	M0
	T2	N0	M0
Stage IIB	T2	N1	M0
	T3	N0	M0
Stage IIIA	T0	N2	M0
	T1	N2	M0
	T2	N2	M0
	T3	N1	M0
	T3	N2	M0
Stage IIIB	T4	N0	M0
	T4	N1	M0
	T4	N2	M0
Stage IIIC	Any T	N3	M0
Stage IV	Any T	Any N	M1

From the American Joint Committee on Cancer's *AJCC Cancer Staging Manual*, 7th edition, 2010; published by Springer Science and Business Media LLC. Used with permission.

Tis: Indicates noninvasive *(in situ)* cancer
mi: Indicates the cancer is <0.2 mm and can only be
   seen by a microscope

T 0-4: Refers to tumor size and spread
N 0-3: Indicates degree of spread to the lymph nodes
M 0-1: Indicates spread to distant parts of the body

within the first five years. More often, it comes later than five years.

Clearly, advances in early detection and treatment have increased survival time. Today, women diagnosed with breast cancer are living longer than did women diagnosed 20 or 30 years ago.

But remember that statistics don't tell the whole story. They only serve to give a general picture and a standard format for doctors to discuss prognosis. Every woman's situation is unique. If you have questions about your own prognosis, discuss them with your doctor or your cancer care team. These individuals can help you find out how these statistics relate, or don't relate, to you.

More information on breast cancer prognosis is provided in later chapters.

Precancerous Conditions

Atypical Hyperplasia 150

Lobular Carcinoma *In Situ* 150

Your Options 152
Watchful waiting 152
Cancer-preventing medications 152
Preventive surgery 152

Sometimes, when doctors check for cancer, they don't find it, but they find a condition that may lead to cancer. One such breast abnormality is a condition called atypical hyperplasia, in which there is an overgrowth of worrisome-appearing cells. Atypical hyperplasia is generally thought of as a precancerous condition — it isn't cancer but women who have it are more likely to develop breast cancer in the future.

Atypical hyperplasia can be further subdivided into atypical ductal hyperplasia — abnormal cells that originate in breast ducts — or atypical lobular hyperplasia — abnormal cells that originate in breast lobules. Another precancerous condition called lobular carcinoma *in situ* (LCIS) is generally viewed as a more extensive version of atypical lobular hyperplasia. It's important to note that while LCIS is called a carcinoma, which means cancer, the exact nature of this condition is still being determined. Most doctors don't consider it a true cancer.

Researchers have many unanswered questions about atypical hyperplasia and LCIS. For instance, it's not clear if some precancerous conditions are actual precursors to cancer — the first steps before cancer development — or if they're cancer markers — indicating an increased risk of breast cancer but not the certainty that cancer will develop.

Atypical Hyperplasia

A woman may receive a diagnosis of atypical hyperplasia (atypia) of the breast after a biopsy is done to evaluate a suspicious spot on a mammogram. It can take two forms — atypical ductal hyperplasia (see opposite page) and atypical lobular hyperplasia, which is different in appearance but not in behavior. Neither of these conditions is considered cancerous, but both represent an increased cancer risk.

A woman with either atypical ductal hyperplasia or atypical lobular hyperplasia has about a four times greater risk of developing breast cancer in either breast, compared with a woman who doesn't have atypia. What does this mean in terms of actual risk? Ten years after a biopsy indicates atypia, about 10 percent of women who receive such a diagnosis will have developed breast cancer; at 15 years, about 15 percent will have developed breast cancer.

And women with atypical ductal hyperplasia and atypical lobular hyperplasia can develop either ductal or lobular breast cancer. In other words, the atypia type doesn't predict the breast cancer type.

At one time, it was thought that having atypia and a family history of breast cancer meant having an even higher cancer risk, but research has shown that's not the case. Scientists believe that development of atypical hyperplasia in the breast is the result of some underlying risk — which may be family history in some women and other factors in other women. So the increased risk of breast cancer associated with a woman's family history has already been factored into the equation when atypia is identified.

When atypical hyperplasia of the breast is found on a needle biopsy, the area is generally treated with surgery to make sure cancer isn't present. Medication also may be an option following surgery. Breast cancer prevention trials evaluating anti-estrogen medications found that women with atypical hyperplasia who received the drug tamoxifen had a much lower risk of developing breast cancer compared with those women who didn't receive the drug. Risk was also reduced with the medication raloxifene (Evista), but to a lesser extent.

Chapter 6 has more information on prevention strategies for women considered at high risk of the disease.

Lobular Carcinoma In Situ

Lobular carcinoma *in situ* (LCIS) is thought to develop within the lobules located at the end of the breast ducts (see opposite page). LCIS usually doesn't show up on mammograms but may be found in breast biopsies done for other reasons.

Over the years, most cancer experts haven't considered LCIS to be cancer in and of itself. Rather, they viewed it as an area of abnormal tissue growth that signals an increased risk of developing invasive breast cancer later on in either breast.

Unlike ductal carcinoma *in situ* (DCIS), discussed in the next chapter, LCIS is much less common. And because it's less common, there hasn't been as much good research on the condition to determine its long-term cancer risk. It's often said that a woman with LCIS has about a 20 to 25 percent risk of developing invasive breast

Atypical ductal hyperplasia

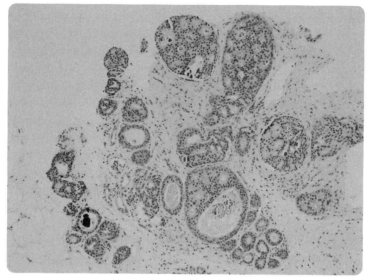

The breast ducts seen in this cross-sectional image no longer have a normal, single layer of cells lining them. Instead, there are too many cells that have an abnormal (atypical) appearance. The dark black spot in the lower left indicates calcification of debris that's collected within the duct.

Lobular carcinoma *in situ* (LCIS)

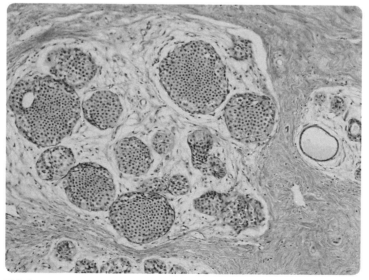

This image shows breast lobules filled with cells that are abnormal (atypical) appearing. A biopsy sample in which similar but less extensive changes were involved would be called atypical lobular hyperplasia.

©MFMER

cancer in either breast over her lifetime, but the data supporting this estimate are relatively weak. In comparison, the lifetime risk of breast cancer for women in general — those who haven't been diagnosed with LCIS — is around 12 percent.

Your Options

In deciding how to treat atypia and LCIS, a number of factors are taken into account, including personal choice.

Watchful waiting

Given the relatively low likelihood of developing invasive breast cancer in the first few years after being diagnosed with these conditions, some women choose the option of close monitoring. This generally involves yearly screening mammograms, monthly breast self-examinations and regular clinical breast exams.

This approach works best in women who have breasts that are relatively easy to examine by clinical examination and mammography, as opposed to women who have lumpy breasts or women whose breast tissue appears very dense on mammograms.

Other women prefer to take preventive measures to reduce their cancer risk. Options include taking cancer-preventing medications or, less commonly, surgically removing both breasts.

Cancer-preventing medications

Two selective estrogen receptor modulator (SERM) drugs are approved to reduce the risk of invasive breast cancer.

One of those medications is tamoxifen. It can be used by both premenopausal and postmenopausal women. Tamoxifen is typically taken for five years. Raloxifene (Evista) also is approved to reduce the risk of invasive breast cancer in high-risk postmenopausal women, including those with atypical hyperplasia or LCIS.

Another type of medication called exemestane (Aromasin) also has been shown to reduce the risk of invasive breast cancer. Exemestane is a type of medication known as an aromatase inhibitor.

These medications do carry some side effects, so the benefits of the drugs need to be weighed against their unwanted effects.

Preventive surgery

Preventive surgery (bilateral prophylactic mastectomy) isn't usually performed in women with atypical hyperplasia. However, it may be considered for women with LCIS.

To obtain the best possible protective benefit from this surgery, both breasts are removed, because LCIS increases your risk of developing breast cancer in either breast. However, there's debate as to whether removing both breasts is justified, considering the majority of women with LCIS won't develop breast cancer.

Ultimately, it's a personal choice, based on a thorough discussion with your doctor. Treatment of LCIS isn't urgent, so you have time to carefully weigh the pros and cons of the procedure.

To learn more about breast cancer prevention strategies, see Chapter 6.

Ductal Carcinoma *In Situ* (DCIS)

Diagnosis	154
Key Factors	154
Treatment Options	155
Surgery	155
Radiation therapy	157
Tamoxifen	159
Making the Decision	160

Ductal carcinoma *in situ* (DCIS) is a common form of breast cancer — it accounts for about 1 in 5 breast cancers diagnosed each year. A diagnosis of DCIS can be confusing for some women. A woman with DCIS may be told that she has stage 0 cancer, but at the same time, she is likely to hear that she needs surgery to remove the cancer and, possibly, additional treatment.

Why such aggressive treatment for a stage 0 cancer? While it's possible that, left untreated, the cancer may never leave the breast duct where it's located, there's also a possibility that it will. Unlike lobular carcinoma *in situ* (LCIS), discussed in Chapter 9, DCIS is more likely to develop into invasive cancer in the future.

The name ductal carcinoma *in situ* also causes confusion for some women. They're not certain what *in situ* means. And because their doctors may use terms like *DCIS* and *stage 0*, they're not certain if what they have is truly breast cancer.

The term *in situ* means located in its natural or normal place. In this case, it means the cancer remains within the breast duct where it originated. Other terms used to describe the condition include *intraductal carcinoma* or *noninvasive carcinoma*. Unlike LCIS, which is considered a risk marker for a later breast cancer, DCIS is generally viewed as early stage cancer.

However, what researchers still don't know, and what they're hoping to learn, is which women with DCIS are more likely to develop invasive or recurrent breast cancer. By knowing those women most at risk, doctors could tailor treatment accordingly.

Diagnosis

DCIS is usually found during mammogram screenings, but it can be difficult to detect. On mammograms, DCIS is often characterized by the presence of tiny groups of calcium deposits called microcalcifications. In some cases, a mass can actually be felt (palpated).

Because of increased mammography screening, the rate at which DCIS is diagnosed has increased dramatically in recent years. DCIS is typically diagnosed either with a core needle biopsy, a procedure that uses a needle to remove a small sample of tissue for examination, or by way of an open excisional biopsy, which involves a small surgical incision to remove a tissue sample. These biopsy procedures are discussed in more detail in Chapter 8.

Fortunately, the prognosis for women treated for DCIS is very good. According to most reports in medical journals, the survival rate is now approaching 100 percent. Different treatment options are available. Ideally, the therapy chosen should be one that neither overtreats, nor undertreats, the condition.

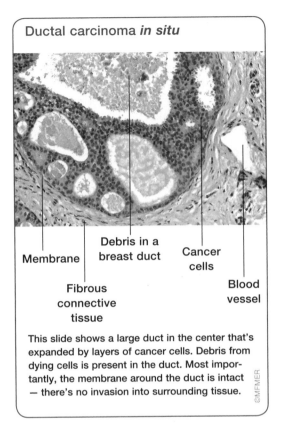

Ductal carcinoma *in situ*

Membrane — Debris in a breast duct — Cancer cells — Fibrous connective tissue — Blood vessel

This slide shows a large duct in the center that's expanded by layers of cancer cells. Debris from dying cells is present in the duct. Most importantly, the membrane around the duct is intact — there's no invasion into surrounding tissue.

©MFMER

Key Factors

Several factors may influence the behavior or aggressiveness of DCIS, although the precise effect of each factor is still being studied. Treatment for each DCIS is generally based on the following factors:

- **Pathologic margins.** If cancer cells extend close to the edge of the tissue samples removed during a biopsy, there's a higher likelihood that some cancer cells have been left behind. In such a situation, a wider excision lumpectomy or a mastectomy may be necessary.
- **Tumor size.** A small tumor has a better chance of being adequately

removed with lumpectomy than does a larger tumor.

- **Grade.** In DCIS, grade refers to the appearance of the control centers (nuclei) of the cells. If, when examined under a microscope, the nuclei of the cells still appear similar to the nuclei of normal cells and very few cells are dividing, the tumor is low grade. If the nuclei are markedly different from the nuclei of normal cells, the cells are dividing rapidly or both, the tumor is high grade. High-grade tumors have a higher rate of recurrence than do low-grade tumors.
- **Cell structure.** Two major subtypes of DCIS are distinguished by the structure of their cells. One type is characterized by large, atypical cells with a central area of dead or degenerating cells (comedo necrosis). The other type is characterized by the lack of these qualities. The presence of comedo necrosis generally signifies a more aggressive DCIS. Tumors with comedo necrosis have a higher rate of recurrence than do DCIS tumors without comedo necrosis.

Women who have high-grade DCIS with comedo necrosis may be advised to have a procedure called sentinel node biopsy (see Chapter 11). This procedure is also sometimes done in women with DCIS who don't have comedo necorsis.

In a sentinel node biopsy, the lymph nodes to which the cancer would most likely spread first are examined for the presence of cancer cells. Because DCIS with comedo necrosis has a higher risk of invasion than do other types of DCIS, studying the sentinel lymph nodes is a way to double-check for any cancer spread to the lymph nodes. If no cancer

is found, chances are the cancer is still confined to the breast.

- **Age.** Women younger than age 40 with DCIS may be at higher risk of recurrence than women age 40 and older.

Treatment Options

Three treatment options are generally considered in women with ductal carcinoma *in situ*:
- Surgery (lumpectomy or mastectomy)
- Radiation therapy (a consideration in women who choose lumpectomy)
- The drug tamoxifen

Surgery

When a woman is diagnosed with DCIS, generally one of the first decisions she has to make is whether to treat the condition with a mastectomy or lumpectomy.

Mastectomy
Mastectomy is the medical term for surgical removal of the entire breast. For the treatment of DCIS, a simple (total) mastectomy is performed rather than a modified radical mastectomy. A simple mastectomy removes the breast tissue, skin, areola and nipple, but not underarm lymph nodes. A modified radical mastectomy removes all these components, including underarm lymph nodes.

Before mammograms were widely used to screen for breast cancer, DCIS was often detected later, when the mass was larger. Because of the size of the tumor, a simple mastectomy was the standard treatment. With regular mammography screening, doctors began identifying cancer

A Gray Zone

Exactly when does ductal carcinoma *in situ* become invasive cancer? Sometimes, it can be hard to tell. There's a continuum of change that occurs at the cellular level between DCIS and a diagnosis of invasive cancer. At times it can be difficult for a pathologist to determine whether a particular breast tumor is a noninvasive cancer or an invasive one.

Some breast tumors labeled as DCIS show some evidence of microinvasion — the beginnings of invasive cancer. In these situations, a surgeon will likely recommend a sentinel node biopsy to provide better assurance that the cancer hasn't spread to the lymph nodes under the arm.

earlier. This, combined with greater use of lumpectomy, made mastectomies less common. In some situations, though, mastectomy may be preferable to a lumpectomy:

- The DCIS area is large compared with the size of your breast. If the area is large, a lumpectomy may not leave you with acceptable cosmetic results.
- There's more than one DCIS area, and it would be difficult to remove all the areas with a lumpectomy.
- Examination of tissue samples removed from the breast shows cancer cells at or near the edge of the tissue specimens. This may mean that there's more DCIS than originally thought, and a lumpectomy may not be adequate.
- You're not a candidate for radiation therapy, which commonly follows a lumpectomy. It may be best to avoid radiation if you're pregnant, you've already received radiation to your chest area or you have a condition that makes you more sensitive to the side effects of radiation therapy.
- You have extremely dense breast tissue, which may make it difficult to detect a recurrence on a mammogram.

- You're a BRCA gene carrier (see Chapter 5) and you and your doctor are concerned about an increased risk of new breast cancers.
- You prefer to have a mastectomy rather than a lumpectomy for any of a number of reasons, including a desire not to undergo radiation therapy.

Breast reconstruction is almost always an option after a mastectomy. It can be done during the same surgery or at a later time. See Chapter 12 to find out more about breast reconstruction.

Lumpectomy

Lumpectomy, also known as breast-conserving therapy, removes only a portion of tissue from your breast. The procedure allows you to keep as much of your breast as possible and, depending on the amount of tissue removed, usually eliminates the need for reconstructive surgery.

When lumpectomy combined with radiation became an accepted treatment for invasive breast cancer, doctors questioned the use of mastectomy for less aggressive conditions such as DCIS. Researchers studied lumpectomy as a potential treatment for DCIS, leading to its widespread use today. Lumpectomy followed by radiation therapy is the most common treatment for DCIS. Although no study has officially compared lumpectomy with removal of the entire breast (mastectomy) for the treatment of DCIS, research suggests that lumpectomy combined with radiation produces survival rates similar to those of mastectomy. Most women with DCIS are candidates for lumpectomy although, as just discussed, in some situations mastectomy may be preferred.

For DCIS, a lumpectomy generally doesn't involve removal of lymph nodes from under the arm because this is a non-invasive cancer and the chance of finding cancer in the lymph nodes is exceedingly small. However, a surgeon may recommend a sentinel node biopsy if there's a large area of DCIS, the area is a mass that can be felt, or the biopsy suggests possible spread. Chapter 11 discusses lumpectomy and lymph node removal in more detail.

Radiation therapy

Radiation therapy after lumpectomy reduces the chance that DCIS will come back or progress to invasive cancer. This was illustrated by a study that randomly assigned women with DCIS to receive either lumpectomy alone or lumpectomy with radiation. After an average follow-up of 15 years, researchers found that women who underwent radiation had less risk of recurrent DCIS and invasive breast cancer in the affected breast (see the table below).

Some doctors have suggested that in the study just mentioned, the amount of normal breast tissue removed with the DCIS tissue may not have been large enough to assure that all the DCIS was removed, leading to the higher risk of recurrence in the lumpectomy alone group. They contend that if larger areas of normal tissue are removed, radiation therapy might not be needed. Nonetheless, this study forms the basis for why radiation therapy is recommended for most women with DCIS who have a lumpectomy.

Radiation therapy uses high-energy X-rays to kill cancer cells or damage them to the point where they lose their ability to grow and divide. Cells that grow out of control, such as cancer cells, are more vulnerable to the effects of radiation than are normal cells and thus are more likely to be damaged.

The two basic types of radiation therapy are external radiation and internal radiation. For treatment of DCIS, external radiation therapy is most commonly used.

Risk of recurrent DCIS and invasive cancer in the same breast

	Lumpectomy alone	Lumpectomy plus radiation
Recurrent DCIS	15%	9%
Invasive breast cancer	20%	11%

Source: Wapnir IL, Dignam JJ, Fisher B, et.al., Long-term outcomes of invasive ipsilateral breast cancer recurrences after lumpectomy in NSABP B-17 and B-24 randomized clinical trials for DCIS. *J Natl Cancer Inst*, 2011;103:478.

3 Women, 3 Choices

The stories that follow highlight three women diagnosed with DCIS and the choices each made regarding her treatment. Each of the women took a different treatment route, feeling it was the best choice in her particular situation.

Geraldine's Story

Geraldine was 68 years old when she was diagnosed with DCIS. The diagnosis came at the same time she learned that she had some abnormal cells in her cervix. After a biopsy of her right breast, where a mammogram detected a small abnormality, she had a double surgery. Doctors removed abnormal tissue in her right breast with a lumpectomy, followed by removal of abnormal cells in her cervix.

After the surgery, Geraldine knew she had some decisions to make. One of them was whether to undergo radiation therapy to the remaining tissue in her right breast. Geraldine wanted to thoroughly study the matter before making a decision. After reviewing the medical literature, Geraldine decided that radiation therapy wasn't for her. She decided to undergo monitoring every six months with mammography. She also has a Pap test regularly to monitor the health of her cervix.

Geraldine's decision not to have radiation was based on several factors:

- The DCIS was very small, about half a centimeter.
- A possible side effect of radiation therapy was damage to her lungs.
- The time and travel involved in receiving radiation for six weeks was fairly extensive.

After weighing the risks versus the benefits, Geraldine felt, with the support of her doctors, that the advantages to be gained from radiation therapy weren't significant enough to outweigh the disadvantages in her situation. Her children worried about her decision but they were supportive. As Geraldine likes to point out, it's her life and she's the one who has to live with her decisions.

Geraldine is quick to emphasize the need to make your own decision and not let others control your life. She continues to do well and sums up, "Do research, put your life in God's hands and make a choice that's good for you."

Cathy's Story

Like Geraldine's, Cathy's DCIS was first detected on a routine mammogram. Cathy was 42 years old at the time. She had had a baseline mammogram at age 38 and thought it would be a good time to have another mammogram. A practicing radiologist, Cathy had ready access to the mammography suite and had her examination while a friend was working in the area. Before long, they were getting extra views of the affected breast. Cathy recognized new clusters of microcalcifications that didn't appear either obviously benign or definitely malignant, but worrisome enough to warrant a biopsy.

A biopsy revealed DCIS with at least three areas of calcifications. Because of this, Cathy opted for a mastectomy. A sentinel node biopsy performed at the same time confirmed that the cancer hadn't spread to the lymph system. This gave Cathy assurance that all the DCIS areas had been removed and that no cancer had spread to the lymph nodes. After a six-month follow-up mammogram and clinical exam of her other breast, she has returned to annual screening of her remaining breast.

Cathy decided against immediate reconstructive surgery in case additional treatment might be needed after her surgery. She wears a prosthesis and is keeping reconstruction as an option when her children are older.

Cathy continues to do well and her advice to other women is to regularly perform breast self-examinations and to have clinical examinations and mammograms on a regular basis.

Agnes' Story

Agnes was 72 years old when a biopsy revealed that she had DCIS. She was given the treatment option of a lumpectomy followed by radiation or a mastectomy. Agnes decided on a lumpectomy with radiation, and she also had a sentinel node biopsy to provide some assurance that the cancer hadn't spread. Agnes' surgery went smoothly, as did the follow-up radiation therapy. She had almost no side effects from her daily radiation sessions.

Standing by to offer Agnes support were two close friends and a sister-in-law with similar cancer experiences. One friend had been disease-free for eight years after undergoing a lumpectomy and radiation, a factor that helped Agnes make her decision.

Agnes has been satisfied with her decision. She also is doing well and she hopes that the future will continue to confirm that her decision was the right one.

See Chapter 11 for more information on radiation therapy.

Tamoxifen

Tamoxifen is a synthetic anti-estrogen hormone that's been shown to be beneficial in the treatment of invasive breast cancer. It's also used as a cancer prevention agent for women at high risk of breast cancer.

Due to this drug's success in treating invasive breast cancer, doctors wanted to know if it might benefit women with DCIS. That question was addressed in a study called the National Surgical Adjuvant Breast and Bowel Project (NSABP) B-24 trial. It involved approximately 1,800 women with DCIS who had undergone lumpectomies and radiation therapy. The women were randomly assigned to receive either tamoxifen or an inactive pill (placebo) for five years. The results of the study led to the Food and Drug Administration's approval of tamoxifen as a treatment for DCIS.

Researchers wanted to know if women taking tamoxifen experienced reduced rates of recurrent DCIS and invasive breast cancer, compared with women taking a placebo.

The table on page 160 shows 15-year follow-up results from the study. All breast cancer events — recurrent DCIS and invasive breast cancer in the same breast and the development of cancer in the opposite breast — decreased by 6 percent in women who received tamoxifen for five years compared with those who received a placebo. The most benefit from tamoxifen use was in the reduction of cancers in the opposite breast.

What the original study didn't address, though, was whether hormone receptor status was an important factor in the study's results. (See Chapters 8 and 11 for more on hormone receptor status.) A group of researchers went back and addressed this issue. They found that 70 percent of the women treated in this clinical trial had positive estrogen receptors in their biopsy specimens and these women benefited from taking tamoxifen, whereas women with negative estrogen receptors didn't. As a result, hormone receptor status is a key factor in determining treatment.

For women who have a mastectomy, there's less reason to use tamoxifen. With a mastectomy, the risk of invasive breast cancer or DCIS in the small amount of remaining breast tissue is almost zero. Any potential benefit from tamoxifen would apply only to the opposite breast.

The bottom line is that tamoxifen is a treatment option to be considered among women with DCIS. However, for some women, it may not provide much benefit.

Discuss the pros and cons of tamoxifen with your doctor. For more information on tamoxifen, see Chapter 11.

Making the Decision

Because not all DCIS is the same, it's important to consider treatment options in the context of your own situation and to make a decision that you feel comfortable with.

If you're trying to decide whether to have a lumpectomy or a mastectomy, Chapter 11 contains a list of several questions to ask yourself that may help you. If you're deciding whether to have radiation therapy after a lumpectomy, discuss the benefits and risks with your doctor.

Finally, if you haven't already, read the stories of three women with DCIS, beginning on page 158. Each of the women made a different choice regarding her treatment, based on her individual circumstances.

Tamoxifen vs. a placebo: A 15-year follow-up of women with DCIS

Issue	Placebo group	Tamoxifen group
All breast cancers	29%	23%
Cancer in the same breast as the original tumor		
All cancers	18%	16%
DCIS	8.3%	7.5%
Invasive	10%	9%
Cancer in the opposite breast		
All cancers	11%	7%
Deaths		
Breast cancer	2.7%	2.3%
All causes	17%	14%

Modified from Wapnir IL, Dignam JJ, Fisher B, et.al., Long-term outcomes of invasive ipsilateral breast cancer recurrences after lumpectomy in NSABP B-17 and B-24 randomized clinical trials for DCIS. *J Natl Cancer Inst*, 2011;103:478.

Chapter 11: Breast Cancer

Treating Invasive Breast Cancer

Treatment Options	162
Surgery	162
Lumpectomy	163
Mastectomy	164
Lymph node removal	165
What to expect	168
Radiation Therapy	171
Radiation after lumpectomy	171
Radiation after mastectomy	172
How radiation works	173
Side effects	175
Decision Guide: Lumpectomy vs. Mastectomy	176
Additional Treatment	179
Who should consider it?	179
Therapy Options	184
Chemotherapy	185
Hormone therapy	188
Anti-HER2 therapy	197
Watchful waiting	199
Decision Guide: Adjuvant Systemic Therapy	196
Clinical Trials	199

After hearing the news and coming to grips with a breast cancer diagnosis, most women have a lot of questions: "What now?" "How do I deal with this cancer?" "Do I have options?" "What's my prognosis?"

The good news is that breast cancer is highly treatable with good results. Survival rates are continuously increasing, and much research is being done to develop better treatment options. But as options increase, so does the information needed to make appropriate treatment decisions. The goal of the next few chapters is to help you become more informed about what's available to treat breast cancer.

This chapter focuses on treating invasive cancer that hasn't spread to other parts of your body, what's known as localized breast cancer (stages I and II). Chapter 13 includes information on the treatment of locally advanced breast cancer (stage III). Treatment for recurrent cancer — cancer that returns after initial treatment — is covered in Chapter 15. Chapter 16 focuses on breast cancer that has spread (metastasized) to distant parts of the body (stage IV).

If you're still grappling with your diagnosis, it's OK to wait awhile before delving into your treatment options. Take the time you need to understand and absorb your situation. This is a life-changing event, and it frequently leads to a time of re-evaluating priorities and life goals. It's also a time to strengthen your connections with family and friends and to gather the support you need for the days ahead.

When you're ready, find a quiet spot to read the following information. Remember that taking a bit of time — up to a couple of weeks — to carefully weigh your options isn't likely to alter the outcome. Thorough consideration of your values, lifestyle and personal priorities can make all the difference in how satisfied you will be with the choices you make. Even if you decide you're more comfortable asking your doctor to decide on your treatment, the knowledge you've acquired may make the process a little less scary.

Treatment Options

The primary goal of treatment for localized breast cancer is to get rid of all cancerous (malignant) cells that are in your body. In general, the two ways of accomplishing this are with locoregional therapy and systemic therapy:

- **Locoregional therapy.** Locoregional therapy is targeted directly at the tumor and the nearby tissue surrounding it. Locoregional therapy includes surgery with or without radiation therapy.
- **Systemic therapy.** Systemic therapy is aimed at treating cancer cells throughout your body. It involves medication that's usually given by mouth or injected into your bloodstream. Systemic therapy includes chemotherapy, immune therapy and hormone (mostly anti-estrogen) therapy.

If you have localized invasive cancer, surgery is usually the first line of treatment. It may be followed by systemic therapy to get rid of any cells that may have split off from the primary tumor and traveled to other parts of your body. This type of additional therapy after surgery is called adjuvant systemic therapy.

The goal of both locoregional therapy and adjuvant systemic therapy is to cure your cancer.

Surgery

Surgery to remove the tumor is usually the first form of treatment for localized breast cancer. In addition to removing the cancerous mass, surgery provides additional information about the type and extent of the cancer that's present. This information can help guide further treatment decisions.

For some women, the most difficult part of surgery is deciding which type of breast surgery to have. In general, two options are available: removal of the tumor only (lumpectomy) and removal of the whole breast (mastectomy). Lumpectomy is often combined with radiation therapy. The combination approach is known as breast-conserving therapy because it allows a woman to receive effective breast cancer treatment and still keep her breast. Making a choice between lumpectomy and mastectomy can be difficult. The following information can help you in the decision-making process. It describes the possible surgical procedures and outlines the pros and cons of each option.

Lumpectomy

With breast-conserving surgery (lumpectomy), only the part of your breast that contains the tumor is removed. This allows as much of your breast to be saved as possible. Because tumors are now detected at an earlier stage and often are smaller in size, and because of the procedure's proven success in research studies, lumpectomy is much more common today than it was in the past.

During a lumpectomy, a surgeon makes an incision large enough to allow removal of both the tumor and a margin of healthy tissue surrounding the tumor. The margin is taken to increase the chance that all of the cancer cells are removed.

As noted in Chapter 8, a lumpectomy can perform dual roles. If you didn't already have a biopsy, tissue from the lumpectomy is used to confirm a diagnosis of breast cancer. In addition, a lumpectomy can serve as a first line of treatment.

Lumpectomy is often followed by radiation therapy to try to eliminate any cancer cells that may remain in the breast. Because breast tissue remains after a lumpectomy, if the procedure isn't

When Lumpectomy May Not Be the Right Choice

Most women with stage I or II breast cancer are eligible for a lumpectomy But in some situations, a lumpectomy may not be recommended. For example:

- The tumor is larger than 5 centimeters (about 2 inches) in diameter.
- The tumor is large relative to the overall size of your breast. You may not have enough breast tissue left after a lumpectomy to achieve an acceptable cosmetic result.
- The tumor is located beneath the nipple, and a lumpectomy would require removing the nipple. For some women, removal of the nipple may not leave an acceptable cosmetic result.
- There are multiple tumors in different areas of your breast.
- There are widespread malignant-appearing microcalcifications on your mammogram.
- You're unable to receive radiation therapy because you're pregnant, you've had previous radiation to your chest area or you have a connective tissue disease, such as systemic lupus erythematosus (SLE) or scleroderma.
- You're at high risk of developing another new breast cancer, and you're considering prophylactic surgery to remove both breasts.

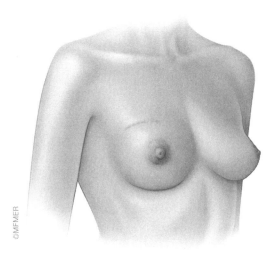

During a lumpectomy, the tumor is removed along with some healthy tissue around the tumor.

followed with radiation treatment, there's a significantly higher chance that the cancer could return. The risk of a cancer recurrence in the breast when radiation isn't used after lumpectomy can range from about 15 to 35 percent, depending on a number of factors. That's why lumpectomy is commonly followed by radiation therapy in the treatment of invasive breast cancer. An exception is in some older women with breast cancer. In this select population, radiation therapy isn't always recommended.

If cancer does return in a breast after a lumpectomy and radiation, then a mastectomy is almost always necessary. However, most women treated with a lumpectomy don't experience a cancer recurrence in the same breast.

A breast-conserving procedure similar to lumpectomy that generally isn't performed in the United States is called a partial mastectomy (quadrantectomy or segmental mastectomy). It removes significantly more tissue than does a lumpectomy.

Mastectomy

Mastectomy is a general term for removal of a breast. A mastectomy may be performed when a lumpectomy isn't possible or when a woman prefers it.

Up until the 1980s, mastectomy was almost always recommended for the treatment of breast cancer. But researchers learned that smaller operations combined with radiation could treat the disease as successfully as a mastectomy. The most important finding of their studies was that survival — the length of time lived after diagnosis — was the same, regardless of the type of surgery chosen: either a lumpectomy with radiation or a mastectomy. In other words, for most breast cancers, it's not necessary to have a mastectomy in order for the treatment to be successful.

During a mastectomy, the surgeon usually makes a single incision across half the chest that allows for removal of the breast and, if necessary, adjacent under-arm (axillary) lymph nodes. Several types of mastectomies may be performed: radical, modified radical and simple (total).

Radical mastectomy

A radical mastectomy is a procedure that's rarely used today. It removes a large amount of tissue, including the breast, some of the chest wall muscles, all the lymph nodes under the arm, and some additional fat and skin. From the early 1900s through the 1970s, this was the standard treatment for women with breast cancer. Today use is generally lim-

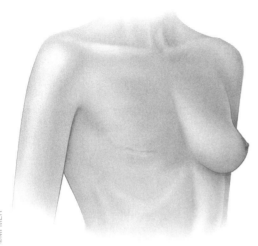

During a modified radical mastectomy, the breast is removed as well as some underarm lymph nodes. Chest muscles are left intact.

ited to cases of locally advanced cancer that's spread to chest wall muscles.

Modified radical mastectomy

During the last three decades of the 20th century, the most common mastectomy used to treat invasive breast cancer was modified radical mastectomy. It involves removing the entire breast, including the skin, areola and nipple, as well as some of the lymph nodes under the arm. It spares the chest wall muscles, thereby leaving a more normal chest wall contour than does radical mastectomy.

Simple mastectomy

A simple (total) mastectomy involves removal of the breast tissue, skin, areola and nipple, but not the lymph nodes. This procedure is generally used when the axillary lymph nodes don't need to be removed, for example, when a sentinel node is examined and shows no sign of cancer cells (see "Sentinel node biopsy," page 166). A simple mastectomy may be used to treat noninvasive breast cancer, such as ductal carcinoma *in situ*, and it's sometimes used to prevent breast cancer in women at high risk of the disease (see Chapter 6).

Lymph node removal

Lymph nodes are small, compact structures where cells of your immune system

---

QUESTION & ANSWER

Q: What are positive margins?

A: When your surgeon removes a cancerous (malignant) tumor, he or she tries to make sure that all the cancer has been removed. The edges of the removed tissue are called the margins. These margins are examined by a pathologist to see if any cancer cells are at the margin or close to it. If cancer cells extend up to the edges of the tissue sample, the sample is said to have positive margins. This means there's a high probability that cancer cells still remain in the area from where the tumor was taken. Additional tissue is usually removed in this situation until cancer-free (negative) margins are obtained.

congregate. They're linked by tiny vessels along the lymphatic system. Lymph nodes are generally clustered in certain areas of your body, such as your neck, armpits and groin. The job of lymph vessels is to drain excess fluid that's not absorbed by blood vessels. Lymph nodes filter out foreign substances, such as bacteria and cancer cells. Lymph nodes are also one of the first lines of defense of your body's immune system, where foreign materials, such as bacteria and cancer, are recognized and your body can mount an immune response. As a cancerous tumor grows, cancer cells may spread to nearby lymph nodes. Some may get past the lymph nodes and travel to other parts of the body.

An early location for breast cancer to spread is the lymph nodes under the arm, called the axillary lymph nodes. That's why women with invasive cancer generally have some of these nodes surgically removed and evaluated. If your surgeon doesn't plan to do this, be sure that you understand why. One reason may be that you have a noninvasive cancer, so there's no reason to believe cancer cells have spread to the lymph nodes.

Surgeons use two methods to examine underarm lymph nodes for cancer cells: sentinel node biopsy and axillary lymph node dissection.

Sentinel node biopsy

Sentinel node biopsy is a procedure designed primarily to reduce the risk of swelling (lymphedema) associated with axillary lymph node dissection. The procedure has become common practice in recent years. It focuses on finding those lymph nodes that are the first to receive

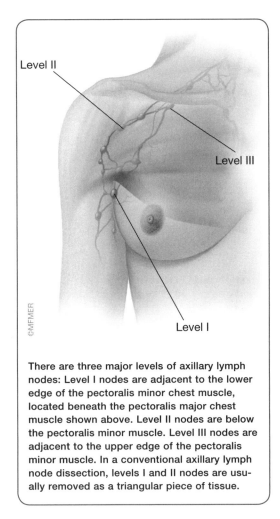

There are three major levels of axillary lymph nodes: Level I nodes are adjacent to the lower edge of the pectoralis minor chest muscle, located beneath the pectoralis major chest muscle shown above. Level II nodes are below the pectoralis minor muscle. Level III nodes are adjacent to the upper edge of the pectoralis minor muscle. In a conventional axillary lymph node dissection, levels I and II nodes are usually removed as a triangular piece of tissue.

drainage from breast tumors (sentinel nodes) and, therefore, the first to collect cancer cells. If these nodes test negative for cancer cells, it's not necessary to remove additional lymph nodes.

Surgeons typically use two methods to find sentinel nodes. One is to inject blue dye in the area of the tumor within the breast. The dye is absorbed in lymphatic channels and travels to a sentinel node or sometimes up to a few sentinel nodes (see the color illustration on page 38). In the early days of the procedure, the dye was injected around the area of the cancer. But later tests showed that no matter where the dye is injected into the breast, it still tends to travel to the same sentinel lymph nodes.

The other frequently used method is to inject a small amount of radioactive solution into the breast and use a special gamma detector to see which lymph nodes accumulate the radioactive solution. At times, both methods are used to better ensure that the appropriate sentinel nodes are removed.

Identification and removal of the sentinel nodes are often combined with lumpectomy or mastectomy surgery. To remove sentinel lymph nodes during a lumpectomy, the surgeon usually makes a separate incision under your arm. During a mastectomy, removal of the breast and sentinel nodes is usually done with a single incision.

Axillary procedures and breast procedures can be paired in any combination. In other words, the type of surgery you choose doesn't affect whether a sentinel node biopsy is done. A lumpectomy can still be done even if cancer is found in the sentinel nodes. You don't have to have a mastectomy.

In some larger medical institutions, tissue that's removed during surgery, such as the sentinel nodes, is examined by a pathologist while the surgery is still taking place. This is done with a technique called frozen section analysis (see page 168). It provides immediate analysis, and the surgeon is notified right away with the results.

However, while the frozen section technique is helpful for analysis of margins and the sentinel node, the tissue

still needs to be stained overnight and re-examined within the next few days to get a definitive assessment. A small percentage of the time, a pathologist finds additional cancer upon re-examination. This could possibly mean further surgery to remove additional lymph nodes.

When cancer is found in the sentinel nodes, the common practice generally was to do an axillary lymph node dissection. This changed in 2011 when a clinical trial was published that showed women with only one or two positive sentinel lymph nodes didn't benefit from removing the rest of the axillary lymph nodes, provided they had had a lumpectomy and would be receiving whole-breast radiation therapy.

If the sentinel nodes are free of cancer cells, the chances of finding cancer in any of the remaining axillary lymph nodes are very small, and no other lymph nodes need to be removed and examined. This spares many women the need for a more extensive operation and it greatly decreases their risk of complications such as lymphedema.

Some side effects of a sentinel node biopsy include possible bruising near the incision, blue-stained urine for a couple of days, pain or tenderness where the dye was injected that may last one or two weeks, and blue-stained breast skin that may persist for weeks or months.

Axillary lymph node dissection

Axillary node dissection is sometimes needed when breast cancer has spread to the axillary lymph nodes. In an axillary lymph node dissection, a surgeon removes multiple lymph nodes under the arm in an attempt to detect and remove any cancer cells that may have traveled away from the primary tumor.

These nodes are examined under a microscope. If the lymph nodes contain cancer, chances are increased that the cancer has escaped and traveled to other parts of the body. Your doctors may recommend additional treatments aimed at destroying these traveling cells. You'll read more about this later on in the chapter.

One of the potential side effects of removing multiple underarm lymph nodes is that the surgery disrupts the lymphatic channels that drain fluid from your arm to the rest of your body. The result can be a buildup of fluid in your arm and hand, causing swelling (lymphedema). The swelling may be mild or extensive.

Other uncommon side effects include recurrent skin infections of that arm, numbness, pain, and a reduced range of motion in the upper arm and chest. These side effects may be temporary or permanent. For more information on lymphedema and other potential side effects, see Chapter 20.

What to expect

Regardless of whether you've had surgery before, the idea of having an operation can be stressful. The information that follows is intended to give you a general idea of what to expect during breast cancer surgery. If you have any questions, be sure to ask your doctors or other members of your health care team. In addition, read any materials that your surgeon or hospital provides on how the procedure you're having is performed and what to expect during recovery.

Mayo Doctor's Idea Changes Surgery

Around the early 1900s, an important discovery took place that brought a significant change to the operating room. Surgeons didn't like having to wait overnight, or sometimes for several days, to receive the results of tissue that was obtained during surgery and sent to pathology for analysis. The surgeons felt that knowing the results while a patient was still under anesthesia could improve procedures and result in better outcomes. In response to this, Mayo Clinic pathologist Dr. Louis Wilson decided to test an idea — and he gave surgeons the tool they were waiting for.

It's said that on a cold winter day in Minnesota, Dr. Wilson set a tissue specimen on an outside windowsill. After the specimen froze, he cut it and examined it under a microscope. The microscopic image of the frozen specimen provided sufficient information to help direct the surgical team. This was the start of Mayo Clinic's practice of frozen section analysis of surgical specimens.

The advantage of a frozen section is that it allows the pathologist to examine the tissue immediately. Today, to perform a frozen section analysis, the specimen is quickly frozen with a freez-

Before surgery

Before your surgery, you'll likely meet with your surgeon and perhaps an anesthesiologist to discuss your operation, review your medical history and determine the plan for your anesthesia — whether you'll receive local, regional or general anesthesia. Local and regional anesthesia don't put you to sleep but numb the area where the surgery is to be performed. You may also receive a mild sedative. In other words, you're conscious for the surgery, but you don't feel any discomfort. With general anesthesia, you're given drugs that make you unconscious and block the memory of the surgery. When receiving this type of anesthesia, people commonly say that you're being put under or put to sleep.

Before your surgery, you may be asked to sign a consent form to allow the surgeon to perform the operation. You'll likely be asked a number of questions about allergies or other chronic problems you may have, medications you're taking and whether you smoke or drink alcohol daily. Some medications — such as aspirin, nonsteroidal anti-inflammatory drugs (NSAIDs) and blood-thinning medications (anticoagulants) — can cause excessive bleeding during surgery. Other medications and herbal supplements may interact with the anesthetics and cause problems. Your doctor may ask you to stop using these medications and supplements for a period of time before and after your surgery.

In addition, you may need to have blood tests and perhaps an assessment of your heart function with an electrocardiogram (ECG). Just before surgery, you'll likely be asked to fast for six to 12 hours.

ing coolant and cut into thin sections. The sections are stained with a colored dye so that the cells can be easily seen. Then they're mounted onto glass slides. A pathologist examines them under the microscope and, within minutes of receiving the specimen, he or she reports back to the surgeon with the findings.

A surgeon may request a frozen section analysis to determine if a sentinel node is positive for cancer or if the tissue margins obtained during a lumpectomy contain cancer cells. If the lymph node or the lumpectomy margins are positive, the surgeon may take additional nodes or tissue during the same surgery to try to remove all of the cancer.

In difficult cases, a pathologist may defer the final diagnosis until conventional tissue processing is complete, which is typically the next day. In some cases, cancer cells aren't detectable on a frozen section, and analysis of a preserved section the following day may reveal that cancer cells are indeed present. In these cases, another surgery may be needed to achieve negative margins or to perform an axillary lymph node dissection.

Although frozen tissue examinations are routine at some medical institutions, it requires expensive equipment and a particular expertise to do them well. That's why they're not done at all institutions.

The day of your surgery you may be admitted to the hospital. A nurse will prepare you for the operation. Your family and friends will be told where they can wait for you.

During surgery

After you receive an anesthetic and when enough time has passed for it to take effect, your surgeon will make an incision in the area of the tumor to remove it and some of the surrounding tissue. The amount of tissue removed depends on whether you've decided to have a lumpectomy or a mastectomy.

After removal of the tissue, the surgeon may also insert one or two plastic drains, about the thickness of a pen, in the location where your breast tissue was removed or under your arm. The tubes help to draw off fluids from the wound and reduce swelling. They're sewn into place and the ends are attached to a small drainage container.

A lumpectomy usually takes less than two hours. Generally, lymph node removal is done during the same operation. A mastectomy that doesn't include breast reconstruction takes one to four hours. If you're having breast reconstruction done at the same time, the surgery is generally longer.

After surgery

After your surgery, you'll go to a recovery room where a nurse checks your vital signs and makes sure you're recovering from anesthesia. You may have an intravenous (IV) catheter in one of your arms to provide access for medications. You'll have a bandage on your incision. If drainage tubes were inserted, a nurse will check that they're draining properly and begin teaching you how to take care of them. This typically involves emptying and measuring fluid and letting your doctor or nurse know of any problems. When drainage slows to less than an ounce of fluid a day — usually after one or two weeks — the tubes are removed.

If lymph nodes were removed, hospital staff will likely try to have you move the affected arm as soon as possible so that it doesn't get stiff. In addition to pain in the breast area, you may experience sensations of numbness and tingling in your underarm. This is because sensory nerves may be cut or stretched during the surgery, though the nerves to the muscles are preserved. Over time, usually several months, some sensation may return. In some cases, a woman may experience decreased sensation that's permanent. This numb area isn't a concern and it generally doesn't affect arm function.

Your surgeon or nurse will give you instructions about how to care for yourself at home. Topics discussed may include how to care for your incision and drains, how to recognize problems such as an infection, when to resume wearing a bra or start wearing a breast prosthesis, which activities you may need to restrict, and how to take your medications. While you're in the hospital, someone also may talk with you or give you information regarding some of the psychological and emotional factors associated with breast surgery.

You'll likely meet with an oncologist after surgery to discuss your pathology results and whether you may need further treatment. You may see your oncologist while you're hospitalized, but it's more common to meet with him or her after you're released from the hospital.

If you've had a lumpectomy, you'll probably leave the hospital the same day as your surgery. In the case of a mastectomy, you're more likely to stay in the hospital overnight. A mastectomy with breast reconstruction may require a longer hospital stay. Breast reconstruction is discussed in the next chapter.

Radiation Therapy

Radiation therapy uses high-energy X-rays to kill cancer cells or to cause them to lose their ability to grow and divide. Rapidly growing cells, such as cancer cells, are more susceptible to the effects of radiation therapy than are cells that grow at a slower rate.

Radiation therapy may be used to treat breast cancer at almost every stage. For primary breast cancer in stages I and II, radiation therapy is commonly used with a lumpectomy, as part of locoregional therapy. In some instances, radiation is also recommended after a mastectomy.

This section discusses radiation therapy as a treatment for early stage breast cancer. Radiation therapy may also be used to treat locally advanced breast cancer (stage III). And in certain situations it's also recommended to control breast cancer that has spread (metastasized) to distant parts of the body (stage IV). Radiation treatment for stages III and IV breast cancer is described in Chapters 13 and 16, respectively.

Radiation after lumpectomy

Radiation therapy is usually recommended after a lumpectomy because with lumpectomy alone there's a relatively high chance of cancer recurring in the

Proton Therapy in Cancer Treatment

Proton therapy is a newer type of radiation therapy that uses energy from positively charged particles called protons to treat tumors. Radiation therapy, which uses X-rays, has long been used to treat cancers and noncancerous (benign) tumors.

Proton therapy has shown promise in treating several kinds of cancer. Studies suggest it may cause fewer side effects than traditional radiation, since doctors can better control where the proton beams deposit their energy, sparing surrounding healthy tissue from harm. Because few studies have directly compared proton therapy radiation and X-ray radiation, it's not yet known if proton therapy is more effective in prolonging lives.

Clinical trials are investigating proton therapy as a treatment for breast cancer, as well as a number of other cancers. Proton therapy currently isn't widely available in the United States. However, Mayo Clinic is developing a Proton Beam Therapy Program on its Minnesota and Arizona campuses.

same breast months to years later. This is called in-breast recurrence.

Without radiation therapy, the risk of an in-breast recurrence after a lumpectomy varies from about 15 to 35 percent, depending on disease characteristics. When radiation therapy is added after lumpectomy, the recurrence rate decreases by about two-thirds.

In some women older than age 70, there's some question as to whether radiation therapy is of benefit. A clinical trial published in 2011 analyzed women older than age 70 who received a lumpectomy followed by radiation. The women who received the radiation had a reduced risk of cancer recurring in the same breast, but there was no difference in survival rates. Your radiation oncologist may discuss this study with you if he or she feels you may be one of those individuals for whom radiation may not be beneficial.

There are also some situations in which radiation may not be appropriate and a mastectomy may be necessary. This may be the case if:

- You're pregnant.
- You've previously had radiation to that breast.
- You have a connective tissue disease, such as lupus or scleroderma.

Radiation after mastectomy

If you've had a mastectomy and you're at high risk of the cancer recurring on the chest wall, your doctor may recommend radiation therapy to reduce your risk. Factors that may put you at high risk of chest wall recurrence include:

- Underarm (axillary) lymph nodes that test positive for cancer cells

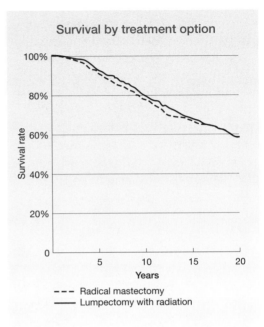

Survival by treatment option

--- Radical mastectomy
— Lumpectomy with radiation

Both mastectomy and lumpectomy with radiation have proved to be equally effective in terms of survival. In a number of clinical trials, women with invasive breast cancer were treated with either mastectomy or lumpectomy with radiation, and the outcomes of their surgeries were compared. After follow-up periods of up to 20 years, survival rates for both groups were found to be virtually identical. The above graph is from one such trial.

Source: *New England Journal of Medicine*, 2002;347:1237.

- A tumor greater than 5 centimeters (about 2 inches) in diameter
- Very narrow margins or margins that test positive for cancer cells
- A tumor that extends to the skin, nipple or chest wall muscles

The value of chest wall radiation therapy for women with just a few positive lymph nodes is controversial. Some studies have shown that radiation after a mastectomy decreases breast cancer deaths but increases deaths from other causes, such as heart-related problems, because radiation can damage the coronary arteries. Some researchers speculate the deaths were related to use of older radiation techniques, and this may no longer be a significant issue. Another study of women who received radiation therapy in the 1970s and 1980s after a mastectomy found that the women were at increased risk of lung cancer. A recent report indicates risk of lung cancer after radiation is higher in smokers than in nonsmokers.

Today, with newer planning and delivery techniques, there's less radiation exposure to the heart and lungs. More recent studies show an increase in survival among women with positive lymph nodes who receive radiation therapy after a mastectomy. Studies are ongoing to more accurately determine who benefits from radiation after a mastectomy. If your biopsy shows cancer spread to the lymph nodes, discuss the potential benefits of radiation with your doctor.

How radiation works

Radiation therapy for breast cancer may be delivered in a couple of ways. Radiation that comes from an external source and is directed to the whole breast and to neighboring lymph nodes is the most commonly used method. This is known as external beam radiation therapy.

Another way of delivering radiation is internal radiation therapy (brachytherapy). In this procedure, small amounts of radioactive material contained in tubes or catheters are placed directly in your breast tissue and allowed to stay there for a few days. This allows only the affected area to receive radiation. External beam radiation and brachytherapy may be used together, with one method following the other, but this is less commonly done.

External beam radiation therapy
External beam radiation therapy generally begins a few weeks after surgery. If you also will be receiving chemotherapy, radiation therapy is typically started three to four weeks after you've completed your chemotherapy treatment. External beam radiation treatment is usually given daily, Monday through Friday, for approximately five to six weeks.

During each visit, you lie flat on a table while a machine moves around you, directing the radiation toward your breast from different angles (see the color illustration on page 39). The procedure is similar to getting an X-ray, but the radiation is more intense. Sometimes, the lymph nodes above your collarbone (supraclavicular lymph nodes), near your sternum (internal mammary lymph nodes) or in your underarm (axillary lymph nodes) also are targeted.

Each treatment is painless and takes just a few minutes. In many treatment centers, you can set up an appointment at the same time each day so that your treatment becomes part of your daily routine. Generally, several health care professionals work together in providing your radiation treatment. Team members usually include:
• **A radiation oncologist.** This person is a doctor who specializes in treatments using radiation. He or she determines the appropriate therapy for you, follows your progress and adjusts your treatment if necessary.

- **A radiation physicist and dosimetrist.** These two people make special calculations and measurements to ensure optimal radiation dosage and delivery.
- **A radiation therapist.** This individual delivers your daily treatments.

Before treatment

Before your first treatment session, you'll go through a simulation process in which a radiation oncologist carefully maps your breast to pinpoint the precise location for treatment. During the simulation, a radiation therapist helps you get into a position that's best suited for targeting the area of the tumor. Sometimes, pads or other devices are used to help you maintain the position.

Using a computerized tomography (CT) scanner, the radiation oncologist identifies the area that needs to be treated. You'll hear noise from the CT equipment as it moves around you. Sometimes, this can be unnerving, but try to relax and remain still during the simulation because this will help ensure consistent, accurate treatments.

After the area to be treated is identified, ink marks or tiny permanent tattoo dots are placed on your skin to provide a reference point for the radiation therapist when administering the radiation. Be sure not to wash the ink marks off until you're allowed to do so. If the marks can't be seen, you may need to go through the mapping process again.

The dosimetrist, radiation physicist and radiation oncologist then plan the dosage of radiation you'll receive and determine how long the beam must be applied to deliver the right amount.

During treatment

After the simulation and planning are complete, you can begin treatment. When you arrive at the hospital or treatment facility, you'll be taken to a special room that's used specifically for radiation therapy. You'll need to remove your clothes above your waist and put on a hospital gown for the session. The radiation therapist carefully helps you into the exact position that you were in during the simulation. The therapist then leaves the room and turns on the machine, called a linear accelerator, that's used for delivering the radiation. Although the therapist isn't in the room, he or she can see you on a television monitor, and the two of you can talk with each other through an intercom.

The treatment itself lasts only a few minutes, but the whole process may take 10 to 30 minutes each visit. The customary schedule for radiation treatments is therapy five days a week for three to six weeks. Occasionally, a boost treatment to the location where the tumor was removed (tumor bed) may be recommended. This typically involves an additional five to eight therapy sessions. Boost treatments are used to further reduce the chances of recurrence in women with stage I or II cancer who are at higher risk. This may include younger women or those in whom cancer cells were found in the tissue (margins) around the tumor that was removed.

After treatment

After the session is over, you're free to go about your regular activities. Generally, no special precautions are necessary.

Internal radiation therapy

Internal radiation therapy (brachytherapy) uses implants of radioactive substances, sealed up in thin wires, catheters or tubes, to deliver a high dose of radiation to a small area of your body, such as to a section of your breast.

The objective of internal radiation is to place the radiation as close as possible to the site where the cancer was removed. This method concentrates the radiation to the site at highest risk of a cancer recurrence and attempts to reduce damage to nearby normal tissue, such as your lungs, heart and normal breast tissue. Internal radiation can be done in a much shorter time than can external therapy — usually three to five days.

During a lumpectomy, or later as a separate procedure, a catheter or another holder for the radioactive material is implanted in the area from where the tumor was taken (tumor bed). The holder is then loaded with seeds of radioactive substances that radiate nearby cells.

In general, internal radiation is given using a high-dose-rate (HDR) machine in which the radiation is delivered for a short period of twice a day, usually over five days.

Side effects

Radiation is a cumulative process. With daily external beam radiation therapy, side effects tend to become more of an issue as treatment continues. Fatigue is the most common side effect. It's a good idea to plan for this possibility so that you can rest whenever you feel the need. Sometimes, putting your feet up for 15 to 20 minutes is enough.

RESEARCH UPDATE

Exploring ways to improve radiation treatment

Doctors and researchers continue to study alternative methods to deliver radiation. The goal of their research is to develop delivery methods that may produce fewer side effects or result in more effective and convenient treatments.

- For women with early-stage breast cancer, researchers are studying the use of external beam radiation to only part of the breast, instead of the entire breast.
- Researchers are studying whether a large, single external beam radiation treatment could be safely and effectively given during a lumpectomy when the incision is still open. The hope is that this could decrease the amount of radiation needed after surgery.
- Researchers are evaluating if giving the boost treatment as a whole-breast treatment, rather than just to the tumor bed, would allow for a shorter, more concentrated course of radiation.
- Scientists are investigating whether internal radiation may be used as an alternative to external beam radiation. Because of the brief treatment period, it may be an option for women who aren't able to receive daily treatments for several weeks.

Decision Guide: Lumpectomy vs. Mastectomy

Deciding between a lumpectomy and a mastectomy isn't always easy. A number of issues need to be considered, including the stage of your cancer, your risk of recurrence, how you feel about having a breast removed and how convenient it is for you to receive follow-up radiation therapy after a lumpectomy.

Many women prefer to keep their affected breast, despite a slightly higher chance of in-breast (local) recurrence. Others prefer mastectomy. Women who feel anxious about the possibility that the cancer might return may be willing to sacrifice their breast for a lower risk of a local recurrence. Neither option is right, and neither is wrong. It's a personal choice.

The table on page 178 lists some of the pros and cons of removing just a portion of your breast (lumpectomy) or all of it (mastectomy). In addition, the following frequently asked questions may help address some of your concerns. Finally, we've included the stories of three women who've undergone breast surgery. They talk about how they decided on their treatments and how they feel about their decisions now.

It's hoped that this information will help you in making your decision. But it's also important that you talk with your doctor about your situation. If you have questions about your diagnosis, treatment or prognosis, be sure to have your doctor explain things to you in detail and make sure that you understand what he or she is saying.

Factors to consider

As you make decisions on the best way to treat your breast cancer, you'll want to weigh each choice against your personal values and with your lifestyle in mind. The following questions may help you work through this process:

How do you generally approach health care?

Are you the type of person who needs to feel that she has done everything medically possible to fight this disease? If so, you may be more comfortable if you're more aggressive in your treatment. If you're less aggressive when it comes to medical intervention, you might prefer to avoid the risks and inconveniences of more aggressive treatment.

Once treatment ends, how much do you think you'll continue to worry?

If you choose lumpectomy and radiation, how will you feel living each day with a breast that once harbored cancer? Despite the scientific evidence that overall survival after mastectomy and lumpectomy with radiation are virtually the same, some women discover that they worry more about recurrence when breast tissue remains. If you still have part of your breast after treatment, will that increase your worry? If so, would removal of the entire breast significantly reduce that worry? These are clearly psychological questions rather than medical ones, but they're worth asking yourself.

How do you feel about losing a breast?
For some women, the loss of a breast is not significant when weighed against their fear of dying of cancer. For others, breasts are closely connected to their self-image. They feel that removing a breast is too great a sacrifice when it doesn't improve overall survival.

How will your choice affect your partner?
Ultimately, the decision is yours to make, but you may want to think about how your choice will affect your partner. This is a difficult area for many couples, and it warrants a frank and open discussion. Whether you choose mastectomy or lumpectomy with radiation, your partner's sexual attitude toward you may be affected. With some couples, the loss of a breast is a permanent, daily reminder of the cancer to both partners. On the other hand, during radiation treatment many women experience fatigue, and some women experience hypersensitivity in their breasts and don't want to be touched. If you opt for breast reconstruction, the resulting change in sensation may alter your sexual practices. Information from your medical team may help you consider these possibilities.

Can your lifestyle accommodate the daily routine of radiation therapy?
Look closely at your support system. Can you meet the Monday through Friday commitment for the three to six weeks needed for radiation treatment? Are you physically able to get to the treatment center each day? Some women need someone to accompany them. Others need help with child care. Some women, regardless if they have a lumpectomy or mastectomy, will need radiation therapy.

How will your choice affect your family?
Again, the decision is yours to make, not your family's. But you may want to consider the time involved and how that will affect your family.
- You'll need time to recuperate from your surgery.
- If you choose radiation, you'll need to commit to appointments Monday through Friday for three to six weeks.

The treatment you decide on will affect how much you can do. Will your family be able to adapt to your treatment demands? Talk through these issues with all members of your family in advance so they'll know what to expect and so that all of you, as a family, can plan how best to meet each person's needs while you're being treated for your cancer.

How will your choice affect your work?
If you work outside the home, can your job accommodate your treatment schedule? Radiation may require a daily weekday commitment for three to six weeks. Ask if you can schedule a regular appointment outside working hours, perhaps on your way to or from work. Talk with your employer about taking time off during the day. Think about the proximity of your workplace to your treatment location and how long you'll need to get there and back. Will your co-workers cover for you if you need additional time off?

Lumpectomy vs. mastectomy: The pros and cons

The following table lists some of the advantages and disadvantages of a lumpectomy with radiation and a mastectomy. For more information on the risk of cancer recurrence and the different types of recurrence, see Chapter 15.

Procedure	Pros	Cons
Lumpectomy with radiation	**Keeping your breast** This can be of great psychological value for some women. **Near-normal appearance** Your breast may appear much the same as before surgery. **Similar cure rate** Despite it being a smaller operation, the cure rate is the same as mastectomy.	**Risk of cancer recurrence** Carries a slightly greater risk of a local recurrence than does a mastectomy. Younger women have higher risk. **Need for a second operation** If all the cancer isn't removed during the first surgery, you may need a second lumpectomy or a mastectomy. **Unsatisfactory cosmetic results** This may happen if you have a large amount of tissue removed. **Need for radiation** Radiation is required, with regular appointments for about three to six weeks. Side effects may include swelling and pain in your breast, fatigue, and a temporary skin reaction similar to a sunburn, as well as long-term skin and tissue changes.
Mastectomy	**Radiation may not be needed** After a mastectomy, many women don't need radiation therapy. **No need for a second operation** Because the entire breast has been removed, there's rarely a need for additional surgery, other than reconstruction, if you so desire. **Reduced risk of cancer recurrence** It usually has less risk of a local recurrence than does a lumpectomy. However, cancer can still recur in the mastectomy scar. The chance of developing a new tumor in remaining chest wall tissue years later is low.	**Loss of a breast** There's often a certain amount of grieving after losing a breast. The surgery may leave a daily physical reminder of your disease, which can be difficult. **Sexual self-image** The absence of a breast can raise issues regarding sexual self-image and feminine identity. **Feeling lopsided** Women with large breasts may feel lopsided. Being lopsided can also cause back pain. Most get accustomed to the feeling; others require breast reconstruction. **Unusual sensations** Rarely, some women experience chronic tenderness and soreness around the scar. **More involved surgical procedure** A larger procedure generally has slightly greater surgical risks.

Other side effects include skin irritation, such as itchiness, redness, soreness, peeling, blistering, swelling, and decreased sensation or hypersensation. Many of these signs and symptoms may be similar to those you've experienced with a serious sunburn. They gradually go away after treatment ends. To reduce skin irritation during radiation, take precautions to avoid exposing the radiated area to direct sun.

A small percentage of women experience more serious problems that may be temporary or chronic, such as swelling in the arm, lung damage, nerve damage, heart damage and increased susceptibility to broken ribs.

Some changes to the breast may be permanent after radiation. These include a difference in skin color, a feeling of heaviness in the breast, changes in the texture of the breast and even changes in breast size.

Internal radiation therapy usually produces fewer skin reactions. However, this form of radiation may cause swelling of your breast and possibly infection at the site of the implant.

If you develop any bothersome signs and symptoms during or after radiation treatment, make sure to discuss them with your doctor.

Additional Treatment

Surgery and radiation therapy are referred to as locoregional therapy because they target cancer cells in one specific area — in this case, the breast. However, doctors can't be certain that all the cancer cells were removed during surgery or destroyed with radiation. There's always the possibility that some cells have been left behind. Or some may have broken off from the primary tumor and traveled to other parts of your body through the bloodstream or the lymph system. These cells may not be detectable early on. But, over time, they can multiply until they reach a size in which they can be seen on an X-ray or felt during a physical examination.

To try to eradicate any microscopic cancer cells, your doctor may suggest additional treatment that travels throughout your entire body. The medical term for this type of treatment is *adjuvant systemic therapy*. The goal of adjuvant systemic therapy is to destroy any cancer cells that might still be in your body to help you remain cancer-free and live longer. Most women with invasive breast cancer are candidates for some form of additional treatment.

Who should consider it?

Several key pieces of information need to be taken into account in determining if you should receive adjuvant systemic therapy. The first of these are called prognostic factors, factors based on the characteristics of your tumor and on your own personal characteristics. Prognostic factors, such as the degree of cancer spread to the lymph nodes, the tumor size, your age and the tumor grade, can help predict the outcome of your cancer (prognosis). Using this information, along with other factors, and keeping in mind the benefits and risks of each type of therapy, you and your doctor can decide on the best plan for you.

Meet Other Women

Each woman is unique, and so is her decision-making process. Sometimes, though, it's helpful to hear other women's experiences. It may offer reassurance regarding the decision you make.

Here are the stories of three women. Each made a different treatment choice, and each is happy with the choice she made. These women don't necessarily represent the most typical treatment decisions, and the stories don't represent the most common treatment paths. They're simply three people sharing their personal experiences.

Jan's Story

Jan received a diagnosis of breast cancer at age 29. She chose to have both breasts removed (a bilateral mastectomy), along with reconstruction, chemotherapy and radiation. This was considered unusually aggressive treatment at the time.

I'm the type of person who wants all the information, and I don't want it sugarcoated. I want members of my health care team to talk to me openly and honestly. Otherwise, you just don't have what you need to make the right decisions.

I was 29 years old and my husband and I had been trying to have a child for some years. On a Friday morning, I went to an infertility clinic for an evaluation. During my basic physical, my doctor found a lump in my right breast. She assured me that it was probably nothing, but she ordered a mammogram just to be sure. The right breast turned out to be fine, but my left breast had some calcifications that concerned the doctors.

Within an hour I saw a surgeon to talk over treatment options, and I saw a plastic surgeon to discuss reconstruction. The surgeon told me that at my age if cancer was found in one breast the risk of it developing in the other breast was 25 to 30 percent. That seemed pretty high to me.

When the biopsy determined it was cancer, I decided to have a double mastectomy. One factor in my decision was knowing that it's easier to get reconstructed breasts to match if you do the same thing to both breasts. A nurse showed me implants and talked about how I would look, which was very helpful. They were using silicone implants then; saline implants were just getting started. This was still Friday. The surgery was scheduled for Monday.

I was actually eager to go to surgery. I could've taken more time to decide, but I understood from the X-ray that it was likely to be cancer. At the same time, I knew this meant at least a delay, if not a change, in my plans to have a child.

On Monday they found a tumor measuring 4 centimeters. All my lymph nodes were benign. Thursday, I was home recuperating.

Shortly thereafter, I saw an oncologist. He reviewed my situation, went over all the test results, talked about where medical science was, discussed ongoing chemotherapy trials and told me there might be some benefit in having radiation or chemotherapy or both. I decided to go for both.

After six weeks of surgical leave, I returned to work from 8 a.m. to 3 p.m. and after work headed for chemotherapy. I had no severe side effects. I tried to remain really upbeat. I thought of therapy as my ally, something that would help me live longer.

Within a few weeks after finishing chemotherapy I began radiation. I went for five or six weeks, every day. I always made it a point to come out of the radiation with a big smile on my face to show other people that it was OK.

I kept a journal throughout the experience, which was really helpful because it gave me a place to record my feelings and let me go back and see where I had been. Occasionally, I still look at it, and it brings back some nice memories. It wasn't all bad. In a way, it was a gift to get this at age 29, because it let me know what was important to me and who was important to me. It brought up spirituality issues and a lot of other things that often don't occur to some people until much later in life.

The decisions I made were the right ones for me, and I'm very comfortable with them. I'm extremely glad I saw different oncologists beforehand. The information I got from them really helped me make intelligent decisions.

Since my diagnosis, I've had three children, so now most of my focus is on being a mom to a beautiful girl and wonderful twin boys.

Colleen's Story

Colleen was 45 when she found out she had breast cancer. After weighing her treatment options, she chose a mastectomy.

A close friend of mine had just been diagnosed with breast cancer, so I decided I should get myself checked, too. I had a history of fibrocystic disease and was accustomed to finding cysts when I checked my breasts. So when I felt a lump in my right breast, I thought it was probably a cyst. A cyst was confirmed by a mammogram and ultrasound. And I was told to watch it and check back again in a year.

More than a year passed. Then, early one morning while I was still in bed, I had this feeling someone was near the bed nudging me to get this lump checked again. When I opened my eyes, no one was there. But I mentioned it to my doctor that day, and that I thought the cyst was bigger. He scheduled me for a diagnostic mammogram and an ultrasound.

The ultrasound showed that the cyst had changed and was growing. The doctor offered me a choice of having a needle biopsy immediately or surgery a week or so later. I opted for the needle biopsy because I could get the results sooner. When they called the next day, they told me I needed another appointment. I had cancer. I met with the surgeon on Monday, and that Wednesday I was in surgery.

The surgeon gave me the option of lumpectomy with radiation or a mastectomy. My husband and I talked. It turned out we felt the same way. I decided I would rather have the mastectomy and not have to deal with any other treatment.

I was OK about making decisions quickly, but I don't think it really hit me until I was waiting to be rolled into surgery. I wound up lying on the gurney with tears rolling down my face. The nurses were very comforting.

They found a stage II cancer, but no lymph nodes were involved. Because the tumor was deeper than they expected, my doctor told me afterward that mastectomy was probably the best call.

My family handled it well. My daughter in college was initially upset but felt better once she learned that lymph nodes weren't involved. One son had just entered Marine boot camp, and we weren't even able to reach him until it was all over. My older son was very involved in supporting me. And my husband was very understanding. Also, my sisters are close and were supportive.

I didn't have a lot of pain waking up. That came later because a rather large nerve was cut. I still have numbness under my arm. I wasn't really prepared for that. And it probably took three years for my hand to get its full strength back. That surprised me the most.

I finished a five-year course of tamoxifen and then went for a follow-up exam every four to six months because my oncologist wanted me checked that often. I'd like to say it didn't bother me but it did. You want to go because you want to hear it's OK. But you don't want to go because you're afraid they're going to find something.

Once you've had a close call with cancer, you always have to be prepared for the worst. I know I could develop cancer again one day, but I also know I'm watched carefully, which means it's more likely to be caught early. I try to enjoy each day because I never know what's ahead.

Rosemarie's Story

Rosemarie was 48 when she noticed a lump. She decided to have a lumpectomy followed by chemotherapy and radiation.

I was just standing, talking with someone, and when I crossed my arms I felt this pecan-sized lump in my breast. I wasn't really worried because everyone told me that if it was cancer, it wouldn't hurt, and this lump felt sore. I called my gynecologist who sent me for a mammogram, and while I was there, they did an ultrasound, too. The radiologist thought I might have a cyst, but when she tried to drain it with a needle, the lump appeared to be solid. Then she told me I needed a biopsy. I was scheduled to take a trip and decided I wanted to do that first, so I didn't have the biopsy until a month or so later.

My gynecologist called a week after that and asked me to come to his office on a Saturday morning and suggested I bring a friend. That's when he told me I had cancer. The section of breast that was removed during the biopsy didn't leave clean margins, so my doctor told me I needed a mastectomy. Mine wasn't an aggressive cancer, so I took some time to think about it.

I wound up seeing a breast specialist on my 49th birthday. He told me I could have a lumpectomy if I chose. That's what I decided to do. I had the surgery on Dec. 26. They removed a bigger section of tissue and 21 lymph nodes, which all turned out to be negative. I wish I had known beforehand about a sentinel node biopsy, because then I wouldn't have had to have so many nodes removed.

The only unexpected part of the surgery was managing the drains. That felt kind of overwhelming, but fortunately my mother came to stay with me and helped.

My oncologist told me that if I had chemotherapy, it would increase my survival chances 20 percent, and radiation would increase those chances another 10 percent. I decided to do both.

I had the chemotherapy first, four treatments, 21 days apart. My biggest fear about chemotherapy was losing my hair, which I did. About 14 days after the first treatment, nearly all of it came off one day in the shower. The few clumps that were left, I just pulled out. For about a week, I wore a wig that I hated. Then I tried new and different ways to wrap scarves around my head. And some days, I just went out without anything. I was more bothered by the loss of my eyelashes and eyebrows than the hair on my head because that's what really makes you look like a cancer patient.

The first seven days after each treatment were really the worst time for me. I felt weak. I didn't really want to get out of bed, and I did feel nauseated, although I never actually threw up. But I kept going to work. For me, being with people helped me deal with having cancer.

Once the chemo ended, I went for radiation. The treatments weren't too bad. I went on my lunch hour. Midafternoon I'd get a little tired. About midway through treatment I did develop a radiation burn on the underside of my breast. That was uncomfortable, and they finally put a bandage on it to block it from rubbing against my bra.

Since my treatment, I've had some problems with lymphedema. I try not to use that arm for lifting, and when I travel, I wear a pressurized sleeve. That part has been frustrating. I also developed costochondritis, a kind of arthritis between the chest and rib bone that my doctor told me is a result of radiation. Some days I can't touch my chest because of pain, and then other days I don't feel a thing.

Being in a support group has helped a lot. You get so much information and so many helpful hints. And when I get an ache or pain, chances are when I check with the group, someone else has had the same thing. So then I don't have to worry.

Now that I've passed the five-year mark, I only see my oncologist once a year. I haven't forgotten I had cancer. I know it can always come back, but I don't let things bother me. It took me a while to get there, but I'm appreciating life more. I look at all the little things that make me happy, and whatever makes me happy, I do.

Some factors to consider when deciding on additional treatment include:

Cancer spread

The degree of cancer spread to underarm (axillary) lymph nodes is an important factor that typically provides substantial information about your prognosis and chances of being cured. As discussed earlier, during surgery the surgeon usually does a sentinel node biopsy or removes some of the lymph nodes under your arm to look for cancer cells that may have spread from your breast. If cancer is found in any of the nodes, there's a greater chance that cancer cells may have spread to other parts of your body.

Tumor size

Tumor size is another important factor in determining your prognosis. Women with smaller tumors usually have better outcomes than do women with larger tumors, especially tumors larger than 5 centimeters (about 2 inches) in diameter.

Your age

Younger women, especially those under age 35, sometimes have a more aggressive type of breast cancer and a poorer prognosis than do older women with otherwise similar tumor characteristics.

Tumor grade

The grade of a tumor refers to how aggressive it looks under a microscope. Tumor cells that resemble normal breast cells are called well-differentiated, or low grade (grade 1). Those that look very abnormal are referred to as poorly differentiated, or high grade (grade 3). Moderately differentiated (grade 2) cells fall somewhere in between. While high-grade cancers have a higher chance of recurring in the first few years after diagnosis, they're often more responsive to chemotherapy. If they don't come back in within five years, the chance of them recurring later on is low.

Cell proliferation

This test measures the percentage of tumor cells that are dividing (proliferating). A higher rate of cell proliferation usually indicates a more aggressive cancer and, thus, a greater need for additional therapy.

HER2 status

The role of certain genes within your body is to help regulate cell growth and oversee cell division and tissue repair. When these genes become damaged (mutated), they're labeled as oncogenes. An oncogene is an altered gene that causes uncontrolled cell growth. Oncogenes produce proteins that can turn normal cells into cancer cells. HER2 is an oncogene associated with breast cancer. If HER2 isn't treated with newer treatments designed to block its expression, the cancer tends to be more aggressive.

Therapy Options

Adjuvant systemic therapy may consist of chemotherapy, hormone (anti-estrogen) therapy, anti-HER2 therapy or a combination of these. Many women with

Prognostic and Predictive Tools

There are tools doctors can use to identify women who may be at increased risk of breast cancer recurrence and, therefore, benefit the most from additional treatment. One computerized tool, called Adjuvant!, takes into account a woman's individual prognostic factors and her overall health to determine how beneficial different treatments might be. It compares her chances of dying of cancer and of being alive 10 years from now if she doesn't have additional treatment and if she does (see page 195).

More recent developments, called gene expression signature tools, look at genetic data in determining prognosis. They're also predictive tools in that they can help predict which type of therapy might be most beneficial. One program, called the 21-gene recurrence score, is designed for women who have estrogen receptor positive cancers. It uses material from the cancer, which is sent to a laboratory to be analyzed to determine if a woman might benefit from chemotherapy in addition to hormone therapy. Women with low scores don't appear to benefit from chemotherapy, whereas women with high scores do.

The downside of this type of test is that it's expensive. However, many insurance companies will pay the cost because it may identify women who don't need chemotherapy, which is more expensive.

hormone receptor positive breast cancer receive two or three therapies. The different treatments work together to help destroy any remaining cancer cells. Hormone therapy is usually given after chemotherapy. Anti-HER2 therapy can be given at the same time (concurrently) as the other two.

Chemotherapy

Chemotherapy is the term for a group of medications that are toxic to cancer cells. The drugs primarily interfere with uncontrolled cell growth, a common characteristic of cancer cells. Unfortunately, chemotherapy drugs can also affect rapidly dividing normal, healthy cells, leading to a number of adverse side effects. However, the drugs don't affect healthy cells nearly as much as they do cancer cells. Most of your normal, healthy cells aren't dividing and, therefore, aren't as susceptible to the effects of chemotherapy medications as are cancer cells.

Chemotherapy is usually given over a period of three to six months every one to three weeks. The medications are most often given intravenously, but some types can be taken orally. At times, two or three different chemotherapy drugs are given at the same time, to attack tumors in a variety of ways. Each treatment session is followed by a period of recovery before the next session begins. For instance, if you received a round of chemotherapy today, you might receive the next treatment in one to three weeks. In the case of breast cancer, chemotherapy usually doesn't require a hospital stay. You can go to an outpatient clinic to receive your treatment.

Some commonly used chemotherapy drugs and drug combinations include:

Cyclophosphamide
Cyclophosphamide (Cytoxan) was one of the earliest chemotherapy agents used as adjuvant systemic therapy. This drug interferes with the growth of cancer cells by blocking their ability to copy their genetic material (DNA). Common side effects include nausea, vomiting, hair loss, lowered blood counts, fatigue, fever, chills and drug-induced menopause.

Doxorubicin
Doxorubicin belongs to the general group of medicines known as anthracyclines. Chemotherapy regimens containing anthracyclines have been found to result in less recurrence compared with regimen that don't include it. Common side effects of doxorubicin include nausea, vomiting, hair loss, lowered blood counts and fatigue. Very rarely, it can cause leukemia or heart damage. With correct dosing, these long-term risks are minimal but they should be taken into account when considering use of doxorubicin.

Epirubicin
Epirubicin (Ellence) is a cancer-fighting medication that works similarly to the drug doxorubicin. It appears to cause less toxicity to the heart than does doxorubicin.

Carboplatin
Carboplatin is a medication that's related to another commonly used drug to treat people with cancer, called cisplatin. Carboplatin is better tolerated than is

Making a Decision

To help you make an informed choice regarding the use of additional treatment after surgery (adjuvant systemic therapy), consider the following steps:

1. Find out and understand what your chances are of being cured without adjuvant systemic therapy.
2. Find out and understand the benefits of adjuvant systemic therapy in terms of increasing your chances of a cure.
3. Find out and understand the risks (side effects) associated with different adjuvant systemic therapy options.
4. Weigh the benefits against the risks.
5. Make an informed personal decision with your health care team.

cisplatin. However, it can cause allergic reactions.

Fluorouracil

Fluorouracil, which is also called 5-fluorouracil, or 5-FU, is an antimetabolite. It interferes with the growth of cancer cells by blocking enzymes necessary for DNA synthesis. Side effects of fluorouracil include mouth sores and diarrhea.

Taxanes

Paclitaxel (Abraxance, Onxol) and docetaxel (Taxotere) come from the group of drugs called taxanes, which disrupt cell division by interfering with the cellular process that separates a dividing cell into two new cells. Side effects of the drugs include muscle aches, hair loss, numbness or tingling in fingers or toes, and lowered blood counts. Allergic reactions also can occur.

Side effects

Chemotherapy can cause both short-term and long-term side effects that may affect your quality of life.

Short-term side effects

Normal, healthy cells located in your blood, hair follicles and digestive tract are some of the most rapidly dividing cells in your body. Many anti-cancer drugs have been designed to target rapidly dividing cancer cells. But they may also damage rapidly dividing normal cells, such as those in your hair follicles, bone marrow and blood, and the digestive tract. This can result in a number of side effects.

Different chemotherapy drugs given at different dosages cause different side effects in each woman. Some women lose their hair and their appetite, and others may experience increased appetite. Nausea, vomiting, diarrhea, lowered blood counts and mouth sores can occur.

The effect of chemotherapy on your blood cells may make you more prone to infection, bruising and bleeding. In addition, you may have less energy during and after your treatment. It's not possible to know ahead of time all of the side effects you may experience. Most short-term side effects go away when your treatment ends.

For example, your hair should grow back after you complete your chemotherapy treatments, although it may return with a different color or texture or both. Chemotherapy doesn't cause long-term harm to your hair.

Medications are available that help block nausea and vomiting caused by chemotherapy. Sometimes, changing the dose of the medications you receive or adjusting your chemotherapy schedule will help counter side effects. If chemotherapy caused your infection-fighting (white) blood cells to drop too low, your doctor may recommend that you avoid people who are sick. He or she may give you a medication with the next chemotherapy cycle to stimulate your bone marrow to make blood cells faster. For more information on managing short-term side effects of chemotherapy, see Chapter 20.

Long-term side effects

A possible long-term side effect of chemotherapy in premenopausal women is ovarian dysfunction. This may cause menstruation to stop (amenorrhea), sometimes permanently. When permanent, this condition is often called chemotherapy-induced menopause. How often this occurs varies with different types of chemotherapy drugs and the age of the woman receiving the medication. Cyclophosphamide tends to produce a higher rate of amenorrhea than do some of the other chemotherapy drugs.

The chances of chemotherapy-induced menopause are much higher for women older than age 40. In younger women, menstruation may stop during chemotherapy and then return after treatment is completed, although in some cases many months later. For the majority of women

Drug Therapy Before Surgery

In some cases, a doctor may recommend that a woman receive anti-cancer treatment before surgery in order to shrink a large tumor and perhaps make it possible to have a lumpectomy instead of a mastectomy. Medication that's given before surgery is called preoperative (neoadjuvant) therapy. Chemotherapy is commonly used, however, hormone therapy and anti-HER2 therapy also may be used before surgery.

In addition, use of chemotherapy before surgery has also been studied in women with relatively small breast cancers. A large clinical trial randomly assigned women with stage II breast cancer to receive either chemotherapy prior to surgery or chemotherapy after surgery. No differences in survival or recurrence rates were noted in the two groups. However, among women who received chemotherapy before surgery, there was a higher probability they could have a lumpectomy rather than a mastectomy because of a reduction in the size of the tumor from the medication.

Because neoadjuvant chemotherapy is effective and because it allows doctors to see how well the drugs shrink tumors, it's being used more frequently, especially in research studies as doctors look for new and better drugs.

Chemotherapy Combinations

Years of evidence suggest that combining chemotherapy drugs decreases the chance that cancer cells will become resistant to them, increasing the chance of a cure. Often, women receiving chemotherapy are given two or more drugs at once.

Drug combinations often are abbreviated using the first letter of each drug. Following are combinations frequently used in adjuvant systemic treatment of breast cancer.

- **AC:** Doxorubicin (*A* is for Adriamycin, a previous brand name) and cyclophosphamide
- **AC + paclitaxel:** Doxorubicin (Adriamycin), cyclophosphamide and paclitaxel
- **CAF:** Cyclophosphamide, doxorubicin (Adriamycin) and fluorouracil
- **CEF:** Cyclophosphamide, epirubicin (similar to doxorubicin) and fluorouracil
- **CMF:** Cyclophosphamide, methotrexate and fluorouracil
- **TAC:** Docetaxel (Taxotere), doxorubicin (Adriamycin) and cyclophosphamide
- **TC:** Docetaxel (Taxotere) and cyclophosphamide

To determine the best combination for you, your doctor looks at a number of factors, including any pre-existing conditions you might have and how well the two of you think that you can manage the side effects of different drugs.

over age 40 — especially those over 45 — chemotherapy will lead to menopause.

Loss of ovarian function may cause several side effects, including menopausal symptoms such as hot flashes, insomnia, mood swings and vaginal dryness. In addition, similar to what occurs in menopause, you may experience a reduction in bone mineralization, leading to osteoporosis and an increased risk of bone fractures. You may wish to have periodic bone density tests and consider treatments to prevent bone loss.

Some medications, such as paclitaxel, can cause damage to nerve endings in your fingers and toes (neuropathy). This can result in numbness, tingling, pain or all three.

In rare cases, chemotherapy with anthracyclines has resulted in heart damage (congestive heart failure) and secondary cancers, such as cancer of the blood cells (leukemia). However, with the dosages of chemotherapy most commonly given for adjuvant chemotherapy, the chance of each of these conditions occurring is generally less than 1 percent.

Hormone therapy

When a breast cancer tumor is estrogen or progesterone receptor positive, or both, hormone (anti-estrogen) therapy often is the most important form of adjuvant systemic therapy. The goal of hormone therapy is to block the effects of the female hormone estrogen, which is known to fuel a majority of breast cancers. Normally, estrogen circulates through your bloodstream and latches on (binds) to certain cell proteins called receptors. Most breast cancer cells also

If You Still Want to Have Children

A breast cancer diagnosis can send ripple effects through your entire life. While you may feel overwhelmed by the decisions you need to make to fight the disease, it's important not to forget about life after breast cancer. Early detection and advances in treatment have improved survival odds. If you're a younger woman, this means that in addition to your treatment, you may wish to think about whether you want to have children, or have more children, in the future.

Why worry about children now — at such a difficult and stressful time? Because cancer treatment can interfere with fertility in many ways. The treatments that work to kill cancer cells also affect other cells, organs and hormones in the body. It's possible that your treatment, especially if you receive systemic therapy such as chemotherapy, could make you infertile, either temporarily or permanently. In young women, chemotherapy is often recommended even for smaller tumors without lymph node involvement, to help ensure successful treatment.

Women who are younger and who receive low doses of chemotherapy are more likely to regain their menstrual periods after treatment. Women who are older are less likely to recover their fertility. If menstruation does return, it may not happen right away.

If you want to have a family or expand your family in the future, you may need to take steps before you begin anti-cancer drug therapy to preserve your ability to have children. If your doctors don't bring up the subject of fertility preservation, let them know as soon as possible about your desire for future children.

The most established option for preserving fertility is through embryo cryopreservation, a procedure in which eggs are harvested from a woman, fertilized with sperm and then frozen for implantation at a later date. Another option that may be considered in single women is oocyte cryopreservation, the freezing of unfertilized eggs. Both of these approaches require approximately two weeks of ovarian stimulation, beginning with the onset of the woman's menstrual cycle. This can be a concern because it may mean a delay in beginning cancer treatment. In addition, the process involves the use of fertility medications to facilitate the growth and development of multiple eggs. It isn't always known what effect, if any, the hormones might have on the cancer. Yet another approach involves harvesting and freezing ovarian tissue, which is implanted back into the ovaries after completion of cancer treatment.

An alternative approach under study involves giving a woman a drug known as a gonadotropin-releasing hormone (Gn-RH) agonist at the same time she receives chemotherapy. The purpose of the medication is to preserve ovarian function by trying to block the harmful effects of chemotherapy on the ovaries. To date, results have been mixed and more study is needed.

These steps can be expensive, so it's important to find out the cost of fertility preservation measures and if your health insurance covers the expense.

make these receptors, and estrogen is believed to help the cancer cells grow and develop.

In one of the laboratory tests performed on your breast tumor, a pathologist — a specialist in diagnosing disease in tissue samples — checks to see if the tumor's cells are hormone receptive positive. He or she checks for both estrogen receptors and progesterone receptors.

If the cancer cells are hormone receptor positive, you may benefit from hormone therapy to control tumor growth. If your cancer cells are hormone receptor negative, hormone therapy isn't beneficial.

Adjuvant hormone therapy may take one of three different approaches:

- Use of anti-estrogen drugs, such as tamoxifen
- In premenopausal women, procedures to shut down the ovaries (ovarian ablation)
- In postmenopausal women, use of aromatase inhibitors

Tamoxifen

Anti-estrogen drugs work by attaching to estrogen receptors in estrogen receptor positive cancer cells and preventing them from binding with estrogen, thereby inhibiting growth of the cancer cells (see the illustration on page 192).

A commonly used anti-estrogen drug for the treatment of breast cancer is tamoxifen. It's probably the most widely studied and, over the past couple of decades, the most widely used anti-cancer medication in the world. The drug has been credited with playing an important role in the reduction in breast cancer deaths.

Tamoxifen was first used to treat advanced breast cancer that had spread to other parts of the body (metastatic cancer). Studies later showed it can also reduce the risk of cancer recurrence and death in women with early-stage breast cancer.

When the worldwide Early Breast Cancer Trialists' Collaborative Group published its third review of all the randomized clinical trial data pertaining to tamoxifen used as adjuvant therapy, data from 37,000 women in 55 clinical trials showed that tamoxifen treatment substantially lowered the rates of cancer recurrence, and it improved 10-year survival in both premenopausal and postmenopausal women with estrogen receptor positive tumors.

Typically, the drug has been taken every day for five years. Research shows that five years of tamoxifen use is better than short-term use in helping women live longer and cancer-free. But the bulk of available evidence suggests that using tamoxifen for more than five years, compared with stopping at five years, doesn't provide any greater benefit and it might increase cancer recurrences and side effects. This may be because when used longer term, the drug may begin to act more like estrogen on breast cancer cells (see "Tamoxifen's Dual Role" on page 193).

Side effects

Tamoxifen's most common side effects are hot flashes and vaginal discharge. The drug is also associated with an increased risk of cancer of the uterus (endometrial cancer or uterine sarcoma). In women who haven't had a hysterectomy, it can increase the rate of uterine cancer threefold. Although this sounds

Hormone Receptor Status

Estrogen, the principal female hormone, is known to influence the growth and development of certain breast tumors. Normal breast tissue cells contain receptors for estrogen and progesterone, another female hormone. Receptors are cell proteins that bind to specific substances in your bloodstream, such as hormones. You might think of receptors and hormones as a lock and key. If the hormone fits with the receptor, it opens the door for the cell to grow.

Many breast cancer cells have hormone receptors for estrogen, progesterone or both. These cancers are called hormone (estrogen, progesterone or both) receptor positive. Breast cancer cells are analyzed in a laboratory to see if they have hormone receptors. Hormone receptor positive cancers may shrink with hormone (anti-estrogen) therapy. Hormone receptor negative cancers don't.

Although the hormone receptor status of your cancer doesn't say much about your chances of a long-term cure, it can tell your doctor whether hormone therapy is likely to help. The hormone receptor status is called a predictive factor, a factor that helps predict what treatment might be useful.

Whether you've entered menopause also is a predictive factor in your treatment decision. During menopause, your ovaries make less estrogen and progesterone until eventually they stop producing them altogether. This may make a difference in the type of therapy you receive. For example, if you've already entered menopause, shutting down your ovaries (ovarian ablation) wouldn't be of much benefit to you, but another class of drugs called aromatase inhibitors may be. You'll learn more about these medications later in this chapter (see page 193).

like a big increase, it means that a postmenopausal woman who uses tamoxifen increases her chance of developing uterine cancer from a 1 in 1,000 chance a year to a 3 in 1,000 chance a year.

About 80 percent of tamoxifen-induced uterine cancers can be cured by removal of the uterus (hysterectomy), which may or may not be followed by radiation.

The most common sign of uterine cancer in postmenopausal women is vaginal bleeding, which in this case is actually uterine bleeding passing through the vagina. If this occurs, a gynecologic

evaluation along with a sampling of uterine (endometrial) tissue should be done. But don't panic if you experience vaginal bleeding while taking tamoxifen. Vaginal bleeding isn't always related to uterine cancer. Rather, it may stem from a noncancerous (benign) cause.

If you haven't yet gone through menopause, you may still continue to get your period. In some women taking tamoxifen, their periods may become irregular or menstruation may stop, but in most premenopausal women taking tamoxifen, the ovaries continue to function. In fact, tamoxifen may cause premenopausal women to produce more estrogen. It's essential that you not get pregnant while taking tamoxifen because the drug could harm the fetus.

Tamoxifen also affects bone density. In postmenopausal women, it helps preserve bone density because it appears that bones react to tamoxifen as an estrogen-like agent. In premenopausal women, though, tamoxifen may actually compete with estrogen in binding with estrogen receptors in bone cells. Because tamoxifen is not as strong of a bone-growth stimula-tor as is estrogen, it can cause bone thinning in premenopausal women.

Tamoxifen can also increase the risk of blood clots. When a blood clot travels to your lungs, it's called a pulmonary embolism. In rare instances, blood clots associated with tamoxifen use can lead to a stroke. Tamoxifen is also associated with increased cataract and other eye problems.

Ovarian ablation

Ovarian ablation is the oldest form of systemic therapy for premenopausal women with early-stage breast cancer. It

Estrogen receptor positive cell

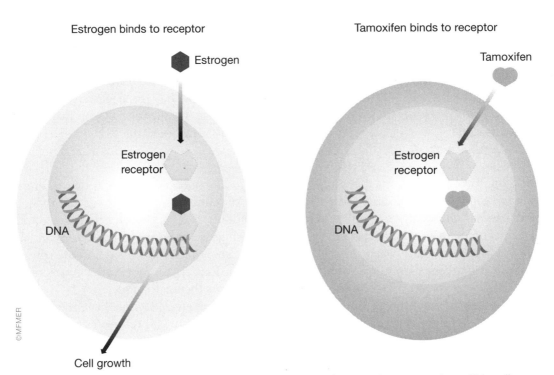

The illustration on the left shows how the hormone estrogen attaches to estrogen receptors within cells, stimulating cell growth. The drug tamoxifen (right) also attaches to estrogen receptors. It prevents estrogen from binding to the receptors, inhibiting the growth of cancer cells.

Tamoxifen's Dual Role

Tamoxifen is used to treat breast cancer because of its anti-estrogen properties. But in some body tissues, it actually behaves like estrogen. Therefore, it's said to be both an estrogen agonist and estrogen antagonist.

What does that mean? It means that tamoxifen works in different ways in different parts of your body. In some breast cells, such as those found in women with estrogen receptor positive breast cancer, it attaches to the receptors in cancer cells and blocks estrogen binding and activity, which means it's functioning as an antagonist. In other tissues, such as in the uterus and bones, tamoxifen attaches to estrogen receptors and promotes cell growth and activity in a way similar to estrogen, meaning it's functioning as an agonist. Because of tamoxifen's estrogen-like effects on the uterus, it slightly increases the chance of uterine cancer. At the same time, it's thought to help maintain bone strength in postmenopausal women.

consists of shutting down your ovaries to reduce the production of female hormones in your body. This may be done with surgery, with radiation or with the use of hormones — luteinizing hormone-releasing hormone (LH-RH) agonists, also known as gonadotropin-releasing hormone (Gn-RH) agonists.

A review of 12 trials of ovarian ablation by surgery or radiation revealed that it improved the 15-year survival rate in premenopausal women. Ovarian ablation wasn't beneficial, though, for postmenopausal women. This, most likely, is because their ovaries had already naturally stopped producing hormones.

Adjuvant ovarian ablation therapy has fallen out of favor, especially in North America, with more interest being given to chemotherapy. However, European oncologists have compared ovarian ablation and chemotherapy, concluding that ovarian ablation may be as good as some types of chemotherapy. This issue continues to be one of much debate. Trials are

under way to see if ovarian ablation in younger women may provide additional benefit when it's combined with chemotherapy, tamoxifen or both.

Side effects
The side effects of ovarian ablation are the same as those of premature menopause, including halting of menstruation, infertility, vaginal dryness, hot flashes and osteoporosis.

Aromatase inhibitors
Although your ovaries are the main source of estrogen, your body produces the hormone in other ways, even after menopause. Your adrenal glands produce several hormones, including androgens. An enzyme called aromatase that's predominant in tissues such as fat, liver, muscle and brain — as well as in normal breast tissue and breast cancer tissue — converts androgens into estrogens.

Medications called aromatase inhibitors work by keeping the aromatase enzyme from converting testosterone to estrogen. The drugs appear useful only in post-menopausal women. In premenopausal women, aromatase inhibitors aren't able to decrease total estrogen production by a significant amount, and therefore aren't effective. That's because the ovaries are still producing estrogen.

Another reason to avoid use of aromatase inhibitors in premenopausal women is that they may induce ovulation, and thus, cause pregnancy.

Aromatase inhibitors include the drugs anastrozole (Arimidex), letrozole (Femara) and exemestane (Aromasin).

Aromatase inhibitors vs. tamoxifen

The aromatase inhibitor anastrozole was studied in one of the largest breast cancer drug trials ever, with more than 9,000 women participating. In this study, postmenopausal women with recently diagnosed, early-stage breast cancer were given anastrozole, tamoxifen or both, which they took for five years. Results of the study suggest that anastrozole is better than tamoxifen in improving disease-free survival — but only by about 5 percent.

While the findings of this study were positive, there was a need for more research — particularly because tamoxifen carries an increased risk of blood clots and uterine cancer. Anastrozole is also associated with a higher rate of some side effects, such as joint and muscle pain, than is tamoxifen. And it also can increase the risk of osteoporosis.

Follow-up results of the anastrozole study are indicating that women who received anastrozole aren't living any longer than women who received tamoxi-fen. The reason may be because anastrozole may cause more heart problems, while tamoxifen may do just the opposite — decrease heart problems.

The other two aromatase inhibitors, letrozole and exemestane, appear to function and produce results similar to anastrozole.

Aromatase inhibitor use after tamoxifen

Other studies of aromatase inhibitors have been developed to find out what happens if the medication is taken after tamoxifen, instead of in place of it.

In one study, 5,000 women who had completed five years of tamoxifen therapy were given either the aromatase inhibitor letrozole (Femara) or an inactive pill (placebo), which they took for another five years. Results showed a significant reduction in new breast cancers among women receiving letrozole, compared with those taking a placebo.

Another study involved more than 5,000 women who had taken tamoxifen for only two to three years. The women were divided into two groups. One group continued to take tamoxifen for a total of five years. Women in the other group switched to the aromatase inhibitor exemestane (Aromasin), which they took for two to three years, for a total of five years of hormone treatment. Results of this study favored the tamoxifen plus exemestane group, indicating a 5 percent reduction in breast cancer recurrences.

Based on what's now known, post-menopausal women who've taken tamoxifen for two to five years might want to consider additional treatment with an aromatase inhibitor.

Tools to Help With Treatment Decisions

Patient Information

Age: | 60

Comorbidity: | Minor Problems ▼

ER Status: | Positive ▼

Tumor Grade: | Grade 3 ▼

Tumor Size: | 1.1 - 2.0 cm ▼

Positive Nodes: | 1 - 3 ▼

➤ Calculate For: | Relapse ▼

10 Year Risk: | 52 | Prognostic

Adjuvant Therapy Effectiveness

Horm: | Aromatase Inhibitor for 5 yrs ▼

Chemo: | 3rd Generation Regimens ▼

Hormonal Therapy: | 56

Chemotherapy: | 43

Combined Therapy: | 75

No Additional Therapy

43.5 alive and without cancer in 10 years

50.1 relapse

6.4 die of other causes

With hormonal therapy: Benefit = 22.8 without relapse.

With chemotherapy: Benefit = 16.7 without relapse.

With combined therapy: Benefit = 32.7 without relapse.

Doctors use online tools to help evaluate the benefits of adjuvant therapy. In this example, a breast cancer patient's information is entered, and the program predicts her risk of a cancer recurrence. Without additional treatment, there's a 43.5 percent chance the cancer won't come back. With hormone therapy, that chance increases to approximately 66 percent (43.5 + 22.8). If she has combined therapy (hormone therapy and chemotherapy), it increases to approximately 76 percent (43.5 +32.7).

Modified from Adjuvant! for breast cancer, version 7.

Decision Guide: Adjuvant Systemic Therapy

Whether you should go ahead with additional treatment for your cancer beyond surgery, or surgery and radiation, isn't always a simple decision. A number of issues need to be considered in determining if it's the best choice for you.

Factors to consider

Following are some frequently asked questions and answers about adjuvant therapy. You'll also find stories of two women who talk about the decisions they made regarding adjuvant therapy and how they felt about it afterward, beginning on page 200. It's hoped that this information will help you in making your decision. If you have questions about your diagnosis, treatment or prognosis, discuss them with your doctor.

Do you want to do everything possible to prevent cancer from coming back?
If so, you may be more comfortable in the long run if you're more aggressive in your treatment choices. If, on the other hand, you generally prefer a less aggressive approach when it comes to medical intervention, you might prefer to avoid the risks and side effects of more aggressive treatment.

Is there evidence that adjuvant systemic therapy helps a woman with cancer like yours live longer?
Adjuvant systemic therapy can help many women, but the benefit gained is different for each woman depending on a number of factors, such as her age, the size of her primary tumor, her lymph node status and her hormone receptor status. With mathematical models of statistical averages, your doctor can help you figure out an estimate of the specific benefits to be gained in your situation.

These tools are discussed on pages 184 and 195. If you want to know this information and your doctor hasn't provided it to you, ask him or her to discuss with you the recurrence and survival odds in your particular case.

Do the benefits of adjuvant systemic therapy appear to outweigh the risks?
Adjuvant chemotherapy, hormone therapy and anti-HER2 therapy can improve cancer-free survival in many women. But there's a price to pay in the side effects that these drugs may cause. Have you weighed the pros and cons? How much importance do you place on the possibility of benefit from these drugs, compared with the potential side effects of the therapy?

Are you still hoping to have children?
Adjuvant systemic therapy can cause your ovaries to stop producing female hormones and may cause infertility. See page 189 for more information on preserving your fertility.

Anti-HER2 therapy

Human epidermal growth factor receptor 2 (HER2) is a protein that appears on the surface of some breast cancer cells. This protein is important to cell growth and survival. Breast cancers that are HER2 positive have a lot of the HER2 protein on the surfaces of their cells. Those that are HER2 negative have little or no HER2 protein.

Approximately 20 to 25 percent of breast cancers have an excess of HER2.

This excess can also occur in other types of cancer, not just breast cancer.

HER2-positive breast cancers tend to be more aggressive than other types of breast cancer, and they're treated with an antibody therapy called trastuzumab. If not treated with medication that specifically targets the HER2 protein, women with HER2-positive cancers have a poorer prognosis than do women with HER2-negative breast cancers. Fortunately, treatments that target the HER2 protein are very effective.

Herceptin improves survival

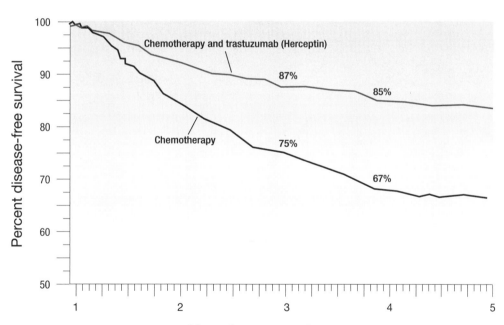

Among women with HER2-positive breast cancer, a change in treatment came about after a study found that women who took the medication trastuzumab (Herceptin) after chemotherapy treatment were 18 percent more likely not to experience a cancer recurrence than women who received only chemotherapy. Disease-free survival four years after the start of treatment increased to 85 percent with trastuzumab use.

Source: Piccart-Gebhart, Martine J., et al. Trastuzumab after Adjuvant Chemotherapy in HER2-Positive Breast Cancer. *New England Journal of Medicine*, 2005;353:1659.

Trastuzumab

Trastuzumab (Herceptin) inhibits the growth of breast cancer cells that depend on excess HER2. Trastuzumab is often used with chemotherapy, but it may also be used in combination with hormone-blocking medications, such as an aromatase inhibitor or tamoxifen.

Studies comparing use of chemotherapy alone and chemotherapy combined with trastuzumab show that breast cancer recurrence is reduced and survival is improved when women with HER2-positive cancers receive both medications in combination (see the graph on page 197).

How long trastuzumab should be given is still being studied. Currently, one year of therapy is recommended. Some data suggest that taking the drug for a longer period of time might be beneficial, while other data suggest benefits of the medication can be seen in as little as three months of use.

Trastuzumab is generally well tolerated, but it has some potential side effects, such as a small chance of congestive heart failure, which can occur in up to 5 percent of women who also took the medication doxorubicin. It can also cause an allergic reaction.

Lapatinib

Lapatinib (Tykerb) is another medication that specifically targets overproduction of HER2. It may be effective for HER2-positive breast cancer that doesn't respond to trastuzumab. Lapatinib is used in combination with the chemotherapy drug capecitabine (Xeloda) and the aromatase inhibitor letrozole (Femara). It's being studied in combination with trastuzumab to see if there may be benefits to combining the two drugs.

Others

Researchers also are studying the effects of other drugs as a possible treatment for

Positive or Negative: Which Is Better?

Given the availability of medications to treat HER2-positive breast cancer, you may wonder if it's better to be diagnosed with HER2-positive or HER2-negative cancer.

It is true that without specific treatment, HER2-positive breast cancers do have a poorer prognosis than do HER2-negative cancers. And they do require additional treatment, which can be expensive and which carries some risk of side effects. Most women, though, tolerate anti-HER2 medications relatively well.

However, because the treatment for HER2-positive breast cancers is effective, treatment, in essence, cancels out the negative prognosis associated with this specific breast cancer. It's not clear, though, if treatment improves a woman's prognosis beyond that of HER2-negative breast cancers.

The bottom line: Having HER2-positive breast cancer is neither better nor worse than having HER2-negative cancer.

QUESTION & ANSWER

Q: What is triple-negative breast cancer?

A: This term refers to breast cancers that have negative estrogen receptors, progesterone receptors and HER2 receptors. Triple-negative breast cancer has received a bad name for itself because, left untreated, the cancer has a poorer prognosis than do hormone receptor positive (estrogen and progesterone) cancers. Even with treatment, it can also have a poorer prognosis than treated HER2-positive cancers.

The good news regarding triple-negative breast cancer is that chemotherapy actually works better against these cancers than it does against hormone receptor positive cancers. In addition, women with triple-negative breast cancer who make it five years without a recurrence have a lower risk of a cancer recurrence later on than do women with hormone receptor positive cancers. This is because when triple-negative cancers recur, they generally do so within five years. Hormone receptor positive cancers, meanwhile, can recur for decades after initial diagnosis.

HER2-positive cancers. The hope is that these medications will add to the benefits seen with trastuzumab, or that they'll be more effective and produce fewer side effects than trastuzumab.

Chemotherapy
Standard chemotherapy agents can be effective in treating HER2-positive breast cancers, although these drugs don't specifically target the HER2 protein.

Watchful waiting

For women with small, node-negative cancers, surgery alone or surgery followed by radiation may provide an excellent prognosis, and additional (adjuvant) therapy may not be needed. Watchful waiting can be a reasonable choice depending on a woman's particular situation. Some women feel there's not enough potential long-term benefit from adjuvant therapy, compared with

its potential risks and side effects. Some women live long, healthy lives after breast cancer surgery without receiving any additional treatment.

Watchful waiting isn't the same as doing nothing. If you decline additional therapy, or it's not recommended, your doctor will encourage you to be vigilant with breast self-exams and mammograms. It's also important to have regular follow-up clinical examinations.

There are some risks with watchful waiting, mainly, an increased risk of cancer spread. However, for women with cancers that have a good prognosis, this increased risk may be very low.

Clinical Trials

A number of new approaches to breast cancer treatment and, in particular, adjuvant therapy, are being studied. The emphasis of breast cancer research is to

Meet Other Women

Here are the stories of two more women, Nancy and Jane. Each made different choices about adjuvant systemic therapy.

Although more than 20 years apart in age, both women were in their 30s (ages 30 and 36) when they received a diagnosis of breast cancer. Their therapy choices were different, but each choice made sense in each woman's case. Remember that you, too, have choices. There's no one right answer for all women.

Nancy's Story

Nancy was 30 years old when she found a lump in her breast. Tests showed that she had a second lump that couldn't be felt. The larger lump was about 2 to 3 centimeters (cm), which is about 1 inch, in diameter, and one sentinel lymph node tested positive for cancer. Nancy looked for the best information she could find about the outcomes of women her age in her situation. She decided to have the AC chemotherapy combination — the A stands for Adriamycin, a previous brand name of the generic drug doxorubicin, and the C stands for cyclophosphamide. Her chemotherapy was followed by tamoxifen hormone therapy. She shared this story four months after she had completed chemotherapy and two months after returning to work. At this time, she had already begun taking tamoxifen.

Before she found the lump, Nancy was, in her words, "At the top of my game … trucking along, doing what I do." She was 30, married, had a healthy baby daughter and had just stopped breast-feeding. She was also a busy doctor in training — a surgical resident. Then she stopped trucking. "I feel like my life was sort of derailed."

She found a lump in her breast through some unusual circumstances. She had recently had some fevers and wondered if she had a viral illness. Because she had just finished breast-feeding her daughter, her doctor had her check for signs of a breast infection, which can occur after breast-feeding. When she went home and did a breast self-exam, she found the lump. She remembers feeling something solid — thicker than other breast tissue — that was about a half-inch to three-quarters of an inch in diameter. Nancy felt no pain, and nothing else seemed different.

A mammogram showed nothing abnormal. So an ultrasound test was done. It showed two lumps, one which Nancy had not felt. Biopsies were done, and both lumps were found to be invasive cancer.

Nancy chose to have mastectomies on both breasts — even though nothing had been found in the other breast. Her age, the unreliability of the mammogram in her case, and the fact that two lumps had been found — one of which no one could feel — all factored in her decision.

Nancy was devastated when she learned that the cancer had spread to a lymph node. She remembers questioning herself. "I thought I had caught it relatively early. How could it have spread already?" Nancy had always thought that if you had cancer and it had spread, you wouldn't feel good. She felt great.

She already knew that adjuvant systemic therapy would be something to consider because of her relatively young age and the size of the cancer. That the cancer had spread to a lymph node pushed the decision even more. "Having the ability to do something more than just the surgery was sort of reassuring to me."

Nancy used statistics to help guide her decision. Her oncologist considered her age, tumor size, lymph node status, and that her tumor cells were hormone receptor positive. These factors helped Nancy and her doctor look at the best estimates of what happens to women like her over time when they choose adjuvant systemic therapy and when they don't. She also carefully analyzed the risks of adjuvant systemic therapy. In the end, she thought she had more to gain than to lose by having both chemotherapy and tamoxifen.

During chemotherapy Nancy endured nausea, anemia, fatigue, hair loss and the knowledge that she may not be able to have more children. Energy was a major issue for her. She returned to a demanding job and was on call every other night. After her chemotherapy, Nancy began taking tamoxifen. The tamoxifen gave her hot flashes at first, but eventually they stopped.

Unfortunately, this was a battle that Nancy would not win. She eventually died of her cancer. But Nancy knew that she had done all that she could to fight what can sometimes be a very difficult disease.

Jane's Story

Jane has had plenty of time to reflect calmly on a health history that could have been devastating. At the time she shared her story, it had been 17 years since she received her first breast cancer diagnosis and 14 years since she received a second diagnosis. Yes, Jane has dealt with breast cancer twice.

Jane wasn't always so cool about her experiences with breast cancer: "I was in my 30s, and the only thing I thought of was that this was a death sentence." She says that once you have cancer, you're always a little paranoid about your health. "In your first year (after the first diagnosis), you worry about every ache and pain. And then in your second year, it has to be more significant to get your attention," she recalls. "Well, the third year I was feeling pretty confident, and then all of a sudden I get another diagnosis. But I did get through that one, too, and now it's 14 years later."

Both times Jane had a lumpectomy and radiation. Both times she declined any adjuvant systemic therapy. Jane says she wasn't convinced about two things. She wasn't convinced that the benefits of adjuvant systemic therapy were proved in people like her with very small tumors and no cancer in the lymph nodes. And, she wasn't convinced that the benefits would outweigh the possible harm — especially in the long term. She says she wasn't very worried about hair loss or nausea or fatigue. It was the possibility that the therapy itself could cause other cancers that gave her the most concern.

A former vice president of an international technical education company, Jane has been comfortable analyzing numbers for years. She once taught a course in statistics. So she wasn't intimidated by statistics when it was time to make this important health care decision. For her, the numbers just didn't stack up in favor of taking adjuvant systemic therapy, so she declined with confidence. And she was determined to make a decision and never look back.

But Jane has also been vigilant. For the first year after her second breast cancer, she saw a surgeon and radiation oncologist every three months. Then she slowly reduced the frequency of those visits. She continues to have annual mammograms. Her doctors carefully compare them with films from past years to scrutinize what might be scarring and what might be something else.

It's not just her breast health that her doctor checks. Jane has had colonoscopy procedures because of her family colon cancer history and her own cancer history.

"I view myself as cured of cancer, but at a higher than average risk of additional problems," she explains. "I'm quite optimistic about my battle with cancer, and I'm really excited and optimistic about what's happening in medical science."

She has become active in breast cancer advocacy work and gets satisfaction from conveying to women that "you can make your own decisions, and you can survive."

find new or improved methods that can successfully treat the cancer and extend a woman's survival with the fewest side effects possible.

Much of what's practiced today in breast cancer treatment is the result of prior clinical trials in which thousands of women participated. Many previous clinical trials have led the way for treatments used today.

If you have breast cancer, you may wish to consider participating in a clinical trial. By taking part, you may be the first in line to receive the potential benefits of cutting-edge breast cancer treatment. It's important to discuss the benefits and disadvantages of participation in a clinical trial with your doctor. For more information on clinical trials, see Chapter 2.

Chapter 12: Breast Cancer

Breast Reconstruction

Immediate vs. Delayed   204

Types   204
Tissue expanders   205
Implants   207
Tissue flaps   207
Prosthetics   209

Issues to Consider   209

A common concern of many women when deciding on surgical treatment for breast cancer is their appearance after surgery. This is especially true of women considering a mastectomy. While you're gathering information about your treatment options, you may also want to gather information on breast reconstruction.

Some women choose not to have any reconstructive surgery after mastectomy. That's OK. Such a decision is perfectly acceptable. In addition, some women decide not to wear an external prosthesis, an artificial breast that's worn in your bra. Many women who take this route are content with this choice.

For women who do choose reconstructive surgery, there are several options available to consider. Breast reconstruction is a surgical procedure designed to restore a more naturally shaped breast mound after mastectomy. Reconstructive surgery, which is generally performed by a plastic surgeon may require a longer recovery than does mastectomy alone. At the same time, some women find reconstructive surgery easier to tolerate than a mastectomy alone because they feel it improves their body image.

Immediate vs. Delayed

Reconstruction may be performed at the same time as a mastectomy (immediate reconstruction), or it can be done later (delayed reconstruction). In general, immediate reconstruction brings the most favorable cosmetic results. In addition, some women feel much better when they wake up from a mastectomy with a reconstructed breast. With immediate reconstruction, a plastic surgeon typically works in tandem with the surgical oncologist who performs the mastectomy.

An important consideration in deciding whether to have immediate or delayed reconstruction is whether you may need radiation therapy to treat your breast cancer. If you may need radiation, you should discuss your reconstruction options with your surgeon before your surgery.

Among women with large tumors and those whose cancer has spread to the underarm (axillary) lymph nodes, radiation therapy is often recommended after mastectomy. Because it can take a day or two after a mastectomy before doctors have a definitive answer as to whether the cancer has spread to the lymph nodes, you may not know before your surgery whether you'll need radiation. For this reason, immediate reconstruction often isn't an option.

As for chemotherapy, you can receive it after immediate breast reconstruction, but you'll need to wait about two to three weeks after your surgery before you can begin treatments. Your surgeon and oncologist will decide when the time is right to begin chemotherapy after surgery.

With delayed breast reconstruction, surgeons generally recommend that you wait several months after completing radiation therapy and chemotherapy before having reconstructive surgery to allow time for healing from your treatment.

Types

If you decide to have breast reconstruction, you have three options to consider:
- Breast reconstruction with implants
- Breast reconstruction with your own tissue, which is called flap (autologous) surgery

---

QUESTION & ANSWER

Q: **Does breast reconstruction make it more difficult to detect a cancer recurrence?**

A: With very rare exceptions, the answer to this question is a strong *No*. This is because the most likely site for recurrence is in the tissue located just underneath the skin (subcutaneous tissue). During reconstruction, the artificial breast mound is placed deep below the subcutaneous tissue, which pushes the subcutaneous tissue upward and closer to the surface. Therefore, recurrent tumors can still be felt during a self-examination or clinical breast examination.

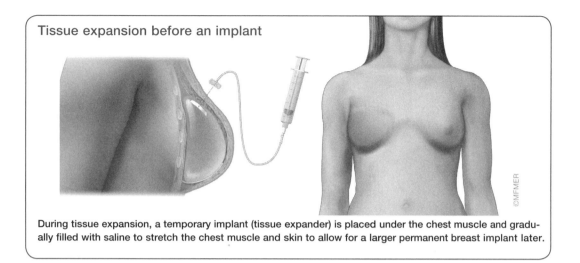

Tissue expansion before an implant

During tissue expansion, a temporary implant (tissue expander) is placed under the chest muscle and gradually filled with saline to stretch the chest muscle and skin to allow for a larger permanent breast implant later.

- No reconstruction, but use of a prosthesis, an artificial breast mound that's worn externally in your bra

Keep in mind that reconstruction may require multiple surgical procedures. Usually, at least two surgeries are required to achieve a correctly positioned and symmetrical breast mound. Some women also undergo areola and nipple reconstruction. In addition, before surgery, steps must be taken to stretch the remaining chest skin so that it can accommodate an implant, a process called tissue expansion.

If you want both of your breasts — your reconstructed breast and your healthy breast — to have a similar size and shape, you might consider surgery on both of your breasts. When breast reconstruction is performed on just one breast, there may be a difference in size and shape compared to your natural, healthy breast. In addition, over time, your reconstructed breast and your natural breast may change in slightly different ways, and they may end up looking even more different from one another.

Tissue expanders

Most women aren't able to simply have an implant placed in their chest wall at the time of a mastectomy. First, they need to undergo a process called tissue expansion to stretch the remaining chest skin to accommodate the implant. The process begins with the insertion of a temporary implant called a tissue expander. The implant can be surgically placed at the time of your mastectomy, or later if you choose to have delayed breast reconstruction. The tissue expander is placed under your chest muscle and skin.

During a series of regular office visits over the next few months, your surgeon or a member of his or her staff will inject sterile saline into your tissue expander to slowly stretch your chest muscle and skin. The filling is done gradually to give the skin covering the implant a chance to stretch between visits.

A few months after the tissue expansion is complete, you'll need a second surgery in which the tissue expander is removed and replaced with a permanent breast

Pedicle TRAM flap surgery

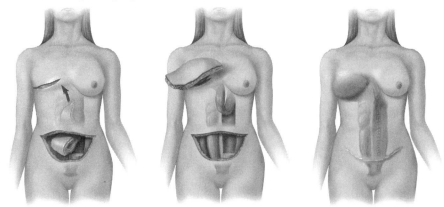

With pedicle TRAM flap surgery, a section of skin, muscle, fat and blood vessels is taken from a woman's abdomen, tunneled underneath the skin, and used to create a new breast mound.

Free TRAM flap surgery

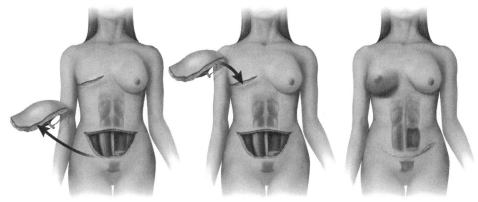

During a free TRAM flap procedure, a surgeon disconnects a section of abdominal tissue — including skin, fat and sometimes muscle — and reattaches the tissue to the chest area, using microsurgical techniques.

Latissimus flap surgery

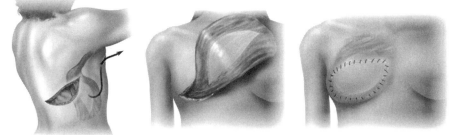

Latissimus flap surgery is performed in much the same way as is TRAM flap surgery, but the section of tissue used to create a new breast mound comes from the back instead of the abdomen.

©MFMER

implant. The permanent implant may be filled with either saline or silicone gel. Your surgeon will discuss these options with you.

Implants

An implant is a breast-shaped device that's placed under the pectoral muscles of the chest wall. This technique may be performed in slender, smaller breasted women who don't have a lot of excess tissue in their abdomens or other parts of their bodies that could be used for autologous breast reconstruction.

The two kinds of implants are saline and silicone. In the 1990s, there were some major concerns regarding silicone implants. At issue was whether the implants caused other health problems. Today, as a result of additional research, these concerns have largely been laid to rest. An advantage of silicone implants, and why they're often used in breast reconstruction, is that they feel more like breast tissue than do saline implants.

An implant may be put in place at the time of the mastectomy or during a later surgery. Implants may cause pain, swelling, bruising, tenderness or infection. There's also a possibility of rupture, deflation and shifting. Another possible complication of implants is capsular contracture, a condition in which tight scar tissue forms around the implant. This causes the breast mound to become excessively firm so that it no longer has the feel of breast tissue. Sometimes, a capsular contracture can cause discomfort. Whether to surgically correct a contracture is an individual decision, often based on the severity of the symptoms.

If you've had radiation therapy or complications such as a blood clot or infection, you may be at a higher risk of capsular contraction. Your plastic surgeon may recommend that you consider another reconstructive option.

A nipple also can be reconstructed using skin from the new breast mound. This is generally done after the reconstructed breast has time to heal and settle. Later, a tattoo may be applied to color the nipple and create an areola.

The entire process takes about four to six months, sometimes longer depending on other treatments you may need.

Tissue flaps

A more complex reconstructive procedure involves using a woman's own tissue. In this type of reconstruction, a section of skin, fat and muscle, along with blood vessels, is taken from one part of the body and moved to the chest to form a breast mound.

Women who choose tissue flaps generally like the idea of using their own tissue to reconstruct their breast. For women who undergo radiation, it also may be the only reconstructive option available. After radiation, it's often difficult to stretch the skin enough to place an implant.

Most often, the tissue is taken from the lower abdomen. This is called a TRAM flap. TRAM stands for transverse rectus abdominis myocutaneous. The rectus abdominis muscle is the "six pack" muscle in the abdomen.

There are two main types of TRAM flap procedures that may be used to reconstruct a breast: the pedicle flap and the free flap. With the pedicle TRAM flap,

Nipple reconstruction

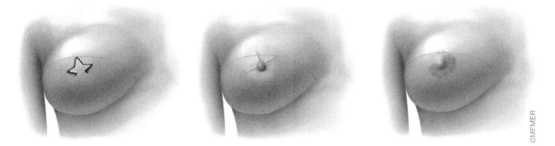

After a reconstructed breast has healed, a plastic surgeon can reconstruct a new nipple and areola.

a surgeon takes the rectus abdominis muscle completely, along with the overlying fat and skin from your abdomen, to construct your new breast. The flap is tunneled under the skin to the chest area, where it's brought through the mastectomy incision.

With the free flap procedure, a surgeon takes only part of the rectus abdominis, along with skin and fat from your abdomen and reattaches the tissue to blood vessels in the chest wall using microsurgical techniques. This is called a muscle-sparing TRAM flap because most of the rectus abdominis muscle is left untouched.

Some women undergo what's called a DIEP flap. In this procedure a surgeon takes only the skin and fat from the abdomen to make a new breast. The DIEP flap is appropriate only in some women and is dependent on the size of the abdominal blood vessels.

For women who don't have enough tissue available on their abdomens for this procedure, the tissue may be taken from the back. This is called a latissimus flap, from the Latin word for the muscle that's

involved in the procedure. The flap is moved to the chest site in the same manner as is done with the pedicle TRAM flap.

In most women, the latissimus flap is too thin to create a natural sized breast. A tissue expander or a breast implant is placed under the flap to create the breast mound. If a tissue expander is used, a second surgery will be necessary to replace the expander with a permanent implant.

In some instances, neither the abdomen nor the back has sufficient extra tissue from which to take a flap. In this case, the tissue may be taken from the buttocks or the inner thigh.

The main advantage of flap reconstruction is that the reconstructed breast mound is made from your own tissue. The mound remains quite soft and, unlike with an implant, contracture doesn't occur. In addition, if the tissue is taken from the abdomen, you get a tummy tuck. However, because the flap is human tissue, it requires an adequate blood supply. If blood supply to the flap is poor, the tissue may not survive. This may lead to significant complications and an unsatisfactory result.

The Do's and Don'ts of Reconstruction

People have many misconceptions about breast reconstruction. It's important to approach the procedure with realistic expectations and to ask questions.

What breast reconstruction can do:
- Give you a permanent breast contour
- Provide symmetry to your breasts so that they look similar under clothing or a bathing suit
- Help you avoid the need for an external prosthesis

What breast reconstruction may do:
- Improve your self-esteem and body image
- Partially erase physical reminders of your disease
- Require additional surgery to correct reconstructive problems

What breast reconstruction doesn't do:
- Make you look and feel exactly the same as before your mastectomy
- Give your reconstructed breast mound the same feeling as your normal breast

Once the reconstructed breast mound has healed, a nipple may be formed using skin from the new breast mound, and a tattoo may be applied to color the nipple and create an areola.

In some instances, tissue flap surgery isn't an option. If you smoke, your doctor may recommend against it because smoking can impair the circulation to the transferred tissue. An abdominal flap may not be an option if you've had previous abdominal surgery.

Prosthetics

Some women choose a prosthesis over reconstructive surgery. A prosthesis is a device that's shaped like a breast and worn in your bra. It's usually made from nylon, rubber, silicone or Dacron fiberfill, and you slip it into a specially designed bra. Immediately after your surgery, you may select from prostheses in a range of shapes and sizes that can be used temporarily. For long-term use, you may want to consider getting a more customized, permanent prosthesis.

Check with your insurance company to see if your insurance will pay for a prosthesis. Sometimes, having a prescription for a prosthesis from a doctor can help with insurance coverage.

Issues to Consider

In making your decision on whether to have breast reconstruction, or what type

Decision Tips

As you think about reconstruction, here are some suggestions to help you in the decision-making process:

- Gather reputable information on breast reconstruction after a mastectomy. Some organizations you might contact include the American Society of Plastic Surgeons, the American Cancer Society and the National Cancer Institute (see pages 413-416 for more information on these organizations).
- Talk with your surgeon before you make your decision and make sure all of your questions are answered. Jot down questions as you think of them so that you can make the most of your visit with the surgeon. Try to establish a relationship with your surgeon that's open, clear and honest.
- Ask to see pictures of the results of different procedures.
- Talk to women who have gone through the various reconstructive procedures. They can give you the personal details that you might want.

of reconstruction to have, consider these issues:

- Will you be able to cope with complications of reconstruction if they occur, such as implant deflation or the need for multiple surgeries to achieve breast symmetry?
- If you choose immediate reconstruction, would a complication such as an infection compromise the start of your chemotherapy or radiation therapy?
- How soon does your surgeon need to know your preferences regarding reconstruction? To make the choice that's most suitable for you, you want to discuss your options with your surgeon.
- Are you doing this for yourself or because of pressure from others? Although you may wish to please your partner or family, you don't want to resent them later on for pressuring you into a procedure you didn't really want.
- Are you having reconstruction to make yourself forget you ever had cancer?

Unfortunately, this usually isn't possible. Even if, physically, you look closer to the way you did before, emotional and psychological aspects of your condition still need to be addressed.

- Have you given yourself enough time to make a decision you're comfortable with? Women are often so overwhelmed after a diagnosis of breast cancer that they just want to have the surgery, get the cancer out and be done with it. This is understandable, but it's usually OK to take a few days to a couple of weeks to think through your decision. Sometimes, a plastic surgeon will recommend delaying reconstructive surgery so that the reconstruction doesn't interfere with your cancer treatment regimen.

If you have questions regarding reconstruction, be sure to consult your doctor or a plastic surgeon. He or she can usually help clarify the issues for you.

Chapter 13: Breast Cancer

Special Situations

Locally Advanced Breast Cancer — 212
Treatment — 213

Women at High Risk of a Second Cancer — 214
BRCA carriers — 214
Hodgkin disease survivors — 215

Bilateral Breast Cancer — 216
Treatment — 216

Unknown Primary Cancers — 216

Metaplastic Breast Cancer — 217

Lymphomas and Sarcomas — 218
Breast lymphoma — 218
Breast sarcoma — 218

Paget's Disease — 219

Breast Cancer and Pregnancy — 220
Treatment — 220
Pregnancy after breast cancer — 222

Breast Cancer in Men — 222
Risk factors — 223
Diagnosis and staging — 223
Treatment — 223
Prognosis — 224

Most women diagnosed with breast cancer have a common type of breast cancer that's still in its earlier stages. Some women, though, develop less common forms of breast cancer. Signs and symptoms of the cancer may not be the same, and — depending on the type of cancer or the situation in which it was diagnosed — the treatment may be different.

Some women also are at higher risk of a second breast cancer than are others, and their treatment recommendations may be different. Breast cancer during pregnancy poses yet another unique situation in which treatment may be altered because of the circumstances.

If you're diagnosed with an uncommon type of breast cancer, are at high risk for a second cancer or are facing unique circumstances, it's important that you see an experienced breast cancer specialist. Talking with someone who's familiar with your condition helps to ensure that you receive an accurate diagnosis and appropriate treatment.

This chapter discusses special breast situations, outlining differences in treatment approaches, compared with those for more common forms of breast cancer.

Locally Advanced Breast Cancer

About 5 to 10 percent of breast cancers are diagnosed as locally advanced breast cancers. Locally advanced breast cancer, which generally falls under the category of stage III breast cancer, refers to larger breast tumors with one or more of the following characteristics:

- Greater than 5 centimeters (about 2 inches) in diameter
- Extensive cancer spread to regional lymph nodes
- Cancer spread to the chest wall or skin, sometimes causing open sores

However, with stage III breast cancer, there's no evidence that the cancer has spread (metastasized) to other parts of the body.

Locally advanced breast cancers sometimes occur in women who may not get medical attention when they first notice a breast lump. This may be because they fear being diagnosed with cancer. Locally advanced breast tumors can also occur because the tumor didn't show up clearly on a mammogram. This is most often the case with a type of breast cancer known as invasive lobular breast cancer. These breast tumors can be very large but not be apparent on breast self-exams, clinical examination or mam-

Inflammatory Breast Cancer

Inflammatory breast cancer is a type of locally advanced cancer that occurs in a very small percentage of women with breast cancer. In addition to spreading to fibrous connective tissue inside your breast, the cancer spreads to lymphatic vessels located in breast skin, causing noticeable skin changes.

Typically, a lump in your breast is the classic sign of breast cancer, but with inflammatory breast cancer, the lump, or mass, may not be apparent. Common signs and symptoms of inflammatory breast cancer include:

- A breast that appears red, purple, pink or bruised
- Swelling that makes your breast feel and appear larger than usual
- A warm feeling in the breast

- Itching
- Ridged or dimpled skin texture, similar to an orange peel — often referred to by the French term *peau d'orange*
- Swelling of lymph nodes in one or more of the following locations: under the arm, above the collarbone, below the collarbone

In spite of its name, inflammatory breast cancer isn't caused by an inflammation or an infection. It occurs as a result of lymphatic drainage channels in breast skin becoming plugged with cancer cells. Inflammatory breast cancer usually spreads rapidly, and skin changes can become apparent in a matter of days to weeks.

Although it's not an infection, inflammatory breast cancer can easily be con-

mography. This may be because they tend to infiltrate into normal breast tissue in a diffuse pattern that can feel like normal breast tissue, rather than forming a large mass.

Treatment

Prognosis is generally less favorable for a stage III breast cancer than it is for a stage I or II breast cancer. However, there's still hope for a cure. Treatment regimens typically include drug treatments (chemotherapy, hormone therapy or both), surgery and radiation.

Instead of performing surgery first, as generally happens with stage I and II breast cancers, for stage III breast cancer, chemotherapy to shrink the tumor is often the first course of action. Usually, an anthracycline medication is recommended, such as doxorubicin or epirubicin (Ellence), and a taxane medication, such as paclitaxel (Abraxance, Onxol) or docetaxel (Taxotere). Chemotherapy is usually given for four to eight cycles over a period of three to six months. In case of a HER2-positive cancer, trastuzumab (Herceptin) may be recommended.

For some women who have strongly positive estrogen (plus or minus progesterone) receptors, hormone (anti-estrogen) therapy may be recommended in place of chemotherapy.

fused with a breast infection (acute mastitis). Breast infections tend to occur in women who are breast-feeding. They typically cause a fever, and they're easily treated with antibiotics. Inflammatory breast cancers don't cause a fever, and they don't respond to antibiotics.

If you have signs and symptoms associated with inflammatory breast cancer, your doctor will likely want to do a breast biopsy. A biopsy can confirm the presence or absence of cancer. In some cases, redness, warmth and swelling of the breast are caused not by an infection or cancer but rather by a previous surgery or radiation therapy that involved the outer breast or underarm. These procedures can cause partial blockage of lymphatic channels. As fluid

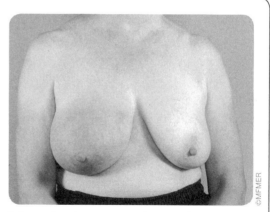

Inflammatory breast cancer is generally characterized by redness of the breast skin and swelling. In this photo, inflammatory breast cancer is present in the woman's right breast. The skin is red, and the breast is swollen (see a color illustration on page 36).

and debris accumulate in the channels, breast tissue may swell (edema) and turn pink in color.

Assuming that the tumor shrinks after initial drug therapy, the next step is usually surgery. A mastectomy is most often performed to remove the tumor. Nearby lymph nodes are evaluated with a sentinel node biopsy and may be removed, depending on the biopsy results. In some instances of locally advanced cancer, a lumpectomy (breast-conserving surgery) may be performed instead of a mastectomy. Lumpectomy isn't an option, though, for inflammatory breast cancer.

After surgery — depending on how much chemotherapy you received before surgery and the response of the cancer to the medication — your doctor may recommend more chemotherapy. He or she also may recommend radiation therapy to destroy any remaining cancer cells in the chest wall area and nearby lymph nodes. If laboratory reports indicate that you have a hormone receptor positive cancer, your doctor may also recommend hormone therapy.

For more information on these types of treatment, and how they're performed, see Chapter 11.

Women at High Risk of a Second Cancer

In situations where breast cancer is identified in a woman at high risk of the disease, treatment decisions tend to be more complex than for a woman at normal risk. That's because women at high risk of breast cancer are also at greater risk of additional new cancers in the same breast or in the other breast.

Groups of women considered at high risk are discussed in Chapter 6. Here we discuss two particular high-risk groups — BRCA carriers and Hodgkin disease survivors — and treatment approaches for them.

You should know that there's no evidence a woman at high risk of developing breast cancer is at a higher risk of the current cancer recurring than is a woman at normal risk with similar cancer characteristics.

BRCA carriers

If you've been diagnosed with breast cancer and genetic tests indicate that you carry a mutation in BRCA1 or BRCA2, you may want to consider surgical removal (mastectomy) of the affected breast, or perhaps both breasts, to decrease the chances of new cancers developing in the same or opposite breast. A mastectomy, however, is not mandatory. If breast conservation is important to you, a lumpectomy with radiation therapy is an option.

If you've been diagnosed with breast cancer and your doctor suspects, but doesn't yet know if you carry an altered BRCA1 or BRCA2 gene, decisions regarding your treatment are more complicated. This is because a formal evaluation of your genetic risk, which typically includes examination of your family history, genetic counseling and possible genetic testing, may take a few weeks.

Some women undergoing genetic testing choose to proceed with a lumpectomy to remove the tumor, along with sampling of the underarm (axillary) lymph nodes to check for cancer spread. They hold off on having more extensive surgery until they've received the results of the genetic tests. Other women choose to proceed with more extensive surgery, such as mastectomy, rather than being faced with the possibility of additional surgery in the future.

Once genetic test results are available, you and your doctor can make decisions regarding other possible treatments to help prevent the development of new breast tumors. Because the BRCA1 and BRCA2 genes also increase your risk of ovarian cancer, you and your doctor may also discuss strategies to prevent development of ovarian cancer.

For more information on the BRCA genes, see Chapter 5. For more information on cancer prevention strategies, including preventive (prophylactic) mastectomy, see Chapter 6. For more information on ovarian cancer, see Chapter 17.

Hodgkin disease survivors

Women who've had Hodgkin disease and received radiation therapy to lymph nodes in their chest as part of their treatment are at increased risk of developing breast cancer. This is especially true among women who received radiation therapy at younger ages.

Factors that play key roles in determining a woman's risk of breast cancer after treatment for Hodgkin disease include:

- **Age.** A female experiencing puberty when she receives treatment for Hodgkin disease is at greater risk because her breasts are exposed to radiation during the time when radiation has the greatest effect on growing breast cells. As a woman matures, her

risk decreases. Women age 30 or older when they receive radiation therapy to the chest area generally have a breast cancer risk similar to that of the general population.

- **Time.** Breast cancer often develops approximately 15 years after radiation treatment for Hodgkin disease. Therefore, a woman treated for Hodgkin disease should begin breast cancer screening about 10 years after her radiation treatments, or even earlier. Some researchers believe screening should begin as early as five years after receiving radiation therapy.

- **Radiation dose.** Older methods of radiation therapy involved higher doses of radiation and wider exposure of the breasts to radiation. The higher the dose of radiation received, the greater the subsequent risk of breast cancer. In recent years, treatment regimens for Hodgkin disease have greatly improved. Now, lower doses of radiation are used that more effectively target lymph node areas, reducing exposure to surrounding breast tissue.

Treatment

For Hodgkin disease survivors who later develop breast cancer, a mastectomy has been the standard treatment. Radiation therapy often isn't possible because normal breast tissues typically can't tolerate additional radiation therapy. However, because lower doses of radiation are now used to treat Hodgkin disease, it may be possible for some women to have a lumpectomy followed by breast radiation therapy, as long as the total amount of radiation they receive is within acceptable limits.

Because there's an increased risk that cancer may also develop in the other breast, some women choose to have prophylactic mastectomy in the other breast, along with mastectomy to the breast affected with the cancer.

Bilateral Breast Cancer

Only a small percentage of women with newly diagnosed breast cancer have cancer in both breasts at the time their cancer is diagnosed. Cancer in each breast is called synchronous bilateral breast cancer. Because breast cancer rarely spreads from one breast to the other in its early stages, the two tumors — one in each breast — are almost always two different breast cancers.

Bilateral breast cancers tend to be more common in women with a strong family history of breast cancer. Having bilateral breast cancer doesn't mean your prognosis is doubly worse. Similar to breast cancer that's confined to one breast, the prognosis for women with bilateral breast cancer depends on the characteristics of the individual tumors, including their size and whether the cancer has spread to the lymph nodes under the arm.

In this situation, prognosis is generally based on the tumor that has the least favorable characteristics.

Treatment

Treatment of synchronous bilateral breast cancer depends on the characteristics — size, grade and lymph node status — of each tumor. Options include a lumpectomy in each breast followed by radiation therapy or a mastectomy of each breast. Sometimes, based on the results of a sentinel node biopsy of each breast, the lymph nodes under one of the arms need to be removed but those under the other arm don't.

If you choose to have a lumpectomy, radiation therapy is also needed. Decisions regarding additional treatment (adjuvant therapy), such as chemotherapy or hormone therapy, are based on the characteristics of the tumors and whether one or both of them carries a high risk of recurrence.

See Chapter 11 for more information on the sentinel node biopsy procedure and adjuvant therapy.

Women who've had one breast cancer and later develop cancer in the other breast are said to have metachronous bilateral breast cancer. Treatment for metachronous bilateral breast cancer is based on the characteristics of the tumor being treated. When treating the second breast cancer, your doctor likely will take into account the type of therapy you received for your first breast cancer, as well as other factors, such as your family history.

Unknown Primary Cancers

Occasionally, a woman will develop an enlarged lymph node under her arm, yet doctors aren't able to find a tumor in her breast. If a biopsy of the enlarged lymph node indicates the presence of cancer, the tissue sample is studied closely under a microscope to determine if the cancer looks like breast cancer. The pathologist needs to make certain — as much as is possible — the cancer in the lymph node isn't something other than breast cancer, such as melanoma or lymphoma. If a different cancer isn't identified, the cancer is considered to be breast cancer and it's treated as such.

The breast located next to the affected lymph node is carefully examined to try and find a hidden tumor. This usually involves a complete physical examination, mammogram and ultrasound exam of the breast. If these aren't helpful, other tests may be used, such as magnetic resonance imaging (MRI) or a positron emission tomography (PET) scan.

If a tumor is found in the breast, a treatment regimen is developed, based on the size and grade of the tumor and number of lymph nodes involved. If no tumor is found and the cancer cells in the lymph nodes appear to be breast cancer cells, both the lymph nodes and the adjacent breast are treated.

In the past, treatment usually consisted of a mastectomy. In approximately half the cases in which a tumor couldn't be identified on diagnostic tests, the pathologist was able to locate cancer cells in the mastectomy specimen removed during surgery. However, even in women in whom no cancerous cells were found in the breast, their cancers generally behaved similarly to breast cancer. Today, an alternative to mastectomy is radiation of the breast with close follow-up screening for any developing tumors.

In virtually all cases, the lymph nodes in the affected underarm area are re-moved (axillary lymph node dissection). Treatment for such cancers also typically includes additional (adjuvant) therapy — chemotherapy, hormone therapy or both.

The prognosis for women with an unknown primary tumor is similar to that of other women with stage II or III breast cancer that has spread to the underarm lymph nodes.

Metaplastic Breast Cancer

Most breast cancers are classified as adenocarcinomas — a subset of carcinomas arising from glands or glandular tissue, such as that in your breasts.

Metaplastic breast cancer is a rare type of breast cancer that undergoes a process of transformation called metaplasia. The cells start out looking similar to adenocarcinomas and then transform into cells that take on a nonglandular growth pattern. This transformation may affect all of the cells within a tumor or only a small portion of them. When viewed under a microscope, metaplastic tumors typically display a mixture of adenocarcinoma-type cells and nonadenocarcinoma-type cells.

As in other breast cancers, the predominant indication of cancer is a lump in the breast. Metaplastic breast cancer is most often seen in women who are older than age 50, although it can occur at a younger age. Generally, this type of breast cancer doesn't spread to the lymph nodes under the arm, and its cells are hormone receptor negative.

In spite of the fact that the cancer generally doesn't spread to the lymph nodes, metaplastic breast cancer is often more aggressive than are adenocarcinomas, and it carries a higher risk of recurrence than do adenocarcinomas.

This type of cancer is generally treated with a lumpectomy or mastectomy. Your doctor may also recommend radiation therapy. Because metaplastic breast cancer is often hormone receptor negative, hormone therapy generally isn't effective. Chemotherapy to help prevent a recurrence would seem to be a logical choice, but experience has shown that this type of cancer often doesn't respond well to chemotherapy. At present, there's no drug therapy regimen that's been shown to be very beneficial against this particular type of breast cancer.

Lymphomas and Sarcomas

As was just mentioned, most breast cancers start in the glandular tissue of the breast, such as the ducts and lobules. A very few breast tumors — about 1 percent — develop in the lymphatic or connective tissues of the breast.

Tumors that originate in the lymphatic tissue are called lymphomas. Those that develop in the connective tissue are called sarcomas. Lymphomas and sarcomas are more likely to develop in other parts of the body than in the breast.

Breast lymphoma

Breast lymphoma is a rare condition. Like carcinomas of the breast, breast lymphoma typically develops into a mass, but its growth is usually more rapid than that of carcinomas of the breast. The lymphoma may also develop into multiple masses or it may occur in both breasts. Occasionally, this type of cancer is accompanied by night sweats, fever and weight loss. A biopsy is needed to confirm the diagnosis.

In general, breast lymphoma is treated with chemotherapy and radiation therapy. Surgery usually isn't an option, other than to establish a diagnosis, if necessary. A combination chemotherapy regimen called R-CHOP (ritaximab, cyclophosphamide, hydroxydaunomycin, Oncovin and prednisone) is often used. A review of breast lymphoma cases at one medical institution found that 11 out of 20 women treated with R-CHOP were still disease-free an average of 80 months (just under seven years) after their diagnoses.

Breast sarcoma

The most common type of breast sarcoma is called a phyllodes tumor. Phyllodes tumors are usually noncancerous (benign), but they can be cancerous. On a mammogram, the tumors appear similar to benign masses called fibroadenomas. Phyllodes tumors tend to occur in women earlier than the age at which most breast cancers tend to occur.

To make an accurate diagnosis, a biopsy is required. If the biopsy reveals a cancerous phyllodes tumor, prognosis is generally dependent on factors such as the grade and size of the tumor and the tissue margins.

The primary treatment for a breast sarcoma is to surgically remove the tumor along with a wide margin of healthy tis-

Radiation Therapy and Sarcoma Risk

Studies and reports of individual cases suggest that radiation therapy to treat breast adenocarcinomas, the most common type of breast cancer, carries an increased risk of development of a later sarcoma in the bone or tissue of the irradiated area.

To further investigate this issue, two groups of researchers reviewed data from the National Cancer Institute's Surveillance, Epidemiology, and End Results (SEER) program. SEER is a database that collects cancer-related information from nine areas in the United States. These areas collectively represent almost 10 percent of the population.

The investigators found that previous radiation therapy does increase a woman's risk of developing a sarcoma. But the increase in risk is extremely small — approximately 1 in 1,000 women over a 15-year period — and it doesn't outweigh the benefits that radiation therapy generally provides in treating breast adenocarcinomas.

sue. Depending on the size of the tumor and its relation to your breast size, your doctor may recommend either a lumpectomy or a mastectomy.

Because cancerous phyllodes tumors — if they do spread — tend to spread through the bloodstream, there's generally no need to examine lymph nodes under the arm. Phyllodes tumors, if they recur, tend to do so locally in the breast or spread to the lungs.

In addition to surgery, chemotherapy and radiation therapy are sometimes considered. However, unlike for treatment of typical breast cancer, there's much less proof that these therapies are effective in treating breast sarcomas.

Paget's Disease

Paget's disease of the breast is a rare form of breast cancer that starts in the breast ducts and spreads to the skin of the nip-

ple and the areola, the dark circle of skin around the nipple. Paget's disease of the breast isn't related to Paget's disease of the bone, a metabolic bone disease.

Paget's disease of the breast is most common in middle-aged women. Signs and symptoms may include:

- Crusted, scaly, red skin of the nipple and areola
- Nipple discharge, such as bleeding or oozing
- A burning or itching sensation in the nipple area
- A lump in the nipple area

Early detection of Paget's disease is important. If you have a lump or skin irritation in the nipple area that persists for more than one or two months, see your doctor. A doctor may be able to diagnose the cancer by testing nipple discharge for cancer cells or with a biopsy of the area.

Because of the underlying breast cancer associated with Paget's disease, a mammogram should be performed to check for any masses or abnormalities in the breast. Paget's disease can be associated with both noninvasive and invasive breast cancer.

Prognosis and treatment for Paget's disease depend on the size of the tumor and whether the cancer has spread to surrounding tissues or lymph nodes. A small, noninvasive tumor may require removal of just the nipple area and some surrounding tissue, followed by radiation therapy. A larger, more aggressive tumor may require a mastectomy.

Breast Cancer and Pregnancy

It's very difficult and emotionally trying when a woman is pregnant and is diagnosed with breast cancer. Fortunately, this is uncommon, occurring in about 1 in 3,000 pregnant women. Women who are told they have breast cancer while they are pregnant usually are in their 30s.

During pregnancy, the ducts and lobules in a woman's breasts multiply, blood vessels swell to allow for increased blood flow and the weight of the breasts can double. This makes the breasts dense and lumpy. As a result, it's difficult to examine the breasts, and mammography has an increased rate of false-negative results, meaning it doesn't detect cancer when cancer is present.

A careful examination of your breasts by your doctor is recommended at your first prenatal visit so he or she can be alert to any abnormalities that might occur later.

If a lump is detected during pregnancy, your doctor may do an ultrasound of your breast to see if the mass is a cyst or solid lump. If mammography or other radiological procedures are necessary, they usually can be done safely by shielding your abdomen and pelvis from radiation. Even if a mammogram comes back normal, but a worrisome mass can be felt, the mass should be biopsied. A biopsy is the surest way to determine if the lump is cancerous or benign. A biopsy is usually done as a needle procedure (see Chapter 8 for a description of biopsies).

If you're breast-feeding when the lump is detected, your doctor may advise that you stop before the biopsy is performed to reduce the risk of complications. Be assured, there's no evidence that cancer can spread to your baby through your breast milk.

Pregnancy itself doesn't appear to worsen your prognosis if you have breast cancer. Most studies indicate that the prognosis for women who are pregnant is similar to that for women at a similar age and with a similar stage of breast cancer who aren't pregnant. But the diagnosis may be delayed because a pregnant woman's breasts are changing, making a cancerous lump more difficult to detect. When detection is delayed, the cancer may be diagnosed at a later stage, decreasing the chances of successful treatment.

Termination of the pregnancy hasn't been shown to improve prognosis and is generally unnecessary.

Treatment

Treatment for breast cancer in a pregnant woman is similar to that for a nonpregnant woman, and is based on such factors as the size of the lump, its grade and the

Laura's Story

Laura was 34 years old, and she and her husband were expecting their second child when she found out that she had breast cancer. Her local doctor suggested termination of the pregnancy, but he also mentioned that he had read some articles in which pregnant women were able to continue their pregnancies while undergoing cancer treatment. Laura and her husband wanted to continue the pregnancy if at all possible, and they sought a second opinion with a cancer specialist.

After much discussion, explanation and careful consideration of the options, Laura, her husband and her doctors decided to continue the pregnancy but to proceed right away with a mastectomy. At the time of her surgery, Laura was five and a half months pregnant.

Unfortunately, Laura's prognosis was very poor. The surgery revealed a very large — 15-centimeter (about 6-inch) — tumor. The laboratory report also indicated cancer cells in 21 of 22 underarm (axillary) lymph nodes.

Knowing that chemotherapy was important to her survival chances, and with the assurance of her medical team that chemotherapy drugs probably wouldn't harm the baby, Laura agreed to have a couple of cycles of chemotherapy while she was still pregnant.

Approximately 10 weeks after her cancer diagnosis, Laura gave birth to a healthy baby girl by way of cesarean delivery. After the baby was born, Laura received additional chemotherapy followed by radiation therapy.

Laura says that the happiness of the pregnancy and the promise of another child made it easier for her to deal with her cancer. "I knew I had to be there to raise my children," Laura says.

After Laura completed her treatment, she met regularly with her doctor, who monitored Laura's health. Laura's doctor was concerned the cancer would recur, but at each checkup Laura reported feeling fine, and there were no indications of a cancer recurrence.

Laura's doctor finally felt comfortable that Laura would be OK when Laura brought with her to one of her checkups, the baby whose life she was determined to save — now a 15-year-old teenager.

extent of lymph node involvement. But modifications may be made to protect the fetus, depending on the trimester you're in. The first trimester is when fetal organ development takes place and is the period of greatest risk. Most medication is avoided during this time, if possible.

Surgery

If the cancer is stage I or II, surgery is usually recommended and is generally safe for both mother and fetus, especially after the first trimester. In the first trimester, anesthesia can be harmful. Traditionally, the procedure of choice has been a mastectomy along with evaluation of the underarm (axillary) lymph nodes with a sentinel node biopsy. The advantage of this option is that mastectomy may decrease the need for radiation therapy, which can be dangerous to a fetus.

Some women diagnosed in the late stages of their pregnancies choose to have a lumpectomy, followed by radiation after delivery of the baby. Even if you're far from delivery, lumpectomy may be an option, followed by chemotherapy after the first trimester and then radiation after the birth of the baby.

Surgery carries a slight risk of miscarriage or preterm labor, but it doesn't increase the risk of birth defects.

Radiation therapy

Radiation therapy generally isn't recommended in pregnant women because of possible risks to the fetus, such as miscarriage, birth defects and childhood cancer. It may also result in poor cosmetic results because of breast changes that occur during pregnancy.

Chemotherapy

In the first trimester, chemotherapy can cause miscarriage and fetal abnormalities, but this risk decreases substantially in the second and third trimesters, making its use an option in later stages of pregnancy. The chemotherapy drug methotrexate should be avoided, though, because it can have toxic effects on the placenta.

The long-term effects of chemotherapy on the child are unknown, but existing data suggest that it doesn't affect later growth and development. Because chemotherapy drugs can come through in your breast milk, breast-feeding isn't recommended during chemotherapy.

Hormone therapy

Hormone therapy generally isn't recommended for a woman who's pregnant, primarily because hormones can influence the pregnancy and may cause side effects in the fetus. After delivery, though, hormone therapy may be used in a woman whose cancer is hormone receptor positive. See Chapter 11 for more information.

Pregnancy after breast cancer

One of the questions related to breast cancer and pregnancy is whether it's safe to become pregnant after being diagnosed with breast cancer. In the past, there was concern about a later pregnancy because during pregnancy levels of female hormones increase, and these hormones are known to influence breast cancer development. The current feeling among doctors is that pregnancy following a diagnosis of breast cancer is generally safe. However, because many breast cancer recurrences tend to happen within the first few years after treatment, most doctors recommend waiting at least five years after treatment to become pregnant.

Sometimes, though, waiting so long may not be an option because doing so may place a woman outside the childbearing age. Ultimately, the decision is a personal one. The most important consideration usually revolves around your own risk of relapse.

Breast Cancer in Men

Breast cancer in men is uncommon. Approximately 1 percent of all breast cancers occur in men, and male breast cancer accounts for less than 1 percent of all cancers that occur in men.

In general, male breast cancer is similar to female breast cancer with a few differences. While hormone levels appear to influence the development of breast cancer in men, just as they do in women, in men, the influence appears to be related, in part, to an imbalance in the hormones estrogen and androgen. Approximately 85 percent of male breast cancers are estrogen receptor positive, and 70 percent are progesterone receptor positive. Men also tend to be older when they're diagnosed.

Risk factors

Factors that might increase a man's risk of breast cancer include:
- A family history of breast cancer, especially having a BRCA1 or BRCA2 mutation
- Testicular abnormalities, such as an undescended testicle, congenital inguinal hernia, inflammation of the testicle, removal of the testicles
- Liver troubles, such as cirrhosis
- Infertility
- Klinefelter's syndrome, a sex chromosome abnormality present at birth
- Radiation exposure
- Age
- Ashkenazi Jewish ancestry

The estimated breast cancer risk, up to age 70, in a man with a BRCA1 mutation is 1.2 percent (about 1 in 100). For a man with a BRCA2 mutation, it's 6.8 percent by age 70 (6 to 7 cancers per 100 men).

Diagnosis and staging

The predominant sign of male breast cancer is a painless breast mass. Other signs and symptoms include nipple retraction, pain or tenderness, an open sore on the nipple, nipple discharge and nipple bleed-

ing. Sometimes, no signs or symptoms are present.

Because men don't have much breast tissue, a mass can usually be easily felt. In some cases, mammography may be helpful in distinguishing between a benign mass and a malignant one. A biopsy is used to diagnose a mass that appears suspicious. If cancer is present, it's staged in the same way as female breast cancer — according to the tumor's size and spread.

Treatment

The standard treatment for male breast cancer is surgical removal of the tumor, if possible. The procedure most often recommended is a mastectomy, which involves removal of the breast tissue and evaluation of underarm lymph nodes (see Chapter 11 for more information). Radiation therapy also may be recommended to reduce the risk of a recurrence in the chest wall or regional lymph nodes.

Because so many male breast cancers are hormone receptor positive, hormone therapy is often recommended. The success of tamoxifen in female breast cancer has led to its use in men. Although no randomized clinical trials have been done to study the benefits of tamoxifen in men, data suggest that it may increase survival. Side effects of tamoxifen may include hot flashes and impotence. For men at high risk of recurrence, chemotherapy may be recommended after surgery.

If the cancer has spread (metastasized) to a distant part of the body, hormone therapy, chemotherapy or both may be recommended. For hormone receptor positive breast cancers, hormone therapy is usually given first.

Before tamoxifen came into widespread use for treatment of male breast cancer, the recommended hormone therapy was androgen ablation, which is essentially the removal of testosterone from the body. This was routinely done by removal of the testicles. Today, men are more commonly given drugs, such as luteinizing hormone-releasing hormone (LH-RH) agonists, to suppress testosterone production. These are the same medications used to suppress ovarian estrogen production in premenopausal women.

If one type of hormone therapy doesn't work, another may be used. If there's no response to any hormone therapies, chemotherapy may be considered.

Prognosis

Survival rates for men with breast cancer are similar to those of women with the same stage of the disease. Unfortunately, in men, breast cancer tends to be diagnosed at a later stage than in women, in part, due to reduced awareness.

As with women, prognostic factors that influence survival in men include lymph node status, tumor size and grade. Whether the cancer has spread to the lymph nodes is usually the most important prognostic factor.

Chapter 14: Breast Cancer

Follow-up and Surveillance

Understanding
Recurrent Cancer   226
Types of recurrences   226
Does early detection help? 227

Follow-up Care   228
Recommended tests   229
Tests that aren't
recommended   230
A look at the research   231

Dealing With Uncertainty   232

Finally, treatment of your breast cancer is over. For the past number of months, the diagnosis and treatment of your cancer has been an active and tangible part of your everyday life. During your treatment, you may have undergone surgery, radiation therapy, drug therapy or a combination of these approaches. You've likely interacted with a team of health care professionals on a regular basis, at times even daily.

But when the flurry of treatment activity is over, you may wonder, "Now what?" Certainly, you're grateful to be done with treatment, but now you may begin to worry about a cancer recurrence and find new concerns taking the place of old ones. Many questions may come to mind. Is there something that you can do to prevent the cancer from coming back or to catch it early if it does? How often should you see your doctor? Will you need to take tests? Which tests are most effective, and how often should you have them?

Monitoring for recurrent cancer is an important component of follow-up care. However, it's only one part of a follow-up program. Other important goals include addressing complications of treatment, meeting physical rehabilitation needs, monitoring your overall health and providing you with psychological support. Addressing all of these needs will help you as you take on what can be a challenging endeavor — reclaiming your life and returning to your "normal" routines (see Chapter 22).

An important point to keep in mind is that while guidelines are established for routine follow-up care after breast cancer treatment, each breast cancer survivor is unique. Just as with diagnosis and treatment, you and your doctor will ultimately decide together what's best for you once your treatment is complete.

Understanding Recurrent Cancer

One of the primary goals of follow-up care is to detect a possible return (recurrence) of your breast cancer. To understand which approach may be the most helpful in detecting a recurrence, it's important to know a bit about recurrent cancer.

When a cancerous tumor is first diagnosed, the cancer is known as a primary cancer. Recurrent cancer refers to cancer that later develops from cells that originally came from the primary tumor. The cells weren't visible at the time of diagnosis, and they weren't eliminated during treatment to remove or destroy the primary cancer. Over time, the cells were able to multiply to a size where they could be found.

Risk of a recurrence is dependent on the size of the original tumor, the number of lymph nodes that contained cancerous cells (lymph node involvement) and other factors discussed in Chapter 11. Women

with a very small tumor and no lymph node involvement have a lower chance of recurrence when compared with women with larger tumors or lymph node involvement.

Types of recurrences

Breast cancer recurrences are divided into three categories — local, regional and metastatic — depending on where the cancer returns.

Local
A local recurrence refers to the regrowth of cancer cells at the site of the original tumor. In women who had a previous lumpectomy, a local recurrence occurs in remaining breast tissue. Among women who had a mastectomy to treat a primary tumor, the cancer may recur locally along the mastectomy scar or in chest wall tissue. With a local recurrence, the cancer cells are still contained within the area where the cancer first began and may be responsive to local therapy such as surgery or radiation.

Sometimes, a new cancer — a new primary tumor — will develop in the other breast. Almost always, this new cancer is not a recurrence but, rather, a second primary cancer. The treatment of this cancer will depend on the characteristics of the cancer: size, lymph node involvement, hormone receptors and other factors discussed in Chapter 11.

Regional
When cancer cells travel from the site of the original tumor and settle in nearby lymph nodes — in the armpit or collarbone area — this is known as a regional

Recurrent Cancer or a New Cancer?

When cancer is detected in a breast that had previously been treated with a lumpectomy and radiation, two possible scenarios need to be considered.

One possibility is that the new tumor stems from cells that were leftover from the original tumor. When the cancer was originally treated, not all the cancer cells were removed or destroyed. This is known as recurrent breast cancer (in-breast recurrence). The other possibility is that the tumor is a new cancer that has developed in the breast. In this case,

the cancer would be referred to as a second, or new, primary cancer.

In some instances, it can be difficult to determine if a new tumor in a previously treated breast is a recurrent tumor or a new primary tumor. Some factors, though, can provide clues. The tumor is more likely to be recurrent cancer if the following are true:

• The new tumor developed less than five years after the original diagnosis.
• The new tumor developed in the same area of the breast as the original tumor.
• When examined under a microscope, the new tumor has an appearance similar to that of the original tumor.

recurrence. With a regional recurrence, the chances of treatment curing the cancer are lower than with a local recurrence, but a cure may still be possible.

Metastatic

In the case of a metastatic recurrence, cancer cells from the original site have traveled to distant parts of the body. The bones, lungs and liver are organs commonly affected by metastatic breast cancer. With metastatic recurrence, a cure generally isn't possible, although effective treatment is available that can prolong survival.

Does early detection help?

The real question regarding tests to detect recurrent cancer is this: Will early detection — identification of recurrent cancer before it produces signs or symptoms — result in a woman living longer or better?

For localized and regional breast cancer recurrences, the answer seems to be yes. Treatments such as mastectomy and radiation may be able to cure the cancer. For regional recurrences, the chance of a cure is lower.

For a metastatic recurrence, no evidence, to date, suggests that early detection of metastatic breast cancer and early initiation of treatment results in longer life expectancy or better quality of life. This can be difficult to understand and accept, but the evidence is strong and consistent. If the cancer cells were able to survive the initial treatment of the disease and they've spread to other tissues, it's highly unlikely that they'll be destroyed with treatment for metastatic disease.

This harsh reality has come to have a significant effect on recommendations for follow-up care after treatment.

Signs and Symptoms to Watch For

Remember that you know your body best, and you know what feels normal and what doesn't.

Most women discover a breast cancer recurrence themselves, before their doctors do. Therefore, it's important to be aware of signs and symptoms that may suggest a recurrence.

If you experience any of the following, talk to your doctor. He or she can evaluate your signs and symptoms further, and together the two of you can decide on the appropriate plan of action.

Signs and symptoms of a breast cancer recurrence may include:

• New, unexplained, persistent pain, such as in your bones, chest or abdomen
• Changes or new lumps in your breasts or surgical scars, or in surrounding tissue
• Unexplained changes in your weight, particularly weight loss
• Any shortness of breath, difficulty breathing or unexplained cough
• Any other persistent, abnormal sensation or occurrence that bothers you

Check your breasts monthly to look for changes. If you have questions, ask your doctor for instructions on how to examine your breasts after cancer treatment.

Follow-up Care

The purpose of follow-up care is to monitor your overall physical and emotional health, respond to complications from your treatment, and watch for indications that your cancer may have returned. Monitoring for recurrent cancer may sound like an involved process, but it includes fewer tests than you might expect.

Years ago, follow-up testing usually involved various blood tests, chest X-rays and bone scans. But recommendations now support limiting testing to medical histories, physical examinations and regular mammograms. Still, a wide range of practices exist: Some women receive a number of tests, and others only a few. This is because some women, and some doctors, don't feel comfortable if they don't take advantage of all the tests available.

Because of these differences, a women may wonder if she's not getting enough tests — if her doctors should be doing more. The truth is, it's not test results that most often lead to a diagnosis of recurrent cancer but rather changes in how a woman feels or the development of a new lump. Tests often used to help identify recurrent cancer — blood tumor marker studies, liver function tests and X-rays — haven't been found to be effective or useful in prolonging survival or improving quality of life.

In the pages that follow, we'll take a look at which tests are recommended by the American Society of Clinical Oncology — an organization that has developed guidelines for follow-up care after breast cancer treatment — as well as which tests this group doesn't recommend.

Recommended tests

The American Society of Clinical Oncology recommends the following steps for routine follow-up care in women who've been treated for early-stage breast cancer and who have no signs or symptoms of cancer.

Medical history

For the first three years after completion of your initial treatment, you'll likely see your doctor every three to six months. Chances are, your visit will begin with your doctor updating your medical history. You'll most likely be asked about your general health since your last appointment, any changes in your body that you may have noticed and any concerns you may have. This is a good time to ask questions about issues such as diet, exercise and hot flashes, as well as questions regarding breast reconstruction or prostheses. You may want to write down your questions and bring them to your appointment.

After the first three years, your checkups may become less frequent. You may need to see your doctor only every six to 12 months for the next two years, and annually after that. If you were treated for noninvasive cancer, such as ductal carcinoma *in situ* (DCIS), your follow-up exams may be less frequent, such as twice a year for the first five years and yearly after that.

Physical exam

After your doctor takes your medical history, a physical examination generally follows. Like a medical history, a physical exam is recommended every three to six months for the first three years after primary treatment, every six to 12 months for the next two years and annually after that. For women who've had a lumpectomy and radiation therapy, breast examinations at six-month intervals may be recommended for up to 10 years.

During your physical exam, your doctor will check for any signs of cancer recurrence. This may include:

- A careful examination of the area where the cancer originally occurred, including the incision site, remaining breast tissue and the chest wall
- A careful examination of your other breast
- An examination of lymph node areas around your armpits, collarbone and neck

Your doctor may also listen to your lungs for any breathing abnormalities and check for liver enlargement and any sign of bone tenderness.

If you've been taking the medication tamoxifen and you haven't had a hysterectomy, your doctor will likely recommend a yearly examination, because tamoxifen slightly increases the risk of uterine cancer.

Mammography

An annual mammogram is recommended for all women who've had breast cancer, with the exception of women who've had bilateral mastectomies. In addition to a medical history and physical examination, this is the only other procedure that's routinely recommended after cancer treatment. A mammogram can detect a local recurrence in the affected breast or a new tumor in the other breast. Studies show there's no advantage to doing mammograms more than once a year, provided no peculiar areas showed up on past mammograms, which might prompt more frequent examinations.

If you've had a lumpectomy, your doctor may want you to have a mammogram of that breast six months after completion of your radiation treatment and yearly after that. If you've had a mastectomy, you still need to have a yearly mammogram of your other breast. In the case of a bilateral mastectomy, there's no need for further mammograms, but a chest wall examination is recommended.

Newer options

Among some women, particularly those with dense breast tissue, a tumor can be difficult to detect with standard mammography. One option for identifying hard-to-find tumors is magnetic resonance imaging (MRI), but the procedure has downsides, including intravenous injection of a dye. While very safe, there is a risk of rare side effects. MRI of the breast can also be overly sensitive, picking up "areas of concern," which upon further testing, aren't cancer. This results in not only unnecessary concern, but added expense due to the need for additional testing.

Another option being studied is called molecular breast imaging (MBI), which is discussed in Chapter 7. This new screening method identifies tumors in dense tissue that often aren't visible with mammography. With MBI, a woman is given an injection of a low-dose, short-lived radioactive agent. This material accumulates in tumor cells more than it does in normal cells. Using a radiation-detecting camera, tumors show up as hot spots on the resulting image.

A Mayo Clinic study comparing MBI with mammography found that MBI detected three times as many cancers in women with dense breast tissue who had an increased risk of breast cancer. Another advantage of the procedure is that there's not as much pressure placed on the breasts as in standard mammography. In addition, the procedure is less expensive than breast MRI.

It's hoped that in the near future this test will be more widely available for use in detecting new and recurrent cancers.

Tests that aren't recommended

For some women — perhaps even you — follow-up visits to the doctor involve a barrage of tests, including some or all of the following:

- A chest X-ray to check for lung abnormalities
- An ultrasound to check for liver tumors
- A bone scan to check for bone cancer
- A computerized tomography (CT) scan or magnetic resonance image (MRI) to look for cancer in the soft tissues and organs of the chest, abdomen and pelvis
- A blood test (blood tumor marker study) to check for certain substances in the blood that may be elevated in people with cancer
- A complete blood count (CBC) to check levels of white and red blood cells and blood platelets
- Liver and kidney function tests to check that these organs are functioning normally

These tests were once more commonly performed in an effort to detect a cancer recurrence before it produced signs and symptoms. But there's no evidence — despite multiple studies — that the tests prolong survival or improve quality of life. That is why these tests aren't recommended by the American Society of Clinical Oncology.

In addition, these tests aren't always accurate — they may miss signs of a recurrence or, just the opposite, suggest cancer is there when none exists. Test results that are wrong or inconclusive can cause a lot of needless stress and anxiety and create the need for additional testing.

A look at the research

A number of investigations have been done to try to assess the role of intensive testing in the routine follow-up care of women with no evidence of breast cancer after treatment. So far, the evidence indicates that such testing doesn't have a significant effect in helping to prolong survival or improve quality of life.

Key studies

The strongest evidence against most follow-up tests comes from two large Italian studies that focused on intensive screening for breast cancer recurrences.

In the first study, 622 women had intensive follow-up testing including regular physical exams and yearly mammograms, plus chest X-rays and bone scans every six months. An additional 621 women followed the same schedule for physical exams and yearly mammograms, but received no other tests. This was known as the clinical follow-up group. The investigators found

that even though cancer that recurred in bone and the lungs was detected earlier in the intensive testing group, there was no difference between the two groups in the detection of metastatic recurrences at other sites or in the detection of local and regional recurrences. And most importantly, there was no improvement in survival 10 years later. The conclusion was that intensive follow-up with chest X-rays and bone scans doesn't offer any survival advantage to women with breast cancer.

In the second study, 655 women had intensive testing consisting of regular physical exams, yearly mammograms and bone scans, liver ultrasounds, chest X-rays, and blood tests every six months. Another 665 women were enrolled in clinical follow-up consisting of regular physical exams and yearly mammograms only. After six years, there was no significant difference in death rates between the two groups. The trial also measured quality of life and found no difference there either.

Blood tumor markers

Tumors can sometimes make unique proteins or other substances that can be measured in the bloodstream. These are usually referred to as tumor markers. To date, there's no ideal tumor marker or combination of markers that's specific for breast cancer, but some markers may suggest the presence of breast cancer. Examples include CA 15-3, CA 27-29 and carcinoembryonic antigen (CEA).

The question arises: Would these blood tests be helpful in detecting recurrent breast cancer? Currently, no available data suggest that the tests are accurate enough to detect a cancer recurrence early enough to improve a woman's chances of survival.

In addition, these substances also exist in healthy people who don't have cancer, meaning that a woman could receive a positive test result, indicating a cancer recurrence when, in fact, there's no recurrence. This is what's known as a false-positive test result. Such tests may also miss certain recurrences.

Finally — even when they work accurately — it appears that blood markers indicate a cancer recurrence only a couple of months before the recurrence would be detected in other ways, such as by a physical examination or the development of signs or symptoms.

As a result, the best use of blood tumor markers is to help diagnose a cancer recurrence when signs and symptoms suggest the cancer may be back.

Imaging tests

Some imaging tests may be better at detecting recurrent breast cancer than is mammography or ultrasound, but these tests haven't been fully evaluated in clinical trials to determine their potential benefits. These include such tests as computerized tomography (CT) scans, magnetic resonance imaging (MRI) and positron emission tomography (PET) scans.

For women who aren't experiencing any signs or symptoms of recurrent cancer, these imaging tests generally aren't recommended because there's no conclusive evidence that they're beneficial.

However, if you do develop signs or symptoms suggestive of a cancer recurrence, your doctor may order an imaging test to help determine if cancer is present, and where.

Dealing With Uncertainty

One of the most difficult aspects of follow-up care after primary breast cancer treatment is dealing with the uncertainty of whether the cancer will come back. Some women feel that testing will help them deal with this uncertainty. When asked, most women say they want to be tested for a possible recurrence. And why not? Learning that your test results were normal can relieve a lot of anxiety and let you breathe a sigh of relief, at least until the next round of testing.

But testing has its pitfalls. Often tests will reveal a slight deviation or small abnormality that may need to be evaluated. And one test often leads to more tests, especially because very few tests are definitive enough to produce certain results by themselves.

For example, the results of your liver function test may come back a few points above the upper normal limit. Your doctor may tell you that this likely doesn't signify a cancer recurrence, but you probably should have it rechecked in a couple of months just to make sure it isn't going up. If the next test shows that the results are slightly higher, you and your doctor will likely want to investigate further and do a more definitive test, such as a CT scan. The CT scan might note a normal liver but suggest a worrisome shadow around the pancreas. An ultrasound might then be obtained, revealing a normal pancreas. You feel great relief when you get all of the results and learn that everything is OK, but waiting for them may have caused a great deal of

Musa's Story

My own love-hate relationship with testing came to a head about two years ago, when my oncologist referred me to a cardiologist because of some minor chest pain I had while exercising. A stress test showed nothing, nor did a thallium stress test, where a radioactive isotope helped with imaging the blood vessels. ...

... "It's probably indigestion," said the cardiologist, unconcerned. But if I wanted a further level of certainty, he told me, there was a new test available, called an ultrafast CT scan of the heart. ... I went ahead with the scan, without a thought in the world about how it might relate to my breast cancer history.

My coronary arteries were, blessedly, completely clear of calcium deposits. But in the report, the radiologist made notations about nodules in my lungs. And there were unexplained "densities" in my liver. ... I remember sitting there with the report in my hand, my heart pounding. I could feel the blood draining from my face. Now what? I had no symptoms, and I felt fine. Or I had until I'd read the test results.

My oncologist thought the nodules would likely be from my smoking history, although I'd quit 25 years before. He recommended an MRI of my liver, to further check the "densities." ... Days later came the definitive answer: I had hepatic cysts, a benign condition that probably would never have caused me any problems. Mixed with a huge sense of relief was a growing conviction that this sequence of tests, and the weeks of anxiety attending them, had probably been unnecessary. Yet once set in motion, the progression of events had been impossible to stop.

Margaret's Story

Margaret Gilseth was diagnosed with breast cancer in 1957. In the decades that followed, she had multiple breast cancer recurrences and, as a result, ran the gamut of testing — blood tests and chest X-rays at almost every doctor's visit. (Read more about Margaret on page 267.) Then she began seeing a new oncologist who relied mostly on medical histories and physical exams. At first, Margaret was worried her doctor wasn't taking good care of her. After talking with him and doing some research, Margaret, an author, wrote an article on follow-up testing, which appeared in an issue of the *Journal of Clinical Oncology*. Following is an excerpt:

We live in a culture that worships technology, and the voice of the testing is more credible than the voice of our doctor. Because testing is frequently performed, we are conditioned to believe that a test will detect an early recurrent cancer and bring hope for our survival. I believe it is imperative that patients be informed of recent research that pertains to their situation. We need to learn to discriminate as new research results are available — to re-examine our myths. ...

... For me reassurance came with new understanding, and that came with learning the truth from my doctor. Routine testing for (recurrent) breast cancer is not very helpful, because it seldom detects cancer before a doctor can, and in those cases in which it does, there is no substantial benefit from early institution of chemotherapy. Nothing can take the place of a good doctor-patient relationship. As I learn to live with insecurity, the minimal assurance given by routine testing becomes irrelevant.

Caring for Your Whole Self

In addition to the physical aspects of follow-up care, it's important to remember the emotional and spiritual components. Adjusting to life after breast cancer takes time and requires the strong support of family and friends. Many women find it helpful to join a support group where they can learn about the experiences of other breast cancer survivors and share their own experiences. Another important aspect of caring for yourself after breast cancer is learning to trust your body to tell you when something is wrong.

For some women, adjusting to life after cancer treatment also means concentrating on those aspects of their lives they can control. This includes eating well, exercising, getting enough rest, and learning to deal with stress and anxiety.

For more information on living with cancer, see Part 3, "Life After a Cancer Diagnosis."

additional and, in the end, unnecessary anxiety.

Musa Mayer, a breast cancer survivor and nationally known breast cancer advocate, illustrates this all-too-common scenario in her book *After Breast Cancer*. On page 233 is an excerpt from the book.

It's also important to remember that just as tests can sometimes find more than you want them to, they can also miss things, such as a cancer recurrence. Negative results aren't a guarantee that no cancer is present.

Chapter 15: Breast Cancer

If the Cancer Comes Back

Types of Recurrence	236
Local recurrence	236
Regional recurrence	236
Metastatic recurrence	236
How Cancer Cells Spread	237
Local Recurrence	238
Recurrence after lumpectomy	238
Recurrence after mastectomy	241
Regional Recurrence	242
Types	242
Signs and symptoms	243
Tests	244
Treatment	244
Prognosis	244
Metastatic Recurrence	244
Signs and symptoms	244
Biopsy	245
Other tests	245
Prognosis and treatment	246

Cancer recurrence refers to the return of cancer. Most women who are treated for early stage breast cancer remain disease-free, but some do experience a recurrence. When a cancer recurs, it means that some cancer cells remained in the body after cancer treatment and these cells have begun to grow.

Recurrence may occur weeks, months, years or even decades after an initial diagnosis. Sometimes, the cancer returns in the same location as the original tumor. Other times, it recurs in a different location. For example, a few cells from a breast tumor may have spread to bone by way of the bloodstream. These cells weren't eliminated during treatment, and eventually they multiplied to a size that could be detected.

For many women, dealing with a cancer recurrence is more difficult than dealing with an initial diagnosis. Recurrence is often a breast cancer survivor's greatest fear. If your cancer does come back, you may feel as if you've lost the battle against the disease and that all your efforts were in vain. But this is not necessarily the case. The treatments you received may have actually delayed the cancer recurrence, giving you additional time you might not have had otherwise.

Although it's true that most breast cancer recurrences aren't curable, for some, there is potential for a cure, depending on where the recurrence is located. Even if a cure isn't possible, treatments can help maintain your quality of life and control the cancer, sometimes for many years.

Types of Recurrence

Breast cancer recurrence is generally categorized by location. It can be local, regional, distant or a combination of these.

Local recurrence

A local recurrence means the cancer redevelops in the same spot, or vicinity, as the primary tumor. For example, if you had a lumpectomy in your right breast and the cancer recurs in that same breast, that's a local recurrence. This type of local recurrence is called an in-breast recurrence.

It's possible that a new primary tumor may develop in the breast of a woman who has had a lumpectomy. A new primary tumor isn't the same as a recurrent tumor, although the two can be difficult to distinguish. A general rule of thumb is that if cancer is found in the same breast 10 or more years after the first tumor, it's considered a new primary tumor. Recurrent cancer tends to develop sooner — usually less than five years from the initial diagnosis. In some cases, a new primary tumor may develop in the opposite breast. This isn't a recurrence either. Rather, it's treated as a new primary breast cancer.

If you've had a breast removed (mastectomy) and cancer appears in your chest wall near where the breast had been, that also is a local recurrence.

Regional recurrence

A regional recurrence means that cancer cells have broken away from the original tumor site and they are appearing in nearby lymph nodes, such as those under your arm, near your breastbone or above your collarbone.

Local and regional recurrences may occur simultaneously. The two are often lumped together and termed local-regional recurrences. In this situation, there isn't any proof that the cancer has spread to more distant parts of the body.

Metastatic recurrence

A metastatic recurrence is when the original cancer cells have managed to travel to other organs or tissues in your body besides your breast, chest area or nearby lymph nodes. This type of cancer is called metastatic because the cancer has been identified in places away from the original tumor site. Other terms that are sometimes used are *systemic* or *distant recurrence*, because the cancer is now affecting more than one part of your body — more than just your breast and the area around it.

Most often breast cancer cells spread to bone. Other sites of metastases include the lungs and liver. Less often, the cancer spreads to the brain or other areas of the central nervous system.

Although it seems logical that a local recurrence would come first, then a regional recurrence and then a distant one, it isn't always this orderly. Many times a distant recurrence will occur without a local or regional recurrence.

How Cancer Cells Spread

The manner in which cancer spreads to your lymph nodes and other parts of your body is a long and complicated process. Most cancer cells don't make the journey, but some of the ones that do are hardy enough to establish themselves in other tissues and survive there.

Normally, the cells that make up the organs and tissues of your body, including your breasts, are held in place by a substance called an extracellular matrix. For cancer cells to travel outside of your breast, they must first break through this extracellular matrix. They appear to do this by breaking down the matrix with enzymes or by altering the adhesiveness of their own cell surface.

Once they're free of this matrix, cancer cells can invade nearby tissues or travel through the lymphatic system or bloodstream to other more distant organs and tissues. Your lymphatic system is a network of channels throughout your body, similar to your circulatory system, but instead of carrying blood, it carries lymphatic fluid and immune cells.

With breast cancer, cancerous (malignant) cells that have broken free of the original tumor may be swept along with the lymphatic fluid that drains from your breast tissue and eventually may end up in your axillary lymph nodes — bean-shaped structures of lymph tissue located under your arm. Some of the cancer cells may be destroyed in the lymph nodes, which are full of scavenging white blood cells that ingest and destroy foreign substances. But some cancer cells may

Is It Now Bone or Lung Cancer?

Breast cancer cells have a different makeup from bone, lung or liver cancer cells. They evolve differently, progress differently and respond differently to various therapies. When breast cancer cells spread to another part of your body — such as your bones, lungs or liver — they're still breast cancer cells, but they're growing in a different area. Breast cancer cells that are found in your bones don't become bone cancer. You still have breast cancer, only now it's called metastatic breast cancer in your bones.

One doctor uses the following analogy to explain this concept: If dandelions are growing in the yard and they go to seed, and the wind spreads this seed to the rose garden, allowing the dandelions to grow in the rose garden, these flowers aren't called roses. They're dandelions that have spread to the rose garden. In the same manner, if breast cancer cells spread within the body and start growing in the bone, they don't become bone cancer, but breast cancer spread to bone.

This is important because breast, bone, lung and liver cancers behave differently and are treated differently. For example, lung cancer cells aren't affected by estrogen in the way that breast cancer cells are. Therefore, lung cancer wouldn't respond to estrogen-related drugs such as tamoxifen, but breast cancer cells in your lungs may.

evade immune cells and survive and multiply in the lymph nodes, or they may travel on within the lymph system.

To get into your bloodstream, cancer cells may burrow their way through a blood vessel wall (see the color illustration on page 35). Once the cells are in the bloodstream, they're swept along with the flow of blood and may be carried to parts of your body far from your breast. Like your lymphatic system, however, your bloodstream is also full of immune cells capable of destroying cancer cells that make their way in. Still, some cancer cells may survive the ride. These cells can become lodged in the smaller branches of your blood vessel network. From there, they burrow their way out of the blood vessel into nearby tissue — such as bone, lung or liver — where they may survive and grow in a different environment from which they originated.

Local Recurrence

Breast cancer can recur in your remaining breast tissue after a lumpectomy and radiation or in your chest wall tissue after a mastectomy. There are some differences between the two, so we'll discuss each separately. Some general factors, though, that might increase your risk of these types of local recurrences include:
- A young age (less than 40) at diagnosis
- A primary tumor that's 5 centimeters (about 2 inches) or more in diameter
- A high tumor grade, indicating markedly abnormal cancer cells
- Cancer cells at the margin of the removed tissue or close to it
- Cancer in the lymph nodes

- Tumors that involve breast skin, such as inflammatory breast cancer, or the chest wall
- Tumors that are triple negative (see page 199)

Some factors that may be in your favor if you have a local recurrence, regardless of your initial treatment, include:
- A long interval — a period of more than five years — from when your cancer was first diagnosed until it recurred. This is called the disease-free interval.
- An isolated local recurrence.

Characteristics such as these are called prognostic factors, which can help predict disease outcome. Keep in mind, though, that these are generalizations about a complex disease, and your individual outcome isn't based solely on such factors. Prognostic factors are mentioned throughout this chapter, but remember they serve only to give you a general picture. Nobody can know absolutely what will happen in your future.

Recurrence after lumpectomy

The risk of a local recurrence after undergoing a lumpectomy and radiation for stage I or II breast cancer is very low. When a recurrence does happen, it's often an isolated local recurrence, meaning the recurrence isn't widespread throughout the breast and there isn't evidence the cancer has spread (metastasized) to distant locations.

Among women whose initial cancer was invasive and who experience an in-breast recurrence, in most cases the recurrent cancer is also invasive. In a small percentage of cases, the recurrent cancer is noninvasive (carcinoma *in situ*). Among women who initially had ductal carcinoma *in situ* (DCIS) and who experience an in-breast recurrence, the recurrent cancer is invasive in about 50 percent of cases.

Signs and symptoms

About one-third of in-breast recurrences are detected by mammography before they can be felt. Another third are detected by self- or clinical examination and another third by a combination of the two. The signs of an in-breast recurrence are generally the same as those of a new primary breast cancer, such as an unusual lump or a new change in your breast skin. But cancer can be a bit subtle the second time around, and sometimes it may be confused with a noncancerous (benign) abnormality. For one thing, surgery can produce changes in your breast, including mass-like areas of scar tissue, lumps of fatty tissue (fat necrosis) and scar tissue around the stitches used to close the incision (suture granulomas). Radiation can also cause scarring and increase decay of fatty tissue, which can make detection of a recurrence more difficult.

Often, breast changes that occur soon after treatment — for instance, within the first year — are benign, and often a result of treatment. However, it's still important to point out the change to your doctor so that it can be monitored.

Occasionally, some women develop a breast infection (mastitis), which is characterized by inflammation, swelling and redness. Mastitis is easily treated with antibiotics, but your doctor will want to make sure that it's not inflammatory breast cancer, a type of breast cancer that involves the skin and has features similar to mastitis.

So what should you watch out for? In general, report to your doctor any changes you notice in your breast, if only for your own peace of mind. Be particularly aware of these signs and symptoms:

- A new, firm lump or nodule in your breast or an irregular area of firmness
- A new thickening in a breast area
- A new pain in your breast
- Dimpling or indentation in your breast
- A skin rash, swelling or inflammation
- Progressive flattening of your nipple or other nipple changes

If you notice any of these signs and symptoms, tell your doctor so that they can be evaluated further.

Tests

If you and your doctor suspect an in-breast recurrence because of results of a mammogram or physical examination, your doctor may use another imaging test, such as ultrasound, magnetic resonance image (MRI), positron emission tomography (PET) scan, or a combination of these, to try to determine whether the suspicious finding is benign or malignant.

You'll likely need a biopsy to confirm the presence or absence of cancer. Because the hormone receptor status of your cancer may change with a recurrence — the cells that survive may be a subpopulation of the original tumor — if cancer is found, the biopsy sample may again be tested for the presence of estrogen and progesterone receptors. The specimen may also be tested for signs of overproduction of the HER2 protein. Both the hormone receptor status and HER2 status are important in determining what types of therapy would be appropriate to treat the recurrent cancer.

Because some women who develop an in-breast recurrence also have distant metastases, other tests will likely be done to determine if the cancer has spread to other parts of the body. These tests may include a chest X-ray and other imaging tests, such as a computerized tomography (CT) scan, bone scan, PET scan or MRI. In addition, a complete blood count and liver function tests, as well as other blood tests may be performed.

Treatment

Treatment for an in-breast recurrence that occurs after a lumpectomy may include surgery, radiation therapy or drug therapy.

Surgery

Assuming there's no evidence the cancer has spread to other locations, an in-breast recurrence is usually treated with a mastectomy. In some cases, a lumpectomy may be done, but using a lumpectomy to treat this type of recurrence is controversial. A lumpectomy carries a higher risk of yet another recurrence that may be more serious.

Because a local breast recurrence may be accompanied by hidden cancer in nearby lymph nodes, your doctor may remove some or all of the lymph nodes under your arm (axillary dissection) during surgery if they weren't removed during your initial treatment.

Radiation therapy

If you haven't had any previous radiation, your doctor will likely recommend it now. However, most women who undergo lumpectomy for their initial cancer also receive radiation. So, a second course of radiation usually isn't be an option.

Not much data exist on the use of repeat radiation in women who received radiation to treat their original tumors. Plus, receiving additional doses of radiation may increase your risk of radiation-related side effects.

Drug therapy

If an in-breast recurrence is so extensive that surgery isn't an option, your doctor may recommend chemotherapy, hormone therapy or both to treat the cancer. Most local recurrences, however, can be treated with surgery.

A decision to use chemotherapy, hormone therapy or both depends on a number of factors, including whether you received either to treat your initial cancer, and what type of treatment you had. Other important factors include your menopausal status, how long it has been since your initial diagnosis (your disease-free interval), details regarding your tumor, such as its hormone receptor status and HER2 status, and whether you have other health problems.

Prognosis

An in-breast recurrence is a sign the disease is still active, and it puts you at an increased risk of other recurrences in distant sites. The risk of metastisis after an in-breast recurrence varies according to a woman's lymph node status at her original diagnosis. Women who were node-positive have a higher risk of later metastisis than women who were node-negative. Other factors that may predict outcome include:

- **Longer time between treatment and recurrence.** The longer the interval between your initial cancer and the recurrence, the better. In general, an interval greater than five years is considered favorable for long-term survival, but some studies have shown that intervals of even two years or more can signify a better outcome than if the recurrence occurred sooner. The sooner a cancer returns, the more likely it is to be fast-growing (aggressive) with a higher risk of spread.

- **Noninvasive recurrence.** A noninvasive cancer recurrence signifies a better outcome than does an invasive one.
- **Isolated recurrence.** Recurrent cancer that's isolated to a small area of the breast is better than is a widespread in-breast recurrence or a regional recurrence involving the lymph nodes.

Recurrence after mastectomy

Among women who have a mastectomy to treat breast cancer, about 5 to 10 percent experience a cancer recurrence in their chest wall tissue, either alone or in combination with other recurrences. Cancer recurrence on the chest wall is more likely in women whose original breast cancer had spread to lymph nodes. A local chest wall recurrence tends to occur within 10 years of initial treatment, but some local recurrences have been reported 15, 25 and even 50 years after a mastectomy.

In about two-thirds of the women who experience a chest wall recurrence after mastectomy, at the time the recurrence is diagnosed there are no indications that the cancer has also spread to distant locations. In the other third, there's evidence the cancer has spread to other areas of the body.

Signs and symptoms

A local recurrence after a mastectomy usually appears as a painless nodule in or under your chest wall skin. It most often develops in or near the mastectomy scar. About half the local chest wall recurrences appear as a solitary nodule, while the rest show up as multiple nodules. Occasionally, a chest wall recurrence may appear as a red, often itchy skin rash.

Among women who've had tissue flap breast reconstruction, a recurrence may develop in the skin near the stitches or in the remaining chest wall skin, but a recurrence in the flap itself is rare. Recurrences isolated to the chest wall muscle also are rare. Benign lumps and fat necrosis, another benign condition, are fairly common with tissue flap reconstruction. If a lump occurs, a doctor may want to do a biopsy to make sure the diagnosis is correct.

Tests

Almost all chest wall recurrences after mastectomy are detected by physical examination. In breast reconstruction using a tissue flap, mammography or magnetic resonance imaging (MRI) may help distinguish between a cancerous mass and a noncancerous mass. A biopsy can confirm the presence of cancer. The biopsy specimen will likely be tested for estrogen and progesterone receptor status and HER2 status.

Again, because of the possibility of distant recurrence, your doctor will likely request other tests also, including a chest X-ray and other imaging tests, such as a CT scan, bone scan, PET scan or MRI. A complete blood count and liver function tests, as well as other blood tests also may be performed.

Treatment

A chest wall recurrence after a mastectomy is typically treated with surgery, if possible, as well as radiation and medication — chemotherapy, hormone therapy or both.

Surgery

If the recurrent cancer is a solitary nodule that can be fairly easily removed, surgery may be done. If the disease is more extensive, surgery usually isn't recommended.

Radiation therapy

If you haven't received radiation before, your doctor will likely recommend it now. Radiation therapy after a mastectomy may provide the most effective local treatment for a chest wall recurrence.

Usually, the whole chest wall area is treated. This may include the area around your collarbone to reach nearby lymph nodes, which are at increased risk of recurrence. Sometimes — especially if some cancer still remains in the chest wall after surgery — an additional boost of radiation is given directly to the area of recurrence.

Chemotherapy and hormone therapy

Medication (systemic therapy) may be recommended after surgery and radiation to reduce the risk of another local recurrence or a metastatic recurrence. There aren't any good studies to direct doctors regarding the use of systemic therapy in preventing additional recurrences, but some studies suggest it can be helpful.

Prognosis

Compared with an in-breast recurrence after lumpectomy, a chest wall recurrence after mastectomy carries a considerably higher risk of eventual spread of the cancer to distant sites. Nonetheless, certain factors may indicate a better prognosis:

- **Longer time between treatment and recurrence.** This is very important. The longer the time between when you were initially diagnosed with cancer and your recurrence, the better the situation.
- **Isolated recurrence.** An isolated chest wall recurrence, particularly a single nodule, often has a better outcome than does a widespread local recurrence.
- **Complete excision.** Removal of the recurrent tumor, with no cancer cells located in the margins of the removed tissue, signifies a better outcome.
- **Estrogen receptor status.** A recurrent cancer that's estrogen receptor positive may respond to hormone therapy, which may improve survival.

Regional Recurrence

After a mastectomy or lumpectomy and radiation, it's possible for cancer to recur in the lymph nodes near the breast that was treated. This is known as a regional recurrence. A regional recurrence can occur by itself, but often it occurs simultaneously with a local recurrence and is referred to as a local-regional recurrence.

Types

Regional breast cancer recurrences are generally divided into one of three categories:
- **Axillary node recurrence.** Cancer is diagnosed in the lymph nodes located under the arm by the treated breast.

- **Supraclavicular node recurrence.** Cancer is present in the lymph nodes above your collarbone. Occasionally, the cancer may also recur in lymph nodes just below your collarbone (infraclavicular lymph nodes).
- **Internal mammary node recurrence.** Cancer is present in a group of lymph nodes located along your breastbone in the center of your chest.

Signs and symptoms

The first sign of a regional recurrence is usually a swelling or lump in the affected lymph nodes, such as those under your arm, in the groove above your collarbone or in the area around your breastbone.

Because your internal mammary nodes are located deep within your chest, a small recurrence in this area is more difficult to detect.

Regional recurrences aren't always accompanied by signs or symptoms. One study found that signs and symptoms occurred in only 30 percent of women with an isolated regional recurrence.

Signs and symptoms that may indicate a regional recurrence include:
- A lump that can be treated or felt in regional lymph nodes
- Swelling of your arm
- Persistent arm and shoulder pain
- Increasing loss of sensation and motor skills in your arm and hand
- Persistent chest pain

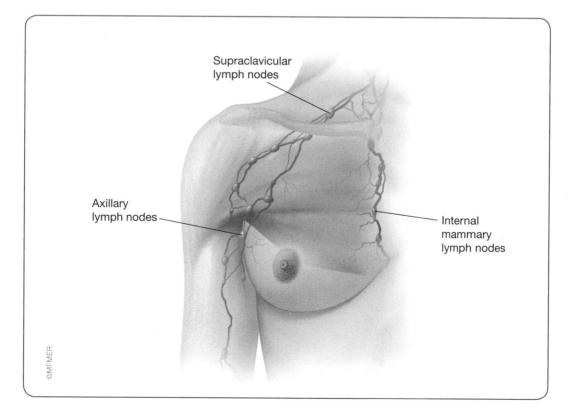

If you experience any of these, tell your doctor so that they can be evaluated.

Tests

A regional recurrence may be detected when your doctor asks you about any new symptoms or while doing a physical examination.

A CT scan, an MRI or a PET scan may be helpful in evaluating a suspected recurrence in regional lymph nodes. A biopsy may be performed.

Because a regional breast cancer recurrence carries a high risk of distant recurrence, your doctor will likely have you undergo other tests to check for spread of cancer to other areas of your body.

Treatment

If it's possible, surgery may be the best option for removing the tumor and controlling the cancer. In some cases, radiation therapy may be used after surgery to further destroy any cancer cells. If surgery isn't feasible, radiation therapy may be used as the primary form of treatment. Other lymph node areas may also be radiated to try to prevent further recurrence.

Because of significant risk of distant recurrence, chemotherapy or hormone therapy may be recommended after surgery, radiation or both to prevent recurrence of the cancer at other sites.

Prognosis

With a regional recurrence, your prognosis generally depends on where the recurrence is located, whether it's isolated, how long it was from the time you were first diagnosed until the recurrence, and certain characteristics of the cancer.

Most women with regional breast cancer recurrences aren't cured. If the cancer has spread to regional lymph nodes, it likely has spread to other parts of the body, too. However, even when a cure isn't possible, with appropriate therapy it's still possible to live for years.

Metastatic Recurrence

When breast cancer cells reappear in parts of your body other than your breast or nearby lymph nodes, the cancer is considered a distant (metastatic) recurrence. Breast cancer most commonly spreads to the bones, lungs and liver. Other sites include the brain, skin, lymph nodes, abdomen and ovaries.

Signs and symptoms

Breast cancer that has spread to other areas of the body usually is detected by way of signs and symptoms.

Breast cancer that has spread to bone may be signaled by bone pain. Breast cancer that has spread to the lungs may produce the following signs and symptoms:
- Persistent, dry cough
- Difficulty breathing
- Shortness of breath
- Chest pain
  Liver metastasis may be signaled by:
- Loss of appetite
- Abdominal tenderness or discomfort
- Persistent nausea, vomiting or weight loss
- Jaundice
  Brain metastasis may be signaled by:

- Severe headaches
- Visual disturbances
- New seizures or symptoms such as weakness, numbness or imbalance
- Persistent nausea not explained by another problem

Biopsy

A diagnosis of metastatic breast cancer needs to be made with as much certainty as possible. Often, this involves a biopsy of a tumor at a distant site. The tissue collected is tested for certain characteristics, such as estrogen and progesterone receptors and HER2 receptors.

In some situations, though, a biopsy is either dangerous or unnecessary. For example, if you have a history of breast cancer and multiple new masses (tumors) occur in your bones or lungs and there's no other explanation for these masses, a diagnosis of metastatic breast cancer can be made with reasonable certainty without the need for a surgical biopsy. However, because breast cancer treatment is dependent upon the characteristics of the tumor cells, sometimes a biopsy is done so that your treatment can be tailored to the characteristics of your cancer.

Other tests

If your doctor suspects your cancer has spread to other areas of your body, he or she may use a number of tests to confirm the presence or absence of cancer cells in these locations.

Laboratory tests

Among women with metastatic breast cancer, laboratory tests may include:

- **Complete blood count.** A complete blood count is a common blood test that's often part of a general physical examination. It measures your red and white blood cells and your platelets.
- **Blood tumor marker tests.** Some cancers produce certain substances (tumor markers) that can be detected in blood. These substances usually are present in low concentrations in healthy individuals. In case of certain cancers, their levels may increase. Some cancer markers associated with breast cancer include CA 15-3 and CA 27-29. A blood test may be done to test for these markers.

  In women who haven't experienced any signs or symptoms of a distant recurrence, blood tumor marker tests generally aren't adequate and specific enough to detect cancer. But they may help confirm a cancer recurrence in women with symptoms.
- **Liver function tests.** When liver cells are damaged, enzymes or other proteins normally found inside the cells leak into blood. Your blood may also contain higher than normal amounts of waste products, because the waste isn't being removed by your liver as it should be.

Imaging tests

Your doctor may use one or more of the following tests to check your lungs, liver, bones and abdomen for any unusual masses or structural abnormalities:

- **X-ray.** Chest X-rays may detect a tumor in your lungs. Bone X-rays may be able to detect cancer that has spread to bone.
- **CT scan.** A CT scan can provide more detailed pictures than can ordinary X-rays. CT scans may be used to examine your head, chest, abdomen,

pelvis and bones for evidence of cancer spread.

- **MRI scan.** Similar to CT, MRI provides views of the inside of your body in cross-sectional slices. But it uses an extremely strong magnet instead of X-rays. An MRI is most useful for detecting cancer that has spread to the brain or around the spinal cord.
- **Bone scan.** A bone scan is a type of nuclear medicine scan. It can provide a picture of your whole skeleton and may be used to check for cancer in your bones. During a bone scan, a small amount of radioactive material is injected into your bloodstream. The material binds to your bone cells. A gamma camera then records the pattern of radioactive absorption in your bones. In areas with bone metastases, generally more of the tracer is absorbed and the area "lights up" on the scan.
- **PET scan.** A PET scan also uses radioactive material injected into your body to produce an image of your body. Tissues using more energy — exhibiting increased metabolic activity — absorb greater amounts of the radioactive material. Tumors are often more metabolically active than are healthy tissues, and they generally appear more prominent on the scan.
- **Liver ultrasound.** An ultrasound exam can often help detect if the cancer has spread to your liver.

Prognosis and treatment

Because metastatic cancer is characterized by the spread of cancer cells throughout the body, systemic therapy — therapy that treats the whole body — is generally the recommended treatment. This may involve use of chemotherapy, hormone therapy or both. Radiation also may be used to relieve cancer-related symptoms, such as pain, in specific locations.

The main goal of treatment for an individual with a metastatic breast cancer recurrence is to have the woman do as well as possible for as long as possible. This concept may be better understood if it's broken down into four parts. The goals of treatment are:

- Experience the fewest symptoms of cancer as is possible
- Experience the fewest side effects as possible from cancer treatment
- Have the best quality of life possible
- Have the longest life possible

In general, metastatic breast cancer isn't considered curable, but the prognosis for individual women can vary widely.

Treatment and prognosis of metastatic breast cancer is discussed in detail in the next chapter.

Chapter 16: Breast Cancer

Treating Advanced Breast Cancer

Determining Prognosis	248
Disease characteristics	248
Personal and treatment factors	249

Treatment Options	250
Treatment goals	250
Hormone therapy	250
Chemotherapy	257
HER2 medications	259
Medications that prevent blood vessel growth	261
New therapies	262

| Monitoring Treatment | 262 |

Localized Treatments	263
Bone metastases	269
Pleural effusions	269
Central nervous system metastases	269

| When Treatment Stops Working | 270 |

When breast cancer spreads to other organs, such as the bones, lungs or liver, it's referred to as advanced breast cancer. Other terms commonly used are *metastatic cancer* or *stage IV cancer*. Some women have advanced breast cancer when they're first diagnosed, but more often it develops when the cancer recurs.

Usually, women with metastatic breast cancer have been through diagnosis and treatment before, when their original tumors were first found. The process of diagnosis and treatment this time has some similarities to that first experience, but it also has some key differences. This chapter focuses on the evaluation and treatment of women with metastatic breast cancer.

Whether or not this is your first experience with breast cancer, you may be thinking that not much can be done for advanced breast cancer. In fact, treatment options are available for breast cancer in its later stages. Even though stage IV breast cancer typically can't be cured, treatment may provide long-term control of the disease. As breast cancer treatments become more and more effective, women are surviving longer with metastatic breast cancer.

Determining Prognosis

Metastatic breast cancer isn't a simple, uniform disease. Instead of viewing it as a single entity, picture it as a spectrum. At one end of the spectrum is a rapidly progressive disease with extensive spread to vital organs. At this end, the disease may be resistant to hormone therapy and chemotherapy. Average survival may be measured in terms of a few months.

At the other end of the spectrum are instances where the cancer follows a long, slow course. Women in this situation generally have cancer spread to bone or soft tissue, but their internal organs aren't affected. At this end, the disease tends to be more sensitive to hormone therapy and chemotherapy. Women with this type of recurrence may live for years or, occasionally, decades. Very rarely, a woman will do well for decades without treatment to halt the disease's progression.

In general, the average length of survival for women who receive a diagnosis of metastatic breast cancer is between two and three years. But survival may vary considerably, based on various tumor behaviors.

In predicting how a woman's cancer will behave and the disease's likely course, doctors rely on a number of factors (prognostic factors). These involve not only characteristics of the disease

but also factors related to the person being treated and the type of treatment received.

Disease characteristics

Characteristics related to the cancer can help determine how it may behave:

Disease-free interval
The disease-free interval refers to the time from initial diagnosis to recurrence. This is often one of the best predictors of how the cancer will act after it has recurred.

Women who develop evidence of metastatic breast cancer early on, while they're still receiving initial treatment for breast cancer or soon after treatment ends, generally have a very poor prognosis. If, on the other hand, metastatic breast cancer becomes apparent 10 to 15 years after the initial diagnosis, the course of the disease is often slow and the prognosis better.

Hormone receptor status
Women with hormone receptor positive breast cancer — estrogen receptor positive, progesterone receptor positive or both — generally have a slower disease course than do women with hormone receptor negative cancers.

HER2 status
In the past, it was generally noted that women with HER2-positive cancers had a poorer prognosis than did women whose tumors were HER2 negative. HER2-positive cancers are more aggressive and less sensitive to hormone treatments.

However, HER2-targeted drugs such as trastuzumab (Herceptin) provide a new

Prognostic factors in metastatic breast cancer

Disease characteristics	Personal and treatment factors
Disease-free period between initial diagnosis and metastatic recurrence	Ability to get around (performance status)
Hormone receptor status	Presence of other medical conditions
HER2 status	Prior treatment
Locations of disease	Age
Extent of disease	

form of treatment for women with HER2-positive cancers. The drugs have greatly improved long-term outcomes.

Locations of disease

Women with metastatic disease that's limited to the skin, lymph nodes or bones generally have a better prognosis, compared with women who have tumors in multiple sites or in the liver or brain. Women with cancer in the lungs or the tissue surrounding them have an intermediate prognosis.

Extent of disease

Women with only small amounts of metastatic disease tend to do better than do women with extensive disease.

Personal and treatment factors

A number of personal and treatment factors also can affect your prognosis, including mobility, other medical conditions, prior treatment and age.

Mobility

Mobility (performance status) refers to your ability to be up and about and to carry on normal activities. Your mobil-

ity helps determine how well you may tolerate certain treatments and how likely these treatments are to help.

Other medical conditions

Conditions such as heart disease, stroke or diabetes can affect your prognosis.

Prior treatment

How well a person with metastatic disease will do may be affected by the extent of the treatment she received when her breast cancer was originally diagnosed.

Your doctor will review your breast cancer history. He or she will also look at the speed at which your cancer has progressed. For example, did the cancer's spread become apparent 10 years after your initial diagnosis? Or did it occur two months after the completion of your initial treatment? These are two very different scenarios that have different effects on prognosis and treatment decisions.

Age

Whether age affects the course of breast cancer after it becomes metastatic is a matter of debate. Some data suggest that particularly young women or older women have poorer prognoses.

Treatment Options

Because the cancer has spread to other parts of the body, treatment for metastatic breast cancer generally involves whole-body (systemic) therapy rather than local therapy, such as surgery or radiation. Several options are available, including:

- Hormone therapy
- Chemotherapy
- Biologically based therapy, such as trastuzumab (Herceptin)
- A combination of therapies
- A clinical trial

You may find that there are easily 10 to 20 different options that may be used to treat metastatic breast cancer. You'll want to work with your doctor to decide which option is most appropriate for you. In addition, if one treatment doesn't work or stops working, you will likely be able to try other treatments.

Treatment goals

When devising a therapy plan, you and your doctor may want to address two important questions:

1. Is being cured a realistic goal among women with metastatic breast cancer?
2. Are women with metastatic breast cancer occasionally cured?

The answer to the first question generally is no. Curing metastatic breast cancer isn't a realistic goal. However, in the majority of women, it can be controlled. This generally means reducing the size of the tumors, controlling symptoms and minimizing toxic effects from the medications. The goal of your treatment is to help you live as well as possible for as long as possible.

This doesn't mean, though, that women have never been cured of advanced breast cancer — meaning that the answer to the second question may be yes. Although being cured typically isn't a goal of metastatic breast cancer treatment, occasionally — maybe 1 to 3 percent of the time — women with metastatic breast cancer will experience a complete remission of their disease that lasts 10 to 15 years or longer. Women with isolated metastatic cancer are more likely to experience a cure than women whose cancer is widespread.

Hormone therapy

It's well known that the female hormones estrogen and progesterone influence the growth and development of a majority of breast cancers. As a result, breast cancers that make receptors for estrogen and progesterone — referred to as hormone receptor positive cancers — can be treated with hormone therapy.

Your menopausal status is often the first thing a doctor evaluates in determining your hormone therapy options. Treatment options are different for premenopausal and postmenopausal women, primarily because of the difference in the levels of estrogen in their bodies. Premenopausal women have high estrogen levels. In postmenopausal women, the ovaries no longer produce estrogen or progesterone, but the adrenal glands and fat tissue still continue to produce some estrogen, although in reduced amounts.

Premenopausal women

There are different ways to moderate the influence of estrogen and progesterone in premenopausal women whose ovaries are

Working Off Of Assumptions

Whether hormone therapy or chemotherapy actually prolongs survival in women with metastatic breast cancer has never been put to a proper scientific test. Doing so would mean that half the participants in the trial would receive drug therapy and the other half would receive no treatment. Because drug therapy appears to benefit the vast majority of women with breast cancer, it's generally considered unethical to conduct a trial that would deny treatment to half the participants.

Based on available information, it appears that women who receive hormone therapy or chemotherapy or a combination of the two do live longer than do women who don't receive such treatment. How much of a benefit is achieved? An average improvement in survival of a year or two appears to be a reasonable estimate. This average includes some women who clearly live many years longer than would have been expected if they had never received such treatment.

still fully functional. Treatment options include ovarian suppression, tamoxifen or both.

Ovarian suppression

One of the oldest methods of hormone therapy is ovarian suppression — keeping the ovaries from producing estrogen and progesterone. This can be done by surgically removing them (oophorectomy), radiating them or using medications.

- **Oophorectomy.** The first description of the use of oophorectomy to treat metastatic breast cancer dates back to 1896 by Sir George Beatson. He had previously noted hormone changes in animals when their ovaries were removed. So he performed an oophorectomy in a young woman with recurrent breast cancer who was willing to try the experiment. Within months, there was a dramatic shrinkage of the young woman's cancer.

For many decades following, oophorectomy became the mainstay of treatment for premenopausal women with metastatic breast cancer, with approximately one-third of the women responding to the therapy.

When medical scientists found a way to identify the presence or absence of estrogen and progesterone receptors on breast cancer cells — indicating whether the cancer was sensitive to hormones — responses could be better predicted. Women with estrogen receptor positive cancers have approximately a 60 percent response rate to oophorectomy, whereas only about 10 percent or less of women with estrogen receptor negative cancers respond to this therapy. The highest response rates to ovarian suppression are generally seen in women who have cancers with both estrogen and progesterone receptors and who experience a long duration between initial treatment and relapse.

Although oophorectomy is a century-old procedure, it's still a viable and effective treatment option.

- **Radiation therapy.** Radiating the ovaries also can cause ovarian suppression, but this method can take weeks to work. Today, it's rarely used.
- **Medications.** Another method of suppressing the ovaries is with a group of drugs called luteinizing hormone-releasing hormone (LH-RH) agonists. These include drugs such as goserelin (Zoladex), leuprolide (Lupron) and triptorelin (Trelstar).

   The medications, generally given by injection once a month, effectively shut off ovarian function. They're used instead of surgery in a large number of women. This means ovarian suppression may be reversible by stopping the medications. However, depending on how close to menopause a woman is and how long she takes these drugs, her ovaries may shut down permanently.

Tamoxifen

The medication tamoxifen is another form of hormone treatment for women with metastatic breast cancer. It differs from drugs used in hormone suppression in that it doesn't prevent the ovaries from producing female hormones. Tamoxifen is a synthetic hormone belonging to a class of drugs known as selective estrogen receptor modulators (SERMs). It works by keeping estrogen from attaching to estrogen receptors on breast cancer cells, thus blocking estrogen's influence on the tumor's growth (see page 192).

Tamoxifen is as effective as oophorectomy among women with metastatic breast cancer, and because it's less invasive than is oophorectomy, it's become a common form of hormone therapy for premenopausal women with metastatic breast cancer. For more information on tamoxifen, see Chapter 11.

Tamoxifen and ovarian suppression

A clinical trial conducted in Europe tested the idea of combining tamoxifen and the LH-RH agonist buserelin to see if the combination would improve treatment results. In the trial, 161 premenopausal estrogen receptor positive women with metastatic breast cancer were randomly selected to receive one of three treatments:

QUESTION & ANSWER

Q: How do you know when you're past menopause?

A: The definition of menopausal status varies. One definition that's commonly used is the absence of any menstrual period for at least 12 months. In some situations, such as if your period has ceased for other reasons, this may not apply. For example, in women whose ovaries are intact but who no longer have a uterus, this definition isn't useful. If your menopausal status is unclear, blood tests may be obtained to help determine your hormone levels. The tests may reveal whether you're premenopausal or postmenopausal, but often the answer isn't clear-cut.

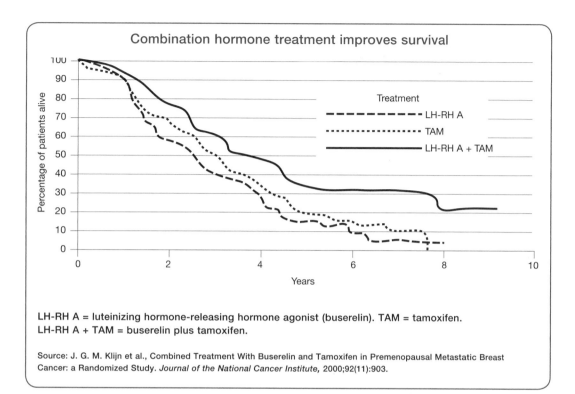

Combination hormone treatment improves survival

LH-RH A = luteinizing hormone-releasing hormone agonist (buserelin). TAM = tamoxifen.
LH-RH A + TAM = buserelin plus tamoxifen.

Source: J. G. M. Klijn et al., Combined Treatment With Buserelin and Tamoxifen in Premenopausal Metastatic Breast Cancer: a Randomized Study. *Journal of the National Cancer Institute*, 2000;92(11):903.

tamoxifen only, buserelin only, or both tamoxifen and buserelin.

After about seven years of follow-up, the results showed an overall benefit in survival for the group that received the drug combination, compared with the group that received only one medication (see the graph above). Average survival with the combination approach was approximately one year greater compared, with the single-drug approach. Thirty-four percent of the participants receiving the drug combination were still alive five years after they started their treatment, compared with approximately 15 percent of the participants who received only one of the drugs. Other similar trials generally reached the same conclusion.

Based on this information, a common approach to treatment for premenopausal women with hormone receptor positive metastatic breast cancer is a combination of ovarian suppression and tamoxifen.

Other options

If the combination of ovarian suppression and tamoxifen isn't effective and your doctor thinks that it's reasonable to consider another form of hormone therapy, several approaches are possible. The drug megestrol acetate (Megace), which is a progesterone medication, and the androgenic agent fluoxymesterone, which is similar to testosterone, have been used. More often, though, doctors are prescribing medications called aromatase inhibitors in combination with continued ovarian suppression. In women who are premenopausal, aromatase inhibitors are effective only when other treatment is included that stops the ovaries from functioning. The drugs aren't effective if your ovaries are still making estrogen.

Postmenopausal women

In postmenopausal women, ovarian suppression isn't necessary because the ovaries have already stopped producing estrogen. However, a number of other treatment options are available to this group.

Treatment for postmenopausal women with hormone-responsive breast cancer has changed dramatically over the past 40 years. Tamoxifen was the first-line agent for many years. However, accumulating evidence shows that, compared with tamoxifen, aromatase inhibitors produce better response rates and they slightly improve survival. Following are hormone therapies used to treat hormone-responsive metastatic breast cancer.

Should You Consider Hormone Therapy?

The goal of treatment for metastatic breast cancer is to have you do as well as possible for as long as possible. Finding therapies with the best response rate and the fewest side effects is important.

Hormone therapy is generally associated with fewer side effects than is chemotherapy. A common initial impression is that chemotherapy is better and more powerful than is hormone therapy and therefore should be used first.

In some situations, though, hormone therapy may have a better chance of fighting the cancer than will chemotherapy. In addition, several studies have shown that people receiving hormone therapy as initial treatment for metastatic breast cancer do as well in terms of survival and life quality as do women who receive chemotherapy as their initial treatment.

Here's an example. A woman with estrogen receptor positive and progesterone receptor positive breast cancer develops a couple of small metastatic tumors in the lungs 10 years after she was initially diagnosed with breast cancer. Chances are that this woman may have a higher response rate to hormone therapy (about 80 percent) than to chemotherapy (60 to 70 percent).

Factors that tend to predict that hormone therapy will be helpful include:

- A positive hormone receptor status
- No prior hormone therapy
- A long disease-free interval between diagnosis of the initial cancer and diagnosis of metastatic breast cancer
- Disease that doesn't involve the liver or brain

In general, hormone therapy is recommended if you have a reasonable chance of responding well to it, and the extent of the cancer is such that you can safely wait a month or two to see if the therapy is working.

High-dose estrogen vs. tamoxifen

Four to five decades ago, the primary form of hormone therapy for postmenopausal women with metastatic breast cancer was high doses of estrogen in the form of a hormone called diethylstilbestrol (DES). Although this sounds strange because estrogen can stimulate cancer growth, in a substantial percentage of women, very high doses of estrogen cause tumors to shrink.

When tamoxifen became available, studies found both methods to be similarly effective. But tamoxifen became the standard treatment approach because it was less toxic than was DES. In some situations, however, high-dose estrogen treatment may still be used.

Aromatase inhibitors

Before the availability of tamoxifen, another type of hormone therapy for postmenopausal women was surgical removal of the adrenal glands — the organs located just above the kidneys. The adrenal glands produce a variety of hormones including androgens. An enzyme called aromatase found in fat cells and breast tissue turns androgen into estrogen. In postmenopausal women, this becomes one of the main sources of estrogen.

Eventually, this surgical procedure was replaced by the invention of a class of medications called aromatase inhibitors, which suppress aromatase enzymes, preventing the conversion of androgen to estrogen. Currently, three aromatase inhibitors are in use, which appear to be equally effective: anastrozole (Arimidex), letrozole (Femara) and exemestane (Aromasin).

In randomized trials comparing aromatase inhibitors and tamoxifen, aromatase

Hormone Withdrawal Phenomenon

Interestingly, one way of shrinking breast cancer tumors is to take away a hormone medication that was previously effective. Although this may seem like a paradox, it does sometimes work.

This type of response was initially observed when high doses of estrogen, in the form of diethylstilbestrol (DES) therapy, were used to treat metastatic breast cancer in postmenopausal women.

In women who received this therapy and experienced tumor shrinkage but later experienced regrowth, stopping the DES therapy caused the cancers to shrink again. This was called DES withdrawal.

What seems to be occurring is that after long exposure to hormone treatment, the cancer cells figure out how to grow during the treatment and are even stimulated by the medication. This same phenomenon has been seen with other types of hormone therapy, including tamoxifen, for women with breast cancer. It also has been seen in men with prostate cancer, another type of hormone-responsive cancer.

What all this means is that sometimes just stopping use of a previously effective hormone medication can in itself be an effective form of treatment.

inhibitors appear to suppress the cancer's growth rate for a longer period of time than does tamoxifen, and they increase average survival times slightly. Based on these studies, doctors usually recommend aromatase inhibitors as initial treatment for postmenopausal metastatic breast cancer that's hormone receptor positive.

However, other factors may influence which medication your doctor recommends first. These include the type of side effects produced by each drug, their cost — currently tamoxifen is cheaper — and whether one of the medications was already used when the cancer was first diagnosed and treated.

Researchers are now studying if it's best to prescribe an aromatase inhibitor with another medication. Results of one trial found that women who received an aromatase inhibitor combined with an investigational medication called everolimus (Afinitor) did better than women who received an aromatase inhibitor alone. However, further study is still needed.

Fulvestrant

Fulvestrant (Faslodex) is an estrogen receptor antagonist that may be helpful for women whose cancer has become resistant to tamoxifen. Whereas tamoxifen works by blocking estrogen, and aromatase inhibitors work by preventing the production of estrogen, fulvestrant works by destroying estrogen receptors in breast cancer cells. Clinical trials involving this

Chemotherapy for Metastatic Breast Cancer

Classes of chemotherapy drugs used to treat metastatic breast cancer include:

Anti-tumor antibiotics
Different from antibiotics used to treat bacterial infections, anti-tumor antibiotics inhibit the ability of cancer cells to multiply by interfering with DNA and by blocking RNA and key enzymes.
- Doxorubicin
- Epirubicin (Ellence)

Mitotic inhibitors
Mitotic inhibitors disrupt division of individual cells by interfering with the specific cellular machinery that separates dividing cells into daughter cells.
- Paclitaxel (Onxol)
- Paclitaxel, protein-bound (Abraxance)
- Docetaxel (Taxotere)
- Ixabepilone (Ixempra)
- Eribulin (Halaven)

medication show its benefits to be similar to those of aromatase inhibitors.

Others

Older hormone therapies also may be considered in postmenopausal women with metastatic breast cancer if other therapies don't work. These include megestrol acetate (Megace) and fluoxymesterone. These therapies can produce side effects. You and your doctor will need to consider the potential benefits and disadvantages of these options.

Chemotherapy

Chemotherapy is most often used to treat metastatic breast cancer when the cancer isn't sensitive to hormone therapy or when the cancer is life-threatening because it has spread so widely or progressed rapidly. Multiple chemotherapy options are available.

Single-agent vs. combination

Chemotherapy refers to a group of drugs that, when ingested or given intravenously, are toxic to cancer cells. Chemotherapy treatment may consist of taking just one drug (single-agent chemotherapy) or a combination of drugs (combination chemotherapy). Combination chemotherapy uses multiple drugs, with each attacking the cancer in a different way. The medications have different side effects, and the combinations are devised to try to increase

Vinca alkaloids

Vinca alkaloids are another form of mitotic inhibitors. They work similarly to taxanes.
- Vinorelbine (Navelbine)
- Vinblastine

Anti-metabolites

Anti-metabolites are medications that block enzymes vital to cancer cell growth by interfering with the synthesis of DNA.
- Fluorouracil, or 5-fluorouracil or 5-FU
- Capecitabine (Xeloda)
- Gemcitabine (Gemzar)
- Methotrexate

Alkylating agents

Alkylating agents interfere with the rapid growth of cancer cells by forming direct chemical bonds with DNA, inhibiting its function.
- Cyclophosphamide (Cytoxan)
- Cisplatin (Platinol)
- Carboplatin (Paraplatin)

destruction of tumor cells and minimize side effects.

Doctors have long debated the merits of using individual chemotherapy agents among women with metastatic breast cancer versus combining two to four agents into a combination chemotherapy regimen. This debate still continues, particularly as new information becomes available from clinical trials.

In general, combination chemotherapy, when compared with single-agent chemotherapy, has a higher chance of causing the cancer to shrink and remain smaller for a longer period of time. But combination chemotherapy also tends to produce more side effects.

A fair amount of evidence also suggests that using medications sequentially — that is, using one drug until it stops working and then using another one —

leads to a similar length of survival and fewer side effects, when compared with combination chemotherapy.

It's generally agreed that women with rapidly progressing, life-threatening disease should be treated with combination chemotherapy, assuming that they're otherwise healthy enough to withstand the side effects of the drugs. Among women with breast cancer that's not as aggressive, many doctors prefer single-agent chemotherapy.

In one study which addressed the question of single-agent chemotherapy versus combination chemotherapy, women participating in the trial received either doxorubicin alone, paclitaxel (Onxol) alone, or a combination of the two drugs. The trial found that no one treatment approach was superior to the other.

Combination Chemotherapy

Chemotherapy drugs are often given in combination in order to fight cancer cells in different ways. Some combinations used for metastatic breast cancer include:

- **AC:** Doxorubicin (*A* is for Adriamycin, a previous brand name) and cyclophosphamide
- **CAF:*** Cyclophosphamide, doxorubicin (Adriamycin) and fluorouracil
- **FAC:*** Fluorouracil, doxorubicin (Adriamycin) and cyclophosphamide
- **CMF:** Cyclophosphamide, methotrexate and fluorouracil
- **AT:** Doxorubicin (Adriamycin) and docetaxel (Taxotere)
- **TC:** Paclitaxel (*T* is for Taxol, a previous brand name) and cyclophosphamide
- **TAC:** Docetaxel (Taxotere), doxorubicin (Adriamycin) and cyclophosphamide
- **TX:** Docetaxel (Taxotere) and capecitabine (Xeloda)
- Gemcitabine (Gemzar) and paclitaxel
- Vinorelbine (Navelbine) and epirubicin
- Ixabepilone (Ixempra) and capecitabine (Xeloda)

*CAF and FAC differ by dose and frequency.

Drug options

An array of chemotherapy drugs may be used to treat metastatic breast cancer. The drugs are grouped into categories based on the mechanism by which they work. Some factors that you and your doctor may consider in deciding which drugs to use include:

- Whether you've already received chemotherapy to treat your cancer, and which drugs you received.
- How you responded to the drugs.
- The side effects of each drug. Each person is affected differently, and some side effects may be more problematic for you than for others.

One of the chemotherapy medications for metastatic breast cancer is called capecitabine. This medication is similar to fluorouracil, one of the older chemotherapy drugs. Unlike many chemotherapy medications, which are given intravenously, capecitabine is given in the form of a pill. It's often used as the first line of treatment for women with metastatic breast cancer.

There are also multiple combination chemotherapy regimens that your doctor may consider when determining your treatment. You may start off with a well-established combination regimen, which usually has a good balance between potency and side effects. If this doesn't work, your doctor may suggest other combinations.

To learn more about chemotherapy medications, see Chapter 11.

Chemotherapy holidays

Once a woman begins chemotherapy for metastatic breast cancer, a question that often arises is how long she should continue to take chemotherapy. Studies involving older chemotherapy drugs suggested the longer the better — the longer chemotherapy was used the longer the cancer stayed under control. Such studies have not been done with newer chemotherapy drugs.

For a woman who is tolerating chemotherapy well, it's reasonable to continue taking the medication as long as it appears to be providing a benefit. If you're having difficulties with side effects from the drugs, your doctor may suggest a chemotherapy holiday — a break from the medication that allows you time to feel better and more fully engage in day-to-day activities. Women with HER2-positive cancers may want to continue their HER2 medications while on a chemotherapy holiday.

HER2 medications

About 20 to 25 percent of women with breast cancer have cancer cells that overproduce a protein called HER2. This protein is normally produced by a gene that regulates cell growth. Certain breast cancers overproduce the HER2 protein. As a result, cells become overstimulated, aiding in the development and growth of a tumor.

Women whose breast cancers are characterized by an overproduction of the HER2 protein are referred to as HER2 positive. For more information on HER2, see Chapter 11.

Herceptin

A drug called trastuzumab (Herceptin) — a type of drug known as a monoclonal antibody — was developed to fight

HER2-positive cancers. The drug works by attaching to HER2 receptors on cancer cells, blocking the action of the receptors. This inhibits the multiplication of HER2-positive cancer cells and, in some cases, is able to shrink the tumor.

Studies show additional benefits when trastuzumab is combined with chemotherapy. In more than half of cases, the drug combination causes tumor shrinkage. One study found that in comparison to women taking chemotherapy alone, those taking trastuzumab and chemotherapy:
• Had slower tumor growth
• Had greater tumor shrinkage
• Maintained their tumor shrinkage for a longer period of time
• Lived longer

Based on this evidence, trastuzumab has become an important part of treatment for women with advanced HER2-positive cancers.

If your tumor is HER2 positive and you're about to start chemotherapy, your doctor likely will recommend that you take trastuzumab. Among women who also have estrogen receptor positive cancer, it's not clear if trastuzumab should be given at the same time as hormone therapy, considering that hormone therapy may work for a considerable period of time.

While it's true that combining hormone therapy with trastuzumab will shrink tumors for a longer period of time, there's no proof that the combination approach will cause women to live longer than if they take the medications one following the other (sequentially).

Other HER2 medications

Other medications have also been developed that attack HER2 receptors. One of them is lapatinib (Tykerb). This medication is generally given when trastuzumab

When to Discontinue Trastuzumab

In general, medications aimed at halting cancer progression are stopped when the disease continues to progress despite use of the drugs. But whether to discontinue trastuzumab (Herceptin) in women who are HER2 positive was unclear and for several years a subject of debate.

In women whose tumors continue to grow while receiving trastuzumab alone, doctors usually continue the medication but add to it a chemotherapy regimen. That's because evidence indicates that chemotherapy combined with trastuzumab works better than chemotherapy alone.

More recent evidence indicates it's also best to continue anti-HER2 therapy in women whose cancer continues to progress while receiving a combination of trastuzumab and chemotherapy. This may be done by combining trastuzumab with a different medication aimed at slowing progression of the disease, or by replacing trastuzumab with another medication that targets HER2 receptors, such as the medication lapatinib (Tykerb).

is no longer effective. At least one study suggests that when lapatinib is combined with chemotherapy it can halt cancer progression in women with metastatic breast cancer for a longer period of time than if the chemotherapy was taken alone.

Another HER2 medication that appears to be of some benefit and is undergoing clinical trials is the drug pertuzumab. In addition, researchers are examining if combining HER2 medications — such as taking trastuzumab and lapatinib together — is more effective than receiving one drug at a time.

Medications that prevent blood vessel growth

For cancers to grow and spread, they need blood vessels to supply them with nutrients and oxygen. Many cancerous tumors send out messages to surrounding tissue cells that encourage new blood vessel growth.

Medications have been developed that aim to stop cancer growth by preventing the growth of blood vessels to tumors. The most common is a drug called bevacizumab (Avastin). It received temporary Food and Drug Administration (FDA) approval after early studies found it effective in shrinking tumors and halting cancer spread when combined with chemotherapy. Recently, though, the FDA revoked its approval of bevacizumab because of potentially serious side effects, including blood pressure problems and some trouble with bleeding and blood clotting. What the future holds in store for this medication is uncertain.

Other drugs that also inhibit blood vessel growth to tumors are under study and may be available in the future.

Deciding on Drug Therapies

As you try to make some decisions about using various drug therapies for treating metastatic breast cancer, it may be helpful to try to address the following questions:

1. What's the goal of the therapy?
2. What's the likely response rate with the therapy? That is, what is the chance that the cancer will shrink? In addition, what is the chance that there will be no evidence of cancer growth for at least six months?
3. In those patients whose cancers shrink or don't grow, what's the average time that this response lasts? This may be called the response duration.
4. Is there evidence that the proposed treatment will prolong the length of your life? If it's expected to prolong survival, what would be the average length of prolonged survival?
5. Will this therapy, on average, improve your quality of life? This is a difficult question to address scientifically, yet some estimates can be made. The effect on quality of life generally depends on how well the therapy works against the cancer, its side effects (toxicities), and the psychological and social considerations of the person receiving therapy.
6. What are the potential side effects of the therapy?

New therapies

New knowledge about the underlying drivers of breast cancer — molecular pathways that allow cancer to start and keep going — has spurred new ideas for drug treatment. Instead of standard chemotherapy, drug manufacturers today are focused on so-called "targeted therapies."

On pages 33 and 40 are illustrations of a cell and its inner workings. The pathways shown in the illustrations are the targets of many new medications. To stop cancer growth, researchers are developing medications that act on:

- Growth factors outside the cancer cell
- Receptors on the cancer cell surface (HER2 is just one example of such a receptor.)
- Message transmitters within the cell that carry a growth signal to the nucleus
- Pathways and checkpoints that control whether or not a cell divides into daughter cells
- A cell's nucleus and its DNA

These new medications use a variety of mechanisms to reach their pathways of interest, as is shown in the diagram on page 29.

As progress in targeted therapies proceeds, there's also interest in testing the medications in women with metastatic cancer to see if a particular drug might be effective. This kind of approach is generally done within a clinical trial. Be sure to ask your doctor if such an approach might be right for you.

Monitoring Treatment

Once you begin treatment, your doctor will frequently monitor the status of your cancer by taking note of how you're feeling, and the results of physical exams and periodic tests.

The most important of these is probably the medical history, which includes how you've felt since your last appointment and any new signs or symptoms you've

---

QUESTION & ANSWER

Q: Are bone marrow transplants ever used to treat advanced breast cancer?

A: In the 1980s and 1990s, there was a lot of enthusiasm about the use of high-dose chemotherapy combined with bone marrow transplantation as treatment for women with breast cancer. The treatment was based on the idea that if some chemotherapy is good, then more should be better. Randomized clinical trials were set up, and women with metastatic breast cancer were randomly assigned to receive either standard chemotherapy or standard chemotherapy followed by high-dose chemotherapy with bone marrow transplantation. The results of these trials didn't suggest any survival benefit in using high-dose chemotherapy with bone marrow transplantation, and as a result, enthusiasm for the treatment has waned considerably.

noticed. Many times this provides the best information for your doctor to determine the effectiveness of treatment. A physical examination is probably the next most important determinant of how you're doing. Various tests can also shed light on how your cancer is responding to treatment. These may include various blood tests and imaging procedures.

After completing his or her assessment, your doctor should be able to place your cancer status into one of three categories:

1. The tumor has clearly shrunk since you started treatment.
2. The tumor has clearly grown since you started treatment.
3. The cancer is stable, a condition often referred to as stable disease.

This last category can be subdivided even further:

- The disease looks like it hasn't changed.
- There's some suggestion that the cancer may be shrinking, but the evidence isn't conclusive. Generally, an oncologist likes to see a substantial reduction in tumor size before indicating a definite response to treatment.
- There's some indication that the cancer is a bit worse, but the status hasn't changed enough to clearly declare it so.

In addition to monitoring your tumor status, your doctor will also look at how you're tolerating the treatment and its side effects. Based on all of this information, you and your doctor can decide whether to continue your treatment. If you decide to stop it, the two of you then need to decide whether to try another form of treatment, and what that treatment should be.

Localized Treatments

Depending on where a cancer has spread and what symptoms it may be causing, a number of treatments may be directed toward specific sites of your body, as opposed to the whole-body (systemic) treatment approaches already described.

Clinical Trials

This chapter discusses the benefits and the risks of treatments for metastatic breast cancer. All this information has become available because of women who have participated in clinical trials. For some of the treatments you may be considering, there may be a clinical trial in which you can participate.

These trials, as a rule, are safe and they provide access to the newest ideas and approaches. They're the best way to continue to identify new treatment options for women with metastatic breast cancer.

You can find out about specific clinical trials by asking your doctor or a member of your health care team or by visiting the National Cancer Institute's website (see page 415). For general information on clinical trials, see Chapter 2.

3 Stories of Advanced Breast Cancer

This book includes many personal stories of women who have survived cancer, who are undergoing treatment or who have taken steps in hopes of preventing cancer. The women discuss why they made the decisions they did and, in many cases, how well they've done.

Unfortunately, though, not all women do well with their cancers. It's important that we tell you not just the good-news stories, but also the ones that didn't have such happy endings.

The pages that follow contain the stories of three women with advanced breast cancer. The first story is of a young woman who died prematurely of a very aggressive cancer. It needs to be noted that this story does not depict a typical case. Rather, it represents one end of the spectrum of metastatic breast cancer. In addition, it illustrates the fortitude of this young woman as she dealt with her disease. If you don't think that you're ready to read this story now, skip over it and consider coming back to it later.

The second story is a hypothetical one that combines parts of several actual cases. The story describes a more typical outcome for a woman diagnosed with recurrent breast cancer. It tells of a woman who does eventually die of her disease, but only after living with it for a relatively lengthy period. We'll call the patient Jane.

The third story is of a woman who amazed her doctors for almost 50 years before she died of breast cancer.

Carol's Story

At the age of 31, Carol was diagnosed with cancer in her left breast. The diagnosis came just a few weeks after she noticed a lump in the breast. Carol decided to have a lumpectomy, and her surgeon removed the lymph nodes under her left arm. The tumor was 2.5 centimeters (about an inch) in diameter — not particularly large — and all the lymph nodes tested negative for cancer. The tumor was also estrogen receptor positive and HER2 receptor negative. Based on the characteristics of her tumor and the laboratory results, estimates were that with just surgery alone, Carol had a 75 percent chance of living disease-free for at least 10 years.

At the time of Carol's diagnosis, for a young woman with a tumor like hers, it was standard practice to recommend chemotherapy after surgery. Carol agreed with the treatment and received the medications doxorubicin and cyclophosphamide. With chemotherapy, Carol's chances of living disease-free for another 10 years increased to an estimated 80 percent.

After completing treatment with doxorubicin and cyclophosphamide, Carol discussed with her doctor the potential benefit of receiving additional chemotherapy with a medication called paclitaxel. Based on the information available at the time, it was estimated that paclitaxel might boost her 10-year survival chances by a couple more percentage points. Because Carol was young and had a young child, she wanted to be aggressive in treating her cancer. So Carol decided to undergo an additional two months of treatment with paclitaxel.

Upon completion of her chemotherapy, Carol met with her doctor to discuss radiation treatment to her left breast. During that visit, her doctor noticed a change in her left breast, which led to further tests. To everyone's dismay, a computerized tomography (CT) scan revealed a large recurrent tumor in her left breast and cancer in some remaining lymph nodes under her left arm and her breastbone (sternum).

Her doctor recommended that Carol begin taking a hormone medication to turn off production of estrogen by her ovaries, as well as the medication tamoxifen. She also received radiation to her left chest wall to try to control the disease, knowing that there was a chance the radiation wouldn't be successful, based on the aggressiveness of her cancer.

During a visit to her doctor a few months later, Carol had more fullness in her left upper breast region. A CT scan showed enlarging tumor masses in the breast and lymph node areas, in addition to spots in her liver, consistent with the spread of breast cancer to the liver.

At this juncture, Carol had to make some tough decisions regarding future treatment. Knowing that there wasn't a chance of curing the cancer, and that the chance of chemotherapy shrinking the cancer was quite small, Carol, with input from her medical team and her husband, decided to try another chemotherapy medication.

Within a month, however, it was clear that not only was the cancer in her liver growing, but it had also spread to her spine, where it was causing considerable pain. To help control the pain, Carol received a course of radiation therapy to her spine. Over the next few weeks, she received even more radiation therapy to new painful sites in her spine, and she had a mastectomy because the tumor in her breast continued to grow and was causing considerable pain. After the mastectomy,

---

Before her death, Carol began writing poetry as a way to cope with her illness. Following is one of her poems:

I had a dream

I dreamed the other night
I married the man I love so
For better, for worse, in sickness, in health
We live, we love, and we grow

I dreamed the other night
A beautiful boy was born
Thanks, praise, adoring him so
We live, we love, and we grow

I dreamed the other night
A cancer crept within
Faith, prayer, strength, hope
We live, we love, and we grow

I dreamed the other night
I was a survivor that had made it through
For better, for worse, in sickness, in health
We lived, we loved, and we grew

Carol Alcalá-Samaniego

Carol decided to try yet another chemotherapy drug, but it was stopped within two weeks because the cancer continued to grow and the drug was causing side effects that only added to her discomfort.

Carol continued to receive supportive care from her health care team to ensure that she was as comfortable as she could be. A little more than a year from when she was diagnosed with cancer, Carol died at home with her extended family present. Despite the relentlessly aggressive course of her disease, Carol lived her life as fully as was feasible. Although they did plan for her likely death, up to the very end, Carol and her husband never gave up hope.

Jane's Story

Jane was diagnosed with breast cancer at the age of 58. On a mammogram, doctors noticed abnormal calcifications in one of her breasts. A biopsy revealed invasive ductal cancer. Imaging tests didn't find any evidence of cancer elsewhere in her body, and Jane was otherwise healthy. After discussing potential treatment options with her doctor, Jane decided to have a lumpectomy, to be followed by radiation therapy.

During her surgery, Jane also had a sentinel node biopsy to check for cancer spread to nearby underarm (axillary) lymph nodes. The test revealed cancer cells in the sentinel lymph node. In light of this finding, other lymph nodes under Jane's arm were removed.

The pathology report following her surgery indicated that Jane had a tumor in her breast that was 2.5 centimeters (about an inch) in diameter and that two of 18 lymph nodes from under her arm contained cancer cells.

Jane's tumor was also found to be estrogen and progesterone receptor positive and HER2 negative.

After her surgery, Jane met with her oncologist who estimated that with surgery and radiation alone, she had about a 50 percent chance of living without a cancer recurrence for the next 10 years. With the addition of chemotherapy and tamoxifen to her treatment regimen, that number increased to 63 percent. Jane chose to have chemotherapy and was given four cycles of the medications doxorubicin and cyclophosphamide. After chemotherapy, she began taking tamoxifen and also received radiation therapy to her breast. She took tamoxifen for five years.

Jane continued to do well for another two years, when she developed back pain. A bone scan revealed metastatic breast cancer in her bones. Jane received radiation therapy to a painful area in her lower back where the cancer had spread. She also started taking the hormone medication anastrozole.

The radiation therapy helped relieve Jane's pain, and for 14 months anastrozole controlled the spread of the cancer. Eventually, Jane developed some shortness of breath caused by fluid around one of her lungs. The fluid was drained and found to contain cancer cells. A surgical procedure was performed to help keep the fluid from re-accumulating. The anastrozole was stopped, and Jane was given another hormone medication. Six months later she developed some pain in her right upper abdomen, and tests indicated that the cancer had spread to her liver.

At this point, Jane and her doctor decided to stop hormone therapy and switch to chemotherapy. The chemotherapy initially shrank the tumors in her liver, but eight months later the cancer began to grow again. She switched to a different chemotherapy medication, which had the same results. The tumors initially regressed, but started to grow again eight months later. A couple more chemotherapy medications were tried over the next three months, but her cancer didn't respond well to them.

Jane discussed the pros and cons of additional treatment with her doctor, and it was clear to both of them, and to her family, that the risk of serious side effects from the medications was greater than any potential benefit they might bring. Jane decided to stop all efforts to control the cancer, and her medical team concentrated on making sure that Jane was as comfortable as possible. Jane received hospice care, and five months later she died in her home with her family present.

Although Jane did eventually die of her breast cancer, she lived for more than 10 years after her initial diagnosis. And, for many of those years, she led a full life, keeping the disease from interfering with her life as much as was possible.

Margaret's Story

To say that Margaret Gilseth lived with breast cancer most of her life is true. Margaret first noticed a lump in her breast when she was 39 years old. That was in 1957. Margaret had a mastectomy to remove her left breast, which was standard procedure at the time. Two years later, a small growth appeared on her incision scar. It turns out, it would be the first of many such tumors.

Initially, the tumors were limited to her left chest wall, but eventually they began to spread across her chest wall and developed in her right breast as well.

Margaret handled each of the recurrences as she did her initial diagnosis. "I took them one at a time, and was glad to get rid of them. And then I went on living each time. I think you make use of each day."

"Getting rid" of her tumors required many major and minor surgeries and radiation therapy. She had more than 25 separate surgical procedures, which removed more than 65 tumor nodules.

To keep new tumors from developing, or at least slow their growth, Margaret received multiple anti-cancer hormone therapies. She did this on and off for well over 20 years. When the effects of one medication began to wear off — signaled by the appearance of new growths — her hormone therapy was changed.

In addition to her strong faith, one of Margaret's biggest allies in her lifelong battle with cancer was a pen and paper, which eventually gave way to a computer.

An English teacher for 25 years, Margaret enjoyed writing and she always kept a journal. Her journal helped her face, and then let go of, her worries and fears. Writing became her therapy. "I always tell people if they have something bothering them — anxieties that persist — there's nothing better than writing."

After her retirement, with more time on her hands, Margaret's writing took on a broader scope. She wrote a novel about the lives of several generations of a Norwegian immigrant family, based, in part, on her own family's experiences. Additional books and collections of poetry followed. Eventually, she wrote a book about her personal battle with breast cancer, called *Silver Linings*.

When she wasn't writing, Margaret found other ways to keep busy. She volunteered at the local nursing home, read to children in the Head Start program and taught Norwegian in community education classes. She and her husband, Walter, traveled when they could, often as part of a volunteer organization. For Margaret, volunteer work was another part of her therapy, another way of coping and carrying on. "I think taking an interest in other people makes a lot of difference. If you just go around thinking about yourself, it can cause you problems."

Over the years, whenever Margaret was facing another surgery or a change in treatment — times when she wondered if "this was the one," the one recurrence that she wouldn't be able to overcome — her son Steve would offer her comfort by telling her in his lighthearted manner that she was going to live to a ripe, old age. It turns out, Steve was right.

Margaret continued to live a full life until she fell on some ice while out walking and broke her hip. After that incident, her breast cancer seemed to become more aggressive. She tried chemotherapy for a short period, but she didn't like it. Almost 50 years after her breast cancer was diagnosed, Margaret died at the age of 88.

So, why did Margaret do so well despite her breast cancer that kept recurring? The oncologist who cared for Margaret the last two decades of her life — Margaret having outlived the 30-year career of her previous doctor — readily admits that he doesn't know. Under the microscope, Margaret's cancer looked like a routine type of breast cancer. Why it acted so differently from 99+ percent of other such cancers is a real mystery. Hopefully, it's a mystery that can one

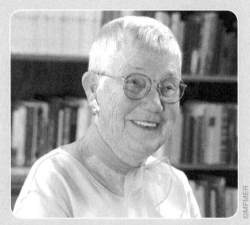

Margaret Gilseth at home in her den, where she kept busy writing and communicating with family and friends.

day be solved to help doctors better understand cancer and better help patients.

Margaret's story is a great reminder to women with cancer and their doctors to never say never, and never say always.

Bone metastases

A group of medications (bisphosphonates) used to treat osteoporosis, a disease that causes bones to become weak and prone to fracture, also is used to treat women with metastatic breast cancer to their bones.

In one study, participants with breast cancer metastasis to bone were randomly assigned to receive a bisphosphonate or an inactive substance (placebo) in addition to their standard cancer treatment. Women receiving the bisphosphonate were less likely to develop subsequent bone fractures or to need radiation therapy to relieve bone pain. Based on this evidence, bisphosphonates are now commonly used in women with metastatic breast cancer in their bones.

In this study, women were given doses of bisphosphonates every month. Other studies are evaluating whether it's best to receive the therapy once a month or once every three months. The results of these studies should be available in the near future.

Because bisphosphonates can cause kidney damage and can lower blood calcium levels, your doctor will likely monitor your kidney function during the course of treatment.

Another side effect of bisphosphonates is a condition called osteonecrosis of the jaw. *Osteo* means "bone" and *necrosis* means "the death of tissue." Jawbone tissues die, leading to a painful lesion which can erode through the gums. The chance of this happening is higher in people with poor dental health or who have been on high doses of bisphosphonates for a long time. Because of this, before prescribing bisphosphonate therapy, your doctor will want to make sure your dental health is as good as it can be.

How long to use bisphosphonates is unclear. There's some evidence people who are on bisphosphonates for a long period of time can actually develop brittle bones that fracture more easily.

Until better data are available, many doctors are now giving less frequent doses of the medication to women who have been on the therapy for a year or more. Newer drugs that act similarly to bisphosphonates also are being studied.

Pleural effusions

At times, cancer can develop in the pleural lining of the lungs, leading to the buildup of fluid around the lungs (pleural effusion). This may require removal of the fluid by draining it with a needle or by a more extensive process in which the fluid is removed either through a chest tube or a surgical procedure. Your doctor may then insert a chemical irritant into the space between the chest wall and lungs (pleural space) to create scar tissue and close up the space. This is done to decrease the chance that the fluid buildup will recur.

Another method for treating the fluid buildup is a procedure in which a catheter is inserted into the pleural space. The catheter contains a mechanism that allows it to be opened and closed, so fluid can be drained as needed.

Central nervous system metastases

If metastatic cancer develops in the brain or around the spinal cord, steroid medications are generally used to try to decrease the swelling and any resulting pain or neurological problems. Sometimes a neurosurgeon may be called upon to try to remove some of the cancer. More often, however, radiation therapy is used to treat the cancer.

Sometimes, radiation is given to the whole brain to treat not only visible cancer but also cancer that may be too small to be seen. This can lead to side effects that may show up months to years later.

Another approach is to treat localized areas of the brain with what's known as radiosurgery, or Gamma Knife treatment. It allows for areas where cancer is present to receive high-dose radiation treatment, without causing as much toxicity to the rest of the brain. Sometimes, the two — localized brain radiation and whole-brain radiation — are performed together.

These new treatment approaches, combined with earlier diagnosis of cancer spread with magnetic resonance imaging (MRI), have improved the prognosis for women with breast cancer whose cancer has spread to the brain.

When Treatment Stops Working

Unfortunately, there are no guarantees that any particular treatment will work. When there's evidence that the disease is progressing despite treatment, it's a reasonable choice to reanalyze what your next step might be — similar to what you and your doctor did when you first learned you had metastatic breast cancer and were deciding on treatment.

With metastatic breast cancer, the value of each subsequent treatment tends to decrease. For example, in a woman who starts off with chemotherapy, the initial response rate might be around 50 to 70 percent, and the benefits may last for an average of 10 to 12 months. If the disease progresses, a second chemotherapy regimen might have only a 30 to 35 percent response rate, with an average response duration of just four to six months.

In addition, studies suggest that some people who receive less chemotherapy in their last weeks of life actually live longer than do those who receive more chemotherapy. It's possible that as the cancer becomes more resistant to chemotherapy and the body becomes less tolerant of its effects, chemotherapy can, in fact, shorten both the quality and duration of life.

There may come a time when it is appropriate for you to say no to further treatment. For some women and their doctors, this may seem like giving up. But this assumption is generally incorrect. If the treatment is more likely to cause troublesome side effects — and not prolong your length of life or improve your quality of life — declining treatment is a reasonable choice. This shouldn't be construed as giving up.

At this point, the goals of your treatment change. The focus of treatment is no longer on controlling the cancer but, instead, on controlling your symptoms and making you as comfortable as possible. This is called supportive care. For additional information on making the transition to supportive care, see Chapter 23.

Chapter 17

Ovarian Cancer: What You Should Know

Your Ovaries	271
What Is Ovarian Cancer?	273
How Common Is It?	274
Risk Factors	275
Preventing Ovarian Cancer	275
Birth control pills	276
Removal of your ovaries	276
Screening Methods	277
Ongoing efforts	278
Recommendations	279
Screening women at high risk	281
Early Warning Signs	281
Nonspecific symptoms	281
Spread of Ovarian Cancer	282
Diagnosis and Treatment	282

You might wonder why ovarian cancer is included in this book. The reason is that breast cancer survivors have an increased risk of ovarian cancer. In addition, women from breast cancer families often have an increased risk of ovarian cancer. In this chapter, we will describe what ovarian cancer is, how common it is, the possibility of screening for it, and some basic information about its staging, treatment and outcomes. Genetic testing for inherited mutations that increase your risk of both ovarian and breast cancers is mentioned in this chapter but discussed more thoroughly in Chapter 5.

Your Ovaries

The ovaries are walnut-sized organs situated in the lower portion of your pelvis on each side of your uterus (see the illustration on page 272). During your menstrual cycle, your ovaries can change in size slightly. After menopause, they shrink to less than half their premenopausal size.

Gynecologic anatomy

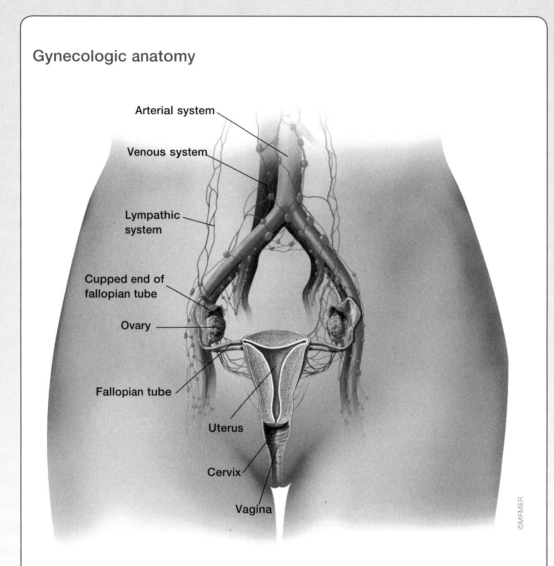

Arterial system

Venous system

Lymphatic system

Cupped end of fallopian tube

Ovary

Fallopian tube

Uterus

Cervix

Vagina

©MFMER

The ovaries, fallopian tubes, uterus, cervix and vagina make up the female reproductive system. Women have two ovaries, one on each side of the uterus. The ovaries — each about the size of a walnut — produce eggs (ova) as well as the hormones estrogen, progesterone and testosterone. Ovarian cancer is a type of cancer that begins in the ovaries or the thin layer of tissue covering them (epithelium). Cancer that develops in the ovaries may spread directly to other structures in the abdominal-pelvic cavity or through lymph channels (lymphatic system) or blood vessels (arterial and venous systems).

The ovaries produce eggs (ova). When a baby girl is born, her ovaries contain all the eggs that she'll need throughout her life. Each month, beginning when a girl reaches puberty and continuing until menopause, the ovaries grow cyst-like structures called follicles. During ovulation, one follicle releases an egg into a fallopian tube, which connects the ovary to the uterus.

The ovaries are also the primary source of the female sex hormones estrogen and progesterone. These hormones influence the development and maintenance of feminine physical characteristics, such as breast development, body shape and body hair. Estrogen and progesterone also help regulate menstrual cycles and pregnancy. At menopause the ovaries stop producing eggs and these hormones.

What Is Ovarian Cancer?

Like other cancers, ovarian cancer results from the loss of control of normal cell growth and regulation. Over time, abnormal cells in an ovary accumulate into a mass of tissue called a growth, or tumor. An ovarian tumor may be noncancerous (benign) or cancerous (malignant). Although benign tumors are made up of cells that are growing in excess numbers, they don't spread (metastasize) to other body tissues. Malignant cells typically spread directly to nearby tissues in the abdominal-pelvic cavity or, less often, they may spread throughout your body by way of your blood vessels or lymphatic system.

While there are several types of cancer that can start in the ovaries, the most common — epithelial ovarian cancer — starts in the epithelial cells that cover the surface of the ovaries. In this book, all references to ovarian cancer are to epithelial ovarian cancer. This is the type that most often develops in breast cancer survivors and breast cancer families. Also, recent research has shown that cells from the cupped end of the fallopian tube that surrounds an ovary (see opposite page) may become cancerous and spread immediately to an ovary, contributing to what we have called ovarian cancer. A closely related cancer called primary peritoneal cancer starts in the cells that line the abdominal cavity (see page 277).

Ovarian cancer causes more deaths than any other gynecologic cancer for two main reasons. First, in its early stages, ovarian cancer produces few — if any — signs or symptoms. And when symptoms do occur, they can easily be confused with those of other conditions. Second, as discussed later in this chapter, there isn't yet an effective test to screen for ovarian cancer. For these reasons, more than two-thirds of women diagnosed with ovarian cancer have advanced-stage disease, meaning that it has at least spread within the abdomen.

However, there is some good news. There's been major progress in unraveling the underlying biology and genetics of ovarian cancer. In addition, some cancers previously considered ovarian cancers actually appear to begin in the fallopian tube. This finding opens up new lines of research for both the causes of ovarian cancer and possible screening techniques to identify the disease earlier.

FASTFACT

Most common cancers among American women

	Type	Estimated number of new cases in 2012
1.	Breast cancer (invasive only)	226,870
2.	Lung cancer	109,690
3.	Colorectal cancer	70,040
4.	Uterine (endometrial) cancer	47,130
5.	Thyroid cancer	43,210
6.	Melanoma	32,000
7.	Non-Hodgkin lymphoma	31,970
8.	Kidney cancer	24,520
9.	Ovarian cancer	22,280
10.	Pancreatic cancer	21,830

Source: American Cancer Society. *Cancer Facts & Figures 2012*. Atlanta, Ga.: American Cancer Society, Inc.

Another bright spot: Ovarian cancers tend to be responsive to chemotherapy — more so than many other types of cancer. With improvements in chemotherapy, there's longer survival for women with ovarian cancer. In the 1970s, the average survival for women with ovarian cancer was about two years. But today, the average survival is closer to four years.

Also, important progress has been made in the ability to identify women at increased risk of ovarian cancer, especially those with hereditary risk. Research has also shown the effectiveness of surgery to prevent the development of ovarian cancer in women who are at high risk. See Chapter 6 for more information on cancer prevention options.

How Common Is It?

The incidence of ovarian cancer — the number of new cases diagnosed each year — is low compared with breast cancer.

There are about 22,000 new ovarian cancer diagnoses made in the United States each year. However, because symptoms are hard to identify and screening options are limited, the disease tends to have a high mortality rate. About 14,000 women in the U.S. die of the disease annually.

To put these figures in perspective, a woman at average risk has about a 1 in 70 (1.5 percent) chance of getting ovarian cancer during her lifetime if she lives to age 80. Compare that with the lifetime risk of breast cancer. About 1 in 8 women (or 12 percent) who live to age 80 will develop breast cancer at some point in their lives.

Ovarian cancer rates are the highest in Europe, the United States and Canada. The disease is more common in Jewish women of Ashkenazi descent (Eastern and Central European). In the United States, the incidence of ovarian cancer is slightly higher among white women than it is among black, Asian-American and Hispanic women.

Risk Factors

The most significant risk factor for ovarian cancer is inheriting a mutation in breast cancer gene 1 (BRCA1) or breast cancer gene 2 (BRCA2). These genes were originally identified in breast cancer families, but they're also responsible for about 10 percent of ovarian cancers.

Women with a BRCA1 mutation have an estimated 39 percent chance of developing ovarian cancer by age 70. Women with a BRCA2 mutation have a 15 percent chance, compared with a 1.5 percent chance for the general population of women. Estimates vary from study to study based on the location of the particular mutation and the features of the women who participated in the studies.

Women of Ashkenazi Jewish ancestry have a higher likelihood of being born with a BRCA mutation than does the general population of women. For women not of Ashkenazi descent, the likelihood of inheriting a BRCA mutation is 1 in 800. For women of Ashkenazi descent, it's 1 in 40. For more information on the BRCA genes and genetic testing, see Chapter 5.

Another known genetic link involves an inherited syndrome called hereditary nonpolyposis colorectal cancer (HNPCC). Individuals in HNPCC families are at increased risk of cancers of the colon and rectum, uterine lining (endometrium), ovary, stomach, and small intestine. The risk of ovarian cancer associated with HNPCC is lower than that associated with BRCA mutations.

Besides these hereditary factors, age is the single greatest risk factor for ovarian cancer. This type of cancer is uncommon in women younger than age 40. In fact, the average age at diagnosis is 60. Other risk factors include never having had children, being of white race, menstruation before age 12, and late menopause. The average age at menopause in the U.S. is 51.

Preventing Ovarian Cancer

Nothing can completely eliminate your risk of ovarian cancer. But, just as certain factors may increase your risk of this cancer, others

BRCA genes increase risk

	BRCA1 mutation carriers	BRCA2 mutation carriers	General population
Risk of developing breast cancer by age 70	54%	45%	8-10%
Risk of developing ovarian cancer by age 70	39%	16%	1.5%

Women who inherit BRCA1 or BRCA2 gene mutations are at significantly higher risk of developing breast and ovarian cancers than are women in the general population.

Data from Sining Chen and Giovanni Parmigiani, Meta-Analysis of BRCA1 and BRCA2 Penetrance. *Journal of Clinical Oncology*, 2007;25:1329.

Prophylactic oophorectomy

Advantages	Disadvantages
Reduces ovarian cancer risk by at least 90 percent	Causes premature menopause and accompanying signs and symptoms
Reduces breast cancer risk up to 50 percent if done before menopause	Increases risk of osteoporosis
	Causes loss of fertility in premenopausal women

---

may reduce it. If you're concerned that you may be at high risk of ovarian cancer, talk to your doctor about your situation.

Birth control pills

Multiple studies show a protective benefit from use of birth control pills. Use of oral contraceptives for three or more years reduces a woman's risk of ovarian cancer by as much as 50 percent, compared with women who have never used them. The protective effect continues for at least 10 to 15 years after you stop taking the pill.

Birth control pills work by suppressing hormones needed for ovulation. These hormones, as well as the inflammation within the ovaries caused by ovulation, may promote the development of cancerous cells. So suppressing ovulation and these hormones with birth control pills may help prevent ovarian cancer.

If you have a strong family history of breast cancer or a known BRCA mutation, talk with your doctor about whether it would be beneficial for you to take oral contraceptives. Along with the benefits, there are some risks. Some studies have suggested that birth control pills may slightly increase breast cancer risk in women at high risk of the disease.

Removal of your ovaries

Women at very high risk of developing ovarian cancer may choose to have their ovaries removed to prevent the disease. This surgery, known as preventive (prophylactic) oophorectomy, is recommended primarily for women who've tested positive for a BRCA gene mutation or women who have a strong family history of breast and ovarian cancer, even if no genetic mutation has been identified. Studies indicate that prophylactic oophorectomy lowers ovarian cancer risk by at least 90 percent. The procedure also reduces the risk of breast cancer if the ovaries are removed before menopause.

Today, it's common practice that both ovaries and the fallopian tubes are removed during the prophylactic surgery. This is technically known as a bilateral salpingo-oophorectomy. The step of removing the fallopian tubes is important because tubal tissue appears to be the source of ovarian cancer in some women.

Prophylactic oophorectomy doesn't completely eliminate cancer risk because despite having both the ovaries and fallopian tubes removed, some women still develop cancer in the cells lining the abdominal and pelvic cavity. This condition, called primary peritoneal carcinoma, behaves much like ovarian cancer (see the box below).

The optimal age at which to have a prophylactic oophorectomy depends on whether you carry a BRCA mutation, the age at which other family members received a diagnosis of breast or ovarian cancer, and whether you have other health risks, such as the bone-thinning disease osteoporosis. Prophylactic oophorectomy isn't an option for a younger woman who wants to maintain her fertility. Many experts recommend that high-risk women have the procedure after age 35 or when they feel that childbearing is complete for them. Women considering the procedure who haven't completed childbearing may wish to talk with a fertility specialist about options for fertility preservation.

The main drawback of prophylactic oophorectomy is that it causes early menopause. Menopausal signs and symptoms include hot flashes, vaginal dryness, sleep disturbances and sexual problems. In addition, premature menopause has been linked to an increased risk of osteoporosis later in life.

The decision to have this preventive surgery is a major one. Before you make a final decision, discuss the pros and cons of the surgery in detail with your doctor. It's key that you have an accurate understanding of your risk of ovarian cancer. Genetic testing may be an option to help define your risk (see Chapter 5).

Screening Methods

As Chapter 7 explains, screening involves looking for a disease before any signs or symptoms appear. Routine screening methods have been developed for several cancers, including mammograms for breast cancer, colonoscopy for colon cancer and the Pap test for cervical cancer. Screening helps save lives by detecting diseases in their early stages, when they're most curable.

There has been extensive research done to test the possible value of screening for ovarian cancer. The bottom line is that doctors don't routinely screen for ovarian cancer. Why not? In a nutshell: Researchers haven't yet found a screening test that's sensitive enough to detect ovarian cancer in its early stages and specific enough to distinguish ovarian cancer from other, noncancerous conditions.

Primary Peritoneal Carcinoma

Closely related to epithelial ovarian cancer is a cancer called primary peritoneal carcinoma. It starts in cells that line the abdominal-pelvic cavity (peritoneum). These cells are very similar to those on the surface of the ovaries (epithelial cells). Under a microscope, peritoneal cancer looks just like epithelial ovarian cancer. It also acts in a manner similar to ovarian cancer and is treated the same way. Women with a family history of ovarian cancer who've had their ovaries and fallopian tubes removed still have some risk of developing primary peritoneal carcinoma.

Ovarian Cysts

Most women have ovarian cysts at some point. Ovarian cysts are fluid-filled sacs in an ovary or on its surface. In women who are still menstruating, cysts typically occur as a normal and expected part of ovulation. Each release of an egg (ovulation) leaves behind a cyst about an inch in diameter. Normally, these cysts disappear without any treatment. In rare cases, though, they persist and grow larger. Some ovarian cancers can have cyst-like components, but most ovarian cysts aren't cancerous and produce few or no symptoms. Unlike malignant tumors, ovarian cysts don't invade neighboring tissue. However, if an ovarian cyst is large, it can cause pelvic discomfort. In some cases, it may interfere with the production of normal ovarian hormones, which could result in irregular vaginal bleeding. If a large cyst presses on your bladder, it may reduce your bladder's capacity, causing you to urinate more frequently.

Developing a good screening test for ovarian cancer is hampered by two key factors:

• Ovarian cancer isn't very common. Compared with several other cancers, including breast cancer, its frequency is relatively low. The more common a disease is, the more beneficial screening becomes. If a disease is uncommon, unless the test is 100 percent accurate — which no test is — it will identify more false-positives than true-positives. False-positives are test results that indicate cancer may be present when it really isn't. False-positives can cause needless worry and expense and the possibility of unnecessary surgery.

• No precancerous (premalignant) stage of ovarian cancer has been identified. With colon cancer, for example, polyps are known to be precursors of cancer. If polyps are discovered during your colonoscopy exam, they can be removed and you'll be monitored more closely. Another example is precancerous changes in the cells of the cervix

that can be detected by a Pap test. The changes are an indicator of possible cancer. For ovarian cancer, there's no recognizable indicator that cancer may be developing.

Ongoing efforts

There are two main tests that have been used for ovarian cancer screening. For both, a major flaw is that they produce too many false-positives. In addition, the tests miss many early cancers. Such results are called false-negatives.

CA 125

CA 125 is a blood test that measures the level of a circulating protein. This protein is produced by a variety of cells, including most ovarian cancer cells, especially in their later stages. Most healthy women have CA 125 levels below 35 units per milliliter of blood. In women with ovarian cancer, the level is often, but not always, elevated. However, measuring a woman's

CA 125 level isn't a reliable screening tool for ovarian cancer, for a couple of reasons:

- Only about 50 percent of women with early-stage ovarian cancer have elevated CA 125 levels. That means the test misses about half of early-stage cancers.
- Several other benign and malignant conditions can cause elevated CA 125 levels. Among them are nonovarian cancers and benign conditions such as endometriosis, ovarian cysts, menstruation, pregnancy and pelvic inflammatory disease. Thus, CA 125 screening can produce false-positives, indicating cancer when it isn't present.

For a woman at high risk of ovarian cancer or for someone who's experiencing signs or symptoms of the disease, a doctor may recommend a CA 125 test. But the test isn't sensitive or specific enough to be used routinely for the general public.

Pelvic ultrasound

Another possible screening method is ultrasound, which uses high-frequency sound waves to produce images of the inside of the body. Although pelvic ultrasound can help find an ovarian mass, it doesn't accurately determine whether the mass is benign or malignant. This is a real problem because benign ovarian cysts are common. This limits the test's effectiveness as a screening tool.

A transvaginal ultrasound can also be done, where an ultrasound probe (about the size of a tampon) is inserted into the vagina. This provides a better view of the ovaries.

Screening research

Recently, the National Cancer Institute studied the possible benefit of screening for ovarian cancer in a multi-institution study involving more than 78,000 women. These women were not known to be at increased risk of ovarian cancer (although about 15 percent of the women had some family history of breast or ovarian cancer). Half of the women were screened each year with CA 125 and ultrasound. The other half had typical medical care without screening. After about 12 years of follow-up, there was no difference in ovarian cancer deaths in the screened group versus the unscreened group. Additionally, there was evidence of harm from screening. Some women in the screened group received false-positive results, which resulted in many unnecessary surgeries.

At this time, a trial of transvaginal ultrasound and CA 125 testing involving more than 200,000 women is ongoing in Britain. The results of this study are expected in the near future.

Current research is focusing on the use of a panel of blood markers, including CA 125, in hopes of finding a better-performing test.

Recommendations

Because of the limitations of screening tests for ovarian cancer, the National Institutes of Health doesn't recommend screening for ovarian cancer among women at average risk of the disease. Experts do recommend, though, that all women have a regular pelvic exam (see the next page). Occasionally, an ovarian mass can be felt on such an examination.

Remember that regular pelvic exams are important to have. They're needed not only for checking the ovaries but also

Pelvic exam

In a pelvic exam, you lie on an examining table with your knees bent and your heels in stirrups. After examining your external genitals, your doctor performs the following:

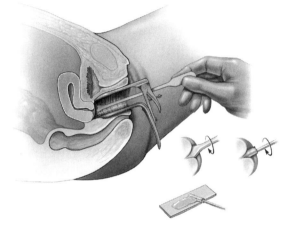

Pap test

To see the inner walls of your vagina and cervix, your doctor inserts an instrument called a speculum into the vagina. When in the open position, the speculum holds the vaginal walls apart so that the cervix can be seen. Your doctor then shines a light inside to look at the walls of the vagina for lesions, inflammation, abnormal discharge and anything else that's unusual. During a Pap test — which is generally included in a pelvic exam — a sample of cells is taken from your cervix.

Vaginal exam

To check the condition of your uterus and ovaries, your doctor inserts one or two lubricated, gloved fingers into the vagina and presses down on your abdomen with the other hand. This allows your doctor to locate your uterus, ovaries and other organs, judge their size, and confirm that they're in the proper position. While exploring the contours of these organs and the pelvis, your doctor feels for any lumps or changes that may signal a problem.

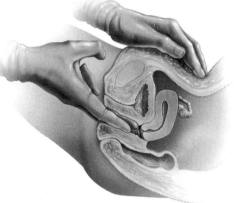

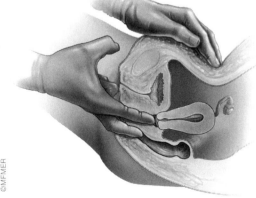

Rectovaginal exam

A rectovaginal exam checks the same organs as the vaginal exam, but from a different angle. For this exam, your doctor inserts one finger into your rectum while another remains in your vagina.

©MFMER

for helping to discover cancer of the uterus, cervix or vagina at earlier an stage. It's recommended that women begin having regular pelvic exams at approximately age 21. Women who've had their uterus removed but still have their ovaries should continue to have pelvic exams.

Screening women at high risk

Screening for ovarian cancer is recommended only for women who are at high risk of the disease. Women at high risk include those who carry breast cancer gene (BRCA) mutations or have a significant family history of ovarian or breast cancer, such as two or more family members with ovarian cancer. Even for this group, there's no good evidence that screening saves lives, but it's the best option available for finding ovarian cancer early, when the chance of a cure is greatest.

For women at high risk of ovarian cancer, doctors recommend a pelvic exam, a CA 125 blood test and ultrasound twice a year beginning at ages 30 to 35, or five to 10 years before the earliest diagnosis of ovarian cancer in the family — whichever comes first. Depending on the results of the tests and a woman's individual circumstances, other tests may also be recommended.

Early Warning Signs

Most of the signs and symptoms of ovarian cancer relate to abdominal bloating or discomfort and other gastrointestinal disturbances. Signs and symptoms that women with ovarian cancer may experience include:

- Abdominal or pelvic pressure, discomfort or pain
- Persistent indigestion, gas or nausea
- Feeling full even after a light meal
- Unexplained changes in bowel habits, including diarrhea or constipation
- Abdominal swelling or bloating, which can cause your clothing to feel tighter
- Changes in bladder habits, including a frequent or urgent need to urinate
- Loss of appetite
- Unexplained weight loss or gain, especially in the abdominal area
- Pain during intercourse
  Less common symptoms include:
- A persistent lack of energy
- Low back pain

Nonspecific symptoms

Because the signs and symptoms of ovarian cancer are associated with many diseases and disorders, they're said to be nonspecific. A woman or her doctor may assume that a more common condition is to blame. In fact, it's not unusual for women with ovarian cancer to be diagnosed with another condition before finally learning they have cancer. The key seems to be having persistent or worsening signs and symptoms. With a digestive disorder, difficulties tend to come and go, or they occur in certain situations or after eating certain foods. With ovarian cancer, there's typically little fluctuation — signs and symptoms are persistent and may gradually worsen.

Researchers have studied whether or not specific symptoms of ovarian cancer are reliable indicators that the disease is present. Unfortunately, there's no one symptom or cluster of symptoms that can clearly point to ovarian cancer, such as the way that a dark, enlarging mole on the skin often signals skin cancer. The reality is that the ovaries are located deep in the pelvis where a problem may go undetected. And the signs and symptoms of the disease, such as abdominal bloating, generally don't occur until after the disease has progressed.

Nevertheless, finding ovarian cancer as early as possible improves the odds of successful treatment. If you're experiencing persistent signs and symptoms, talk to your doctor. If you've already seen a doctor and received a diagnosis other than ovarian cancer, but you're not getting relief from the treatment, schedule a follow-up visit with your doctor or get a second opinion.

In particular, don't ignore persistent abdominal bloating or discomfort. Unusual bloating may indicate that ovarian cancer has spread to your upper abdomen, causing a buildup of fluid, a condition known as ascites. A pelvic examination, a CA 125 blood test, and an ultrasound exam or computerized tomography (CT) scan may help to rule out ovarian cancer as the cause of your symptoms.

Understand that your odds of developing both breast cancer and ovarian cancer are generally low. But because there are links, especially for women with a genetic susceptibility, it's important to be vigilant. Get an accurate estimate of your risk. If a screening schedule is recommended by your doctor, stick to it. And be watchful for any warning signs.

Spread of Ovarian Cancer

As the tumor grows on the surface of the ovary and becomes larger, it can shed cells like seeds directly into the abdominal-pelvic cavity. The shed cells can become implanted on the surrounding tissues and organs, such as the membrane that lines the abdominal-pelvic cavity (peritoneum), diaphragm, fallopian tubes, uterus, bladder, spleen and liver. The seeded cells then form new tumors in these sites. One of the most common sites for this spread is the fatty apron that covers the stomach and intestines (omentum). Seeding within the peritoneal cavity is the most common way ovarian cancer spreads.

As the disease spreads, it may cause fluid to collect in the abdominal cavity. The tumor nodules themselves may cause formation of excessive fluid. Or a collection of tumors may interfere with normal fluid drainage from the abdominal cavity. This abnormal fluid collection is known as ascites. In some women, several quarts of excess fluid may accumulate.

Diagnosis and Treatment

Ovarian cancer is often diagnosed with a concerning ultrasound or CT scan and abdominal or pelvic surgery that's based on worrisome symptoms. It's very important that this surgery be performed by a gynecologic oncologist. A gynecologic

Ovarian cancer stages

Stage I

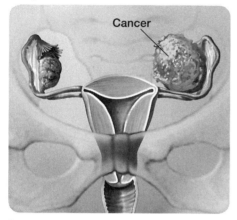

Stage I cancer is confined to one or both ovaries.

Stage II

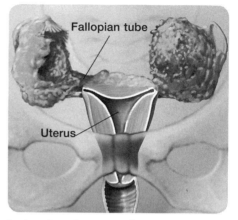

In stage II ovarian cancer, the cancer has spread from one or both ovaries to another organ in the pelvis. This may include the uterus, fallopian tubes, bladder, rectum or pelvic sidewalls.

Stage III

Stage IV

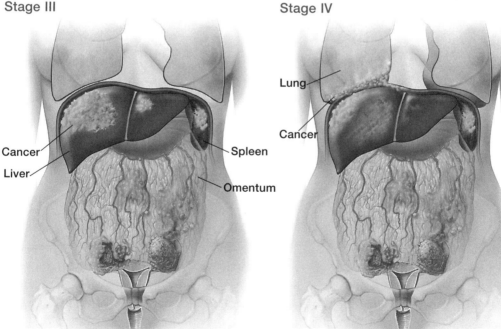

The cancer is in one or both ovaries and has spread beyond the pelvis to the surface of organs in the upper abdomen or to the lymph nodes.

The cancer is found outside the abdominal-pelvic cavity, such as the area surrounding the lungs. The cancer may have spread to the interior of the liver or spleen.

©MFMER

Ovarian cancer spread

Ovarian cancer typically spreads when the tumor sheds cancerous (malignant) cells into the abdominal-pelvic cavity (seeding). These cells can then implant in the lining of the abdominal-pelvic cavity (peritoneum) or on the surface of other organs. Ovarian cancer may also spread to lymph nodes in the groin and pelvic area or to lymph nodes near the aorta. Less commonly, the cancer may travel to other parts of the body by way of the bloodstream.

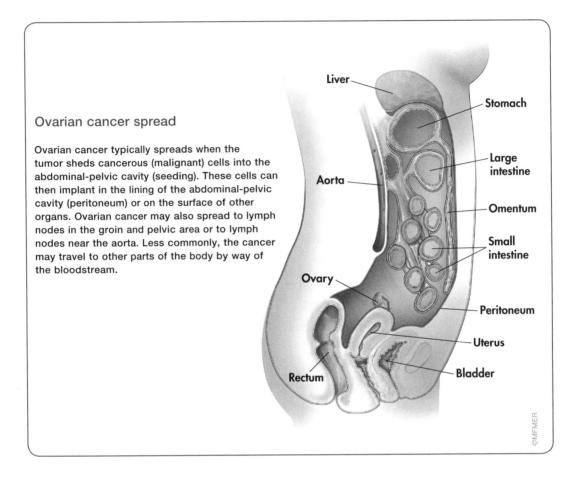

oncologist is a surgeon with extensive training in the care and treatment of women with cancers of the reproductive tract.

The goal of surgery is to remove as much of the ovarian cancer as possible. Numerous studies have shown that the more effective this initial surgery, the better the outcome. If you've been told that you may have ovarian cancer or another type of gynecologic cancer, ask for a referral to a gynecologic oncologist.

Based on the results of your surgery and laboratory tests, your doctor or team of doctors gathers all of the infor-mation needed to classify the stage of your cancer — or how far the cancer has spread. Staging is a key factor in determining your prognosis and the treatment approaches that will be used. The stages of ovarian cancer are shown on page 283.

After surgery, you'll likely receive combination chemotherapy with a platinum agent and a taxane. This is done to try to destroy cancer cells that may have remained. You might consider taking part in a clinical trial aimed at improving upon standard chemotherapy. Such trials are available in most centers that specialize in treating ovarian cancer.

Pat's Story

Pat Goldman's journey from survivor to activist began when she was 50 years old. On a November day, she saw a gynecologist because she had had some breakthrough spotting between her regular periods. The doctor did an endometrial biopsy, which found nothing, and an ultrasound, which revealed gallstones. The doctor told her that everything seemed to be fine and recommended regular checkups.

Early the following year, Pat got a call from a resident at the hospital where she had had the ultrasound. The resident had seen Pat's ultrasound and suspected that she might have adenomyosis, a noncancerous (benign) thickening of the outside of the uterus. Pat was offered a free magnetic resonance imaging (MRI) scan as part of a study the resident was conducting on diagnosing adenomyosis.

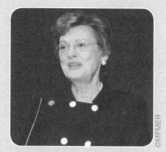

Pat Goldman speaking at a meeting of the Ovarian Cancer National Alliance, the ovarian cancer awareness organization she helped establish.

Pat had the test, and the resident confirmed that she had the condition. "I was not the aggressive or informed consumer prior to my ovarian cancer diagnosis that I am today," she reflects. "When the resident said that was what I had, I accepted it, never asked for a written report or copy of the pictures. With today's knowledge, I certainly wouldn't have accepted a phone diagnosis. I would have insisted on seeing her, the records and my gynecologist for a follow-up."

Pat was told she may need a hysterectomy, but it wasn't urgent. Over the next few months, she experienced more discomfort. "I'd roll over in bed and feel a twinge," she recalls. "In the car, driving over bumps made my stomach hurt." She went up two dress sizes and could no longer fit into her pants because she was so bloated.

By the following July, Pat was so uncomfortable that she could barely eat. She went back to her regular doctor and had another ultrasound. This time it showed a mass. She was referred to a gynecologic oncologist. Pat had surgery and was diagnosed with stage II ovarian cancer.

"I was devastated … because the only thing I knew was that Gilda Radner had it, and she died," Pat says. "First you expect you're going to die, then you have to figure out how to live."

That wasn't easy at first. After she finished her treatment, she kept expecting to have a recurrence, even though her surgeon told her that her relatively early stage at diagnosis improved her odds. Pat even postponed needed hernia surgery, figuring she was going to have another operation for cancer anyway, so she could take care of everything at once. Meanwhile, she began educating herself about ovarian cancer. She read a lot and looked for a support group. To her disappointment, she couldn't find one. She told a friend involved with a breast cancer organization, who said, "You can't do this alone. You're going to have to find others."

Gradually, Pat connected with other ovarian cancer survivors. She and a few other women in the Washington, D.C., area put a notice in *The Washington Post* announcing a meeting on ovarian cancer advocacy. To their surprise, 30 people showed up. They formed a group called the Ovarian Cancer Coalition of Greater Washington.

From there, Pat, representing the Washington group, and leaders from six other organizations established the Ovarian Cancer National Alliance (OCNA). From the beginning, OCNA's foremost goal has been to raise awareness of ovarian cancer among the public, physicians and policymakers. As Pat's experience demonstrates, ovarian cancer often goes undetected or misdiagnosed at an early stage. Alliance members have worked to promote earlier detection. As Pat and her colleagues continue to say today, "Until there's a test, awareness is best."

Chapter 18

Uterine Cancer: What You Should Know

The Uterus	287
Uterine Cancer Basics	288
How common is it?	289
Causes	289
Risk Factors	289
Age	289
Race and ethnicity	290
Hereditary nonpolyposis colorectal cancer	290
Obesity	290
Reproductive risk factors	291
Other factors	292
Putting risk in perspective	293
Can It Be Prevented?	293
Warning Signs	293
Diagnosing Uterine Cancer	294
Health history	294
Physical exam	294
Pelvic exam	295
Ultrasound	296
Biopsy	297
Dilation and curettage	297
Determining the Extent of the Cancer	299
Imaging tests	299
Surgery	299
Uterine cancer staging	300
Treatment Options	300
Surgery	300
Radiation therapy	300
Systemic therapy	300
Estimating survival	300

There are several important links between breast cancer and uterine cancer. These include the role of female hormones in promoting both of these diseases and the breast cancer drug tamoxifen's link to uterine cancer risk. In addition, there are shared risk factors.

Of the gynecologic cancers, uterine cancer is the most common. About 50,000 women are diagnosed with uterine cancer each year in the United States. Fortunately, approximately 80 to 85 percent of these women are cured with current treatments.

Most cases of uterine cancer are discovered before the cancer has spread outside the uterus, when chances of a complete cure are the greatest.

The Uterus

The uterus is the hollow organ where a baby grows and develops during pregnancy. When you're not pregnant, it's about the size and shape of an upside-down pear.

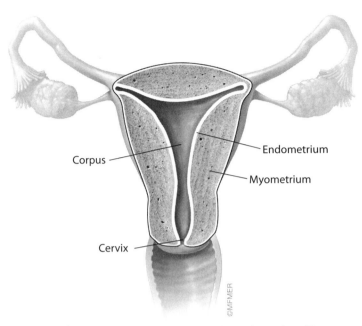

The body of the uterus (corpus) has an inner lining known as the endometrium. The myometrium is a thick layer of smooth muscle tissue.

The uterus has two main parts. The lower, neck-like portion that extends into the vagina is called the uterine cervix. The upper, larger portion of the uterus is called the uterine corpus. The uterine corpus is also known as the body of the uterus.

The body of the uterus has an inner lining known as the endometrium. A portion of this thick, blood-rich lining is what's shed each month during your menstrual period. If fertilization has occurred, this is where the fertilized egg attaches and develops during pregnancy.

The myometrium — a thick layer of smooth muscle tissue — makes up the wall of the uterus. This tissue contracts during menstruation as well as during childbirth to help push the baby through the birth canal.

Uterine Cancer Basics

Cancer can start in either the uterine corpus or the uterine cervix. In this book, the term *uterine cancer* is used to refer to cancers of the uterine corpus. This chapter focuses on the most common form of cancer to affect the uterine corpus, endometrial cancer, which accounts for about 95 percent of all uterine cancers. Cervical cancer begins in the cervix and will not be addressed in this book because it doesn't have a link to breast cancer.

There are two major subtypes of uterine cancer. Endometrioid cancer is the most common form, making up 80 to 85 percent of all cases. This type of cancer, often referred to as type I, is often preceded by a condition called atypical hyperplasia. In this condition, there's an increase in the number of tissue cells (hyperplasia) in the endometrium and the cells begin to take on abnormal features (atypia).

Type II uterine cancers include both papillary serous carcinoma and clear cell cancer. These types are less common and behave more aggressively.

How common is it?

Uterine cancer is the fourth most common cancer among American women, after breast cancer, lung cancer and colorectal cancer (see the table on page 290). It most often occurs after menopause — age 60 is the average age at diagnosis.

Uterine cancer is more common among white women than among black women and other ethnic and racial groups in the United States. However, deaths from uterine cancer are higher among minorities. The reasons for these trends aren't well understood.

Causes

Healthy cells grow and divide in an orderly way to keep your body working normally. But sometimes this tightly regulated process goes awry. Cells keep dividing even when new cells aren't needed. At a very basic level, this is cancer.

In uterine cancer, cancerous (malignant) cells develop in the inner, glandular lining of the uterus. Why these cancer cells develop isn't entirely known. Scientists believe that increased exposure to the female hormone estrogen plays a key role in the development of the most common subtype — endometrioid cancers. Excess estrogen given to laboratory animals produces increased cell growth in the endo-

metrium (endometrial hyperplasia), as well as cancer.

Does this mean that estrogen causes uterine cancer? Yes and no. Although estrogen appears to be an important factor in the development of uterine cancer, exactly what occurs to cause the cancer isn't known. One possible explanation is called the unopposed estrogen hypothesis. According to this theory, when the cells of your endometrium are exposed to estrogen that's not offset (opposed) by the hormone progesterone, these cells start dividing and accumulating more quickly. This sets the stage for an increased number of DNA replication errors — genetic mistakes, if you will. These mistakes can ultimately result in completely transformed, malignant cells.

Scientists have identified several factors that are associated with increased estrogen levels, as well as other factors that seem to increase the risk of uterine cancer. And new risk factors continue to emerge.

Risk Factors

When it comes to cancer, there are many different kinds of risk factors. Some, such as age, race and family history, can't be changed. Others, such as obesity and smoking, can be.

Age

As you get older, your risk of uterine cancer increases. About 95 percent of cases of uterine cancer occur in women age 40 or older, with most occurring in women between ages 50 and 70. As mentioned earlier, the average age at diagnosis is 60.

FAST FACT

Most common cancers among American women

	Type	Estimated number of new cases in 2012
1.	Breast cancer (invasive only)	226,870
2.	Lung cancer	109,690
3.	Colorectal cancer	70,040
4.	Uterine (endometrial) cancer	47,130
5.	Thyroid cancer	43,210
6.	Melanoma	32,000
7.	Non-Hodgkin lymphoma	31,970
8.	Kidney cancer	24,520
9.	Ovarian cancer	22,280
10.	Pancreatic cancer	21,830

Source: American Cancer Society. *Cancer Facts & Figures 2012.* Atlanta, Ga.: American Cancer Society, Inc.

Race and ethnicity

Compared with black women and women of other ethnic and racial minorities in the United States, white women have about twice the risk of uterine cancer. However, black women who get uterine cancer are more likely to have advanced-stage disease at the time of diagnosis. Perhaps because of this, black women are almost twice as likely to die of the disease, once diagnosed, as are white women.

Hereditary nonpolyposis colorectal cancer

Uterine cancer occurs in select families that have an inherited predisposition to develop colorectal cancer. This is called hereditary nonpolyposis colorectal cancer (HNPCC) or Lynch syndrome. It's caused by defects in certain genes responsible for repairing errors in DNA.

After colorectal cancer, uterine cancer is the most common form of cancer in families with HNPCC. In women in these families, 30 to 60 percent will develop uterine cancer in their lifetimes, usually in their 40s.

If several of your family members have had colorectal cancer or uterine cancer, genetic counseling and testing is recommended. Research has shown that prophylactic hysterectomy essentially eliminates the risk of uterine cancer in women in HNPCC families. For women who may not be finished having children, heightened screening options can be considered.

Obesity

Obesity, roughly defined as being 30 pounds or more overweight, is a major risk factor for uterine cancer. Scientists estimate that it could account for about 25 percent of all cases of the disease. The heavier a woman is, the higher her risk.

What's the link between obesity and uterine cancer? Your ovaries produce most of the estrogen in your body. However, fat tissue also can change some hormones — those produced by the ovaries and adrenal glands — into estrogen. Thus, having excess fat tissue can increase your estrogen levels, increasing your risk of uterine cancer. If you're obese and have been through menopause, you're at even higher risk of uterine cancer. Your fat cells are making estrogen, but your ovaries are no longer making progesterone to oppose the estrogen.

Reproductive risk factors

Your ovaries produce the two main female hormones, estrogen and progesterone. In your menstruating years, the balance between these two hormones changes during each month. These shifts help the lining of your uterus to thicken in case it needs to nourish a fertilized egg or to shed tissue through menstruation if an egg isn't present.

When the balance of the female hormones estrogen and progesterone shifts more toward estrogen, your risk of developing uterine cancer increases. That's because estrogen stimulates growth of the cells lining your uterus, while progesterone shuts off this growth. In fact, high lifetime exposure to estrogen appears to be the main risk factor for developing uterine cancer.

Any factor that increases your exposure to estrogen over time, especially if it's not offset (opposed) by progesterone, leads to an increased risk of uterine cancer.

Early onset of menstruation and late menopause
If you had your first period before age 12 and continue to have periods after age 50, you're at greater risk of uterine cancer than are women who menstruate for

fewer years. Studies suggest women who go through menopause in their mid- to late 50s have an increased risk of uterine cancer.

Early menstruation is less of a risk factor if you also experience early menopause. Likewise, late menopause isn't a risk factor for uterine cancer if you got your first period later in your teens.

Never having been pregnant
During pregnancy, the balance of female hormones shifts more toward progesterone, which helps protect you from uterine cancer. If you've never been pregnant, you don't get the benefit of this protection. As a result, your risk of developing uterine cancer is higher than that of women who have had children.

Endometrial hyperplasia
Often, uterine cancer evolves from a condition called endometrial hyperplasia, in which cells lining the uterus overgrow and cause it to thicken. There are four main types of endometrial hyperplasia: simple, complex, simple atypical and complex atypical.

Simple hyperplasia, the most common type, refers to an excess of normal-appearing cells. It's very unlikely to develop into uterine cancer. It can go away on its own or with hormonal treatment. Complex hyperplasia refers to an increased thickness of the endometrium, similar to simple hyperplasia, but the cells — though they appear normal — are more crowded and have a more complex structure.

The term *atypical* signifies that the excess cells appear abnormal. Simple atypical hyperplasia and complex atypical hyperplasia refer to endometrial cells that are enlarged and whose center (nucleus) is irregular in size, shape or composition. These conditions are more serious.

Studies have shown progression to uterine cancer in 1 percent of women with simple hyperplasia, 3 percent of women with complex hyperplasia, 8 percent of women with simple atypical hyperplasia and 29 percent of women with complex atypical hyperplasia.

Heavy menstrual periods, bleeding between periods and bleeding after menopause are common signs of endometrial hyperplasia. Treatment includes hormone therapy and follow-up exams, or removal of the uterus (hysterectomy).

Estrogen therapy after menopause

In the past, doctors commonly prescribed the hormone estrogen to treat symptoms of menopause, without also prescribing a synthetic form of the hormone progesterone (progestin). Studies show that taking estrogen alone after menopause, without also taking a progestin, increases a woman's risk of uterine cancer.

As a result of these and other findings, hormone replacement therapy (HRT), or menopausal hormone therapy, as it's also called, now generally consists of estrogen combined with a progestin. (If a woman has had a hysterectomy, it's safe to take estrogen alone.)

This combination therapy poses no increased risk of uterine cancer. Recent studies, though, have shown that some combination hormone therapies may increase the risk of developing other health problems, including blood clots and breast cancer. Use of hormones after menopause should be determined on an individual basis.

Other factors

Your risk for uterine cancer is also dependent on these health factors.

Breast cancer or ovarian cancer

If you've had breast cancer or ovarian cancer in the past, you may be at increased risk of endometrial cancer. Some of the same risk factors for breast cancer and ovarian cancer also increase your risk of endometrial cancer.

Tamoxifen use

Tamoxifen is an anti-estrogen drug used to treat breast cancer. It's also used to help prevent breast cancer in women who have a high risk of developing it. Although it acts as an anti-estrogen on breast cancer cells, it acts like estrogen on some tissues, including the uterus. It can cause your uterine lining to grow, increasing your risk of uterine cancer.

Among women who take tamoxifen to treat or prevent breast cancer, about one in 500 (0.2 percent) will develop uterine cancer each year.

Women taking tamoxifen who haven't had a hysterectomy are advised to have a yearly pelvic examination and report any unusual vaginal bleeding to their doctors. Studies haven't shown that women taking tamoxifen should be screened for uterine cancer.

Diabetes

Uterine cancer is more common among women who have diabetes. Because type 2 diabetes (formerly called noninsulin-dependent diabetes) is common among women who are overweight, many doctors think that obesity, not diabetes, actually increases a woman's risk of uterine cancer.

However, some studies have compared women who are both overweight and diabetic with those who are overweight but not diabetic. They've found that the risk of uterine cancer is higher among women who have both conditions. This evidence is further bolstered by data from women with type 1 diabetes, the type in which the pancreas doesn't produce insulin. These women have higher rates of uterine cancer even though their diabetes isn't caused by obesity.

Putting risk in perspective

Having one or even several risk factors for a particular condition doesn't mean that you'll develop it. Most women who have known risk factors for uterine cancer never get the disease. At the same time, many women who develop uterine cancer have no major risk factors for it. In most cases, doctors can't explain why one woman develops uterine cancer and another doesn't.

If you're at higher risk of uterine cancer, it's particularly important to have a yearly pelvic exam and to be aware of signs and symptoms of the disease.

Can It Be Prevented?

Unfortunately, most cases of uterine cancer happen for reasons that are unknown or beyond a woman's control. However, if there's a risk factor in your life that can be modified, do so. For obese women and those with diabetes, weight loss and better control of diabetes can help to reduce

risk. A healthy diet and exercise also appear to be protective against developing uterine cancer. If a woman who still has her uterus wishes to take hormone replacement therapy, a combination of both estrogen and a progestin should be taken. Also, combination birth control pills (which contain both estrogen and a progestin) can reduce your risk of uterine cancer, even if used years earlier.

Warning Signs

Most uterine cancers develop over years. Often, cancer follows the development of a less serious uterine condition, such as endometrial hyperplasia.

Signs and symptoms of uterine cancer may include:
- Vaginal bleeding or spotting after menopause or during the time around menopause (perimenopause)
- Heavy menstrual periods or bleeding between periods
- A watery pink or white discharge from the vagina
- Pain in the lower abdomen or pelvic area
- Pain during sexual intercourse

Abnormal vaginal bleeding is the most common sign of precancerous hyperplasia and uterine cancer. It may be that your signs and symptoms are associated with a noncancerous condition, such as a vaginal infection, uterine fibroid or uterine polyp. But it's still important to bring them to the attention of your doctor right away.

If you begin having especially heavy menstrual periods, have bleeding between periods or have bleeding after menopause, talk with your doctor. Because this warning sign is easy to notice, uterine cancer is often detected early, when it's most likely curable.

Diagnosing Uterine Cancer

If your primary care doctor suspects that you have uterine cancer, you may be referred to a gynecologist, a doctor who specializes in conditions affecting the female reproductive system.

A gynecologist or your primary care doctor will likely perform a general physical examination, including a pelvic exam, and talk with you about your signs and symptoms, risk factors and family medical history. He or she may then request one or more tests and procedures needed to make an accurate diagnosis, including a transvaginal ultrasound exam, endo-metrial biopsy and a minor surgical procedure called dilation and curettage (D&C).

Health history

The first part of an evaluation for uterine cancer typically is a discussion of your health history, including any risk factors for the disease.

You may also have other medical problems that need to be evaluated to determine their effect, if any, on your treatment. Be sure to tell your doctor about any medical problems you have, including those you've had in the past. Also tell your doctor about any medications or herbal supplements you're taking.

Physical exam

The next step is often a complete physical examination. A thorough exam allows

Screening for Uterine Cancer

When doctors and scientists talk about screening people for cancer, they're referring to something very specific. Screening for cancer means testing people for early stages of a disease, even though the people being tested have no signs or symptoms.

Some cancer-screening tests are relatively simple, such as a Pap test, which is used to check for cervical cancer. Others are more involved, such as a colonoscopy exam to detect the early stages of colon cancer.

Unfortunately, in the case of uterine cancer, there's no effective screening test yet available.

With uterine cancer, scientists have studied whether techniques used to diagnose the cancer, such as endometrial biopsy and transvaginal ultrasound, might be worthwhile as screening tests. But results suggest that they're not. In one study of 800 women with no signs or symptoms of uterine cancer, endometrial biopsy detected only one case of uterine cancer. Screening by way of endome-

your doctor to feel for suspicious lymph nodes or areas within the pelvis where cancer may have spread. As part of your assessment, your doctor may order some tests. A blood test called a complete blood count (CBC) measures red blood cells, white blood cells and blood platelets. Often, women with excessive blood loss from uterine cancer have a low red blood cell count (anemia). Other routine blood and urine tests may be done to make sure you don't have undetected health problems.

Pelvic exam

During a pelvic exam, you lie on your back on an examining table with your knees bent. Usually, your heels rest in metal supports called stirrups (see the illustration on page 280).

Your doctor begins by examining your external genitals to make sure they look normal — no sores, discoloration or swelling. The internal examination is next. To see the inner walls of your vagina and your cervix, your doctor gently inserts an instrument called a speculum into your vagina. When the speculum is placed in the open position, it holds your vaginal walls apart so that your cervix can be seen. Your doctor then shines a light inside to look for lesions, inflammation, signs of abnormal discharge and anything else unusual. Looking at your cervix also helps your doctor determine whether a cervical problem might be causing your bleeding.

Your pelvic exam may or may not include a Pap test — a test in which your doctor takes a sample of cells from your cervix by gently scraping it with a small spatula and brush. Because uterine cancer begins inside the body of the uterus, not the cervix, it rarely shows up in the results of a Pap test.

trial biopsy isn't even recommended for women taking tamoxifen — a known risk factor for uterine cancer.

The current recommendation of the American College of Obstetricians and Gynecologists is to perform an endometrial biopsy only if a woman develops abnormal bleeding. A yearly pelvic exam can find some cancers of the female reproductive system, but it's not a very effective way of finding early uterine cancers. A Pap test can detect some early uterine cancers, but only a relatively small number. It's a much better tool for detecting cervical cancer.

In the absence of a routine screening test for uterine cancer, your best defense against the disease is to be informed. Familiarize yourself with its signs and symptoms, especially if you've gone through menopause or have known risk factors for the disease. Above all, if you have any abnormal vaginal bleeding or spotting, make an appointment to see your doctor.

After removing the speculum, your doctor checks the condition of your uterus and ovaries. This is done by inserting one or two lubricated, gloved fingers into your vagina and pressing down on your abdomen with the other hand. Usually, this is followed by a rectovaginal exam, done with one finger in your vagina and another in your rectum. This allows your doctor to locate your uterus, ovaries and other organs, judge their size, and confirm that they're in the proper position. While exploring the contours of these organs, your doctor feels for any lumps or changes in the shape of your uterus that may indicate a problem.

You may be apprehensive about having a pelvic exam. Many women are. During the exam, try to relax as much as you can by breathing slowly and deeply. If you tense up, your muscles may tighten, which can make the exam even more uncomfortable. Let your doctor know if you're experiencing a lot of discomfort. Remember, a typical pelvic exam takes only a couple of minutes.

Ultrasound

Ultrasound may be used to examine the uterus, fallopian tubes and ovaries. The procedure is done with a device called a transducer that's placed either on your abdomen (transabdominally) or within the vagina (transvaginally). For viewing the uterine lining, transvaginal ultrasound is most often used.

In a transvaginal ultrasound exam, a small transducer about the size of a tampon is inserted into your vagina. The transducer uses sound waves to create a video image of your uterus. This test helps your doctor evaluate the size and shape of your uterus and look for abnormalities in your uterine lining. Increased thickness of the uterine lining or tissue buildup can be a predictor of endometrial cancer. In some cases, transvaginal ultrasound images can help determine if a tumor is present and if it extends into the muscular wall of the uterus (myometrium).

Sometimes, sterile saline water is inserted into your uterus by way of a thin tube during the ultrasound test. The saline water enhances the image, making any abnormalities of the uterine lining more visible on video. This procedure is called a saline infusion sonogram (sonohysterogram). With a more detailed picture of your uterine lining, your doctor is better able to determine whether your problem might be related to a noncancerous condition, such as an endometrial polyp or uterine fibroid.

Ultrasound is an important imaging tool when evaluating a woman for one of several gynecologic diseases, including uterine cancer. Its advantages are that it's safe, relatively inexpensive and noninvasive. It can detect a suspected uterine cancer and, sometimes, provide information about whether the cancer has spread through the muscular uterine wall or to the cervix.

But ultrasound also has limitations. Transvaginal ultrasound isn't a definitive test. It can't indicate for certain if something is cancerous or noncancerous. It can only highlight abnormalities in your uterine lining that look suspicious. To know for sure whether you have cancer, your doctor must obtain a sample of tissue from your endometrium, through either an endometrial biopsy or a D&C.

Biopsy

An endometrial biopsy is a procedure in which your doctor removes a small piece of tissue from your uterine lining so that it can be examined under a microscope. It's a commonly performed diagnostic test for uterine cancer.

An endometrial biopsy is typically done in your doctor's office and usually doesn't require anesthesia. However, in some women who've gone through menopause, the opening into the cervical canal has closed off. The canal needs to be reopened, and, for this, anesthesia is usually required.

During an endometrial biopsy, your doctor uses a speculum to open your vagina. He or she then threads the biopsy instrument — a flexible tube about the diameter of a thin straw — into your vagina, through the cervix and into the uterus. This biopsy instrument removes a small sample of your uterine lining, either through suction, scraping or both. The tissue is then sent to a laboratory, where a pathologist examines it under a microscope to determine whether cancer cells are present.

You may need a few minutes of rest after an endometrial biopsy, but you'll probably be able to drive yourself home and resume your normal activities right away. Before you leave your doctor's office, be sure to ask when and how you'll get the results of the biopsy.

After a biopsy, you may experience cramping, similar to menstrual cramping. And you may have some spotting for a day or two, requiring the need to wear a panty liner. If you experience heavy bleeding, call your doctor. Also call if you have any signs or symptoms that suggest infection, such as pain in your vagina or lower abdomen, foul-smelling vaginal discharge or fever.

Dilation and curettage

In certain situations, a doctor wants to remove and examine the majority of cells that line the uterus. This minor surgical procedure is called dilation and curettage (D&C).

For the procedure, your doctor dilates your cervix and scrapes endometrial tissue from the entire inside of your uterus using a thin, spoon-like surgical

---

QUESTION & ANSWER

Q: Is a biopsy painful?

A: You may feel some pain during an endometrial biopsy, something similar to menstrual cramps. Some women may also have cramps and vaginal bleeding for a few days after a biopsy.

To reduce your discomfort, your doctor may recommend that you take an over-the-counter pain reliever about an hour before the biopsy. If you have pain after the procedure, your doctor may prescribe one or two doses of a pain reliever.

Endometrial biopsy

D&C procedure

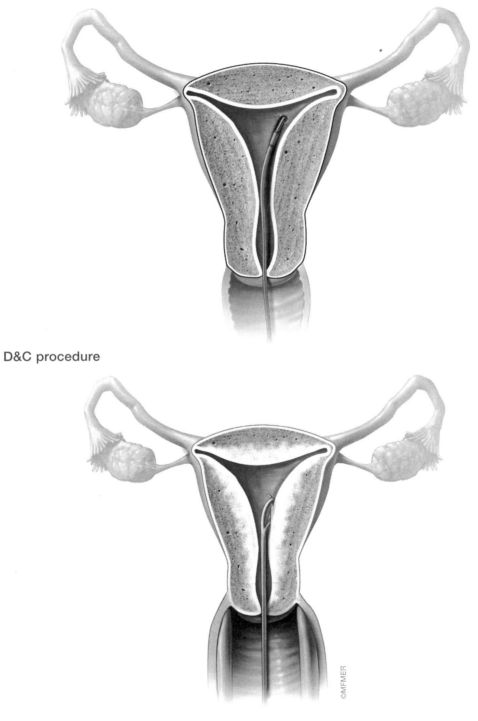

instrument called a curet, a low-pressure suction device or both. The tissue that's removed is then sent to a pathologist for analysis.

A D&C usually takes less than an hour. You may have either general anesthesia, in which you're fully sedated, or conscious sedation, in which you're drowsy but awake.

As part of your D&C, your doctor may also insert a thin, telescope-like instrument through your vagina and cervix, directly into your uterine cavity. This procedure is called a hysteroscopy. Unlike endometrial biopsy or D&C, hysteroscopy allows your doctor to see the inside of your uterus.

Having a D&C generally doesn't require an overnight hospital stay. Most women go home the same day. You may experience some vaginal bleeding for a few days afterward, and you may have some cramps or back pain. But most women usually can resume normal activities almost immediately. However, you shouldn't have sexual intercourse or use tampons until your cervix returns to normal and your endometrium is completely healed, which usually takes two weeks.

Determining the Extent of the Cancer

If laboratory tests show that you have cancer, the next step is to determine if the cancer is confined to the uterine lining or if it has spread. This is known as staging. Staging typically involves imaging tests, followed by surgery. To stage your cancer, you'll likely be referred to a gynecologic oncologist — a surgeon who specializes in treating cancers of the female reproductive system.

Imaging tests

Imaging tests help provide your doctor an "inside view" of your internal organs. Imaging tests may be used to help determine if cancer has spread beyond the uterus to neighboring structures or, rarely, to the lungs or liver.

Common imaging tests used to stage uterine cancer include a chest X-ray (to check the lungs), computerized tomography (CT) scan and magnetic resonance image (MRI).

Surgery

The purpose of surgery is twofold. It's used to determine how far the cancer has spread. Surgery is also used to remove the cancer.

Surgery may be performed in a minimally invasive fashion using laparoscopic or robotic surgical methods. After accessing the abdomen, a surgeon views and feels the pelvic and abdominal areas for signs of disease, looking especially to see whether any tumors or suspicious lesions are outside the uterus. The surgeon also takes samples of fluid from the abdominal-pelvic cavity (peritoneum) and often removes lymph nodes from the pelvis to test for cancer cells. This process of examining the uterus, pelvic organs and abdominal cavity for signs of cancers is referred to as surgical staging.

During the same procedure, the surgeon generally removes the cancer as well.

Uterine cancer staging

Based on the results of surgery and laboratory tests, your doctor gathers all the information needed to classify the stage of your cancer — the extent to which the cancer has spread.

Staging is the most important factor in selecting a treatment for uterine cancer. The four stages of uterine cancer are shown on the next page.

Treatment Options

How uterine cancer is treated depends mainly on the stage of the disease and the type of cells present. Other factors, such as your age and health, also play a role in determining the best treatment plan.

Surgery

Surgery is the most common treatment for uterine cancer. Most women diagnosed with uterine cancer will undergo a hysterectomy. In this procedure the surgeon will typically remove the entire uterus (including the cervix), as well as the fallopian tubes and both ovaries. This full procedure is known as a total hysterectomy and bilateral salpingo-oophorectomy.

If your uterine cancer is discovered early, then removing the uterus often eliminates all of the cancer. This is why following up on early warning signs is so critical.

Radiation therapy

If your doctor thinks that you're at high risk of developing recurrent cancer in the pelvis or neighboring lymph nodes, he or she may suggest radiation therapy after a hysterectomy. Radiation therapy may also be recommended for a tumor that's fast growing or one that has invaded deeply into the muscle of the uterus.

Either external beam radiation or internal radiation (brachytherapy) may be used, depending on the extent of the cancer. Your doctor can advise on the best approach for you.

Systemic therapy

Some uterine cancers — such as those showing signs that they may have spread outside the uterus — may require treatment that goes throughout the body. This is known as systemic therapy.

One type of systemic therapy that may be used is hormone therapy, such as an oral medication used to suppress uterine cancer cells that rely on estrogen to help them grow. In other circumstances, chemotherapy may be recommended. With chemotherapy, drugs enter your bloodstream and then travel through your body, killing cancer cells.

Estimating survival

In general, the chances of surviving uterine cancer are quite good. Most women do — about 85 percent. Your chances of surviving uterine cancer depend on the stage and type of your tumor. Endometrioid cancer, the most common form of uterine cancer, is often diagnosed at an early stage. The more aggressive papillary serous and clear cell uterine cancers are often diagnosed at a more advanced stage.

Uterine cancer stages

Stage I

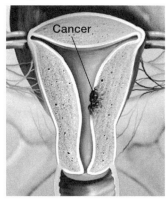

Cancer is limited to the endo-metrium and myometrium.

Stage II

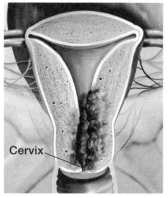

Cancer extends to the cervix.

Stage III

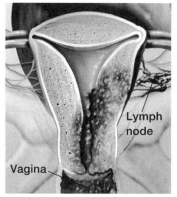

Cancer has spread through the muscle wall of the uterus or to the vagina or nearby lymph nodes.

Stage IV

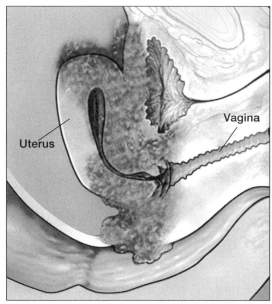

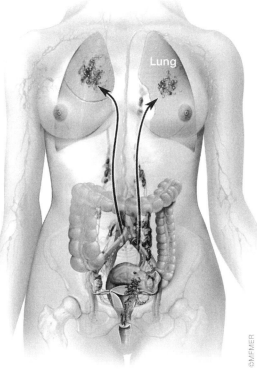

Cancer has spread to the rectum or bladder (side view above) or to sites outside of the pelvis, such as the lungs (right).

©MFMER

Keep in mind that your chances of developing both breast cancer and uterine cancer are low. But even so, it's important to know your risks and take any warning signs seriously.

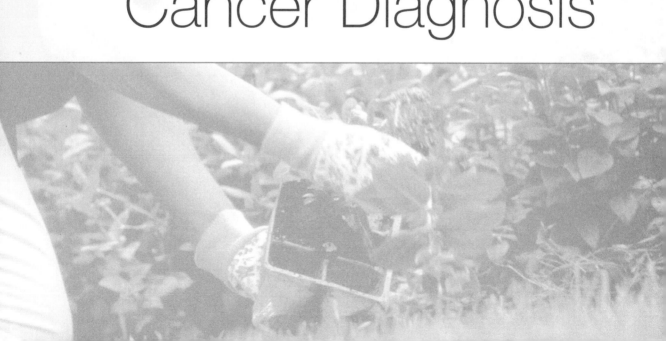

PART 3:

Life After a
Cancer Diagnosis

Chapter 19:

Life After a Cancer Diagnosis

Feelings and Emotions

Making the Journey	305
Absorbing the diagnosis	306
Going through treatment	307
After treatment is over	309
Tips for the Trip	311
Self-help strategies	311
Communicating With Family	315
When cancer becomes a barrier	316
Seek help	317
Communicating With Children	317
Some helpful tips	317
Communicating With Friends	322

Receiving a diagnosis of cancer may be one of the most difficult challenges you'll ever face. The feelings that follow can be very powerful. While most people have known someone who's been diagnosed with cancer, hearing these words spoken to you personally can be devastating.

Although cancer remains a serious illness, knowledge of cancer and its treatments has advanced significantly in the past few decades. Increasingly, cancer is about survivorship — dealing with the initial diagnosis, making decisions about treatment, and managing the treatment's side effects and aftermath. It's also about finding strength and resiliency during your initial care and a balance in life after your active treatment is complete.

Making the Journey

Everyone responds differently to a diagnosis of cancer, and women diagnosed with breast cancer are no different. All sorts of feelings and emotions — disbelief, fear, anger, anxiety, sadness — can arise. How could this happen to me? I don't have time for this right now. Did I do something wrong? I want to go away and hide. Will I die? Is this a punishment? What about my family?

Many women wonder whether their feelings are normal at this point. Trust that these are all common emotional responses. There is no standard set of "normal feelings" when facing a crisis such as cancer. Feelings are what they are.

As you go through your diagnosis, treatment and recovery, you'll likely experience a variety of emotions. Some feelings may overwhelm you, causing you to burst into tears or get angry about simple things. Others may surprise you, making you laugh when you thought humor was long gone.

Some women find it helpful to reframe their thoughts and think of cancer as an unexpected journey — an act of traveling from one physical, emotional and perhaps even spiritual place to another. The diagnosis begins the journey with the destination being the completion of treatment and learning to live in a new landscape of survivorship.

Absorbing the diagnosis

When you learn that you have cancer, it's not uncommon to react with disbelief. You can't believe this is happening to you. You may wonder if your doctor has the diagnosis right or if your test results got mixed up with someone else's. You might find yourself walking around in a dream-like state, unable to concentrate or make decisions. Or you may avoid dealing with the diagnosis completely and carry on as if nothing has happened.

Another common feeling is being scared. You might start to imagine all

sorts of outcomes — some of which may be true and others not. For many women, their first thought is will I die from this? You may be scared of the treatment procedures ahead of you and their side effects, such as nausea and pain. You may be scared for your partner and your family. You may wonder if life will ever be the same or if you'll ever be able to enjoy life again. You may worry that you won't be able to handle all that lies ahead of you. These fears and concerns are reasonable. The first few days to weeks after learning that you have cancer is often a highly stressful time, and your feelings may be new and unfamiliar.

Handling decisions

In practical terms, you may be faced with multiple decisions regarding treatment, even though you may still be reeling from the diagnosis.

A typical first reaction for many women once they learn they have breast cancer is to have surgery as quickly as possible to remove the cancer. But you may have a choice in the type of surgery you receive, such as mastectomy or lumpectomy, as well as various breast reconstruction options. In some cases, the first treatment offered isn't surgery, but rather treatment to shrink the cancer's size, such as chemotherapy or hormone (anti-estrogen) treatment. Some women may be offered the option of participating in clinical research trials.

Having to make choices such as these can often add to your stress. How can you know what is the right thing to do when there are so many options offered? First, try to slow down and take a deep breath. When facing a decision point, focus on the present and what needs to be done in the short term. Break larger issues into steps and focus on the first step. For instance, if surgery is offered as the initial treatment, ask questions about the procedure, what you may need to do beforehand and the estimated recovery time.

Start assessing your resources. Ask who is on your health care team. The team often includes an internal medicine physician, a surgeon, medical oncologist, radiation oncologist, nurses, psychologists, social workers, chaplains and research staff. The team is there to meet your needs, so don't be afraid to ask for the help you need.

You'll probably find it helpful to bring at least one other person, such as a family member or trusted friend, with you to your appointments. He or she can take notes, listen to the conversation and help you think of additional questions to ask.

Going through treatment

Once decisions have been made and treatment is under way, your initial feelings of shock and disbelief may fade. Now you're focused on getting through treatment and doing what needs to be done. Although you may have adjusted to your diagnosis at this point, it's not uncommon to feel anxious or nervous about your upcoming procedures and their side effects, to worry about whether your treatment will get all of the cancer, and to wonder if your body will undergo any permanent changes. Again, these feelings are normal.

Having a good relationship with your oncologist and other members of your team can go a long way toward helping you deal with some of the fears and

concerns that can fuel your anxiety. Your doctor can clarify test results, explain procedures and help provide you with realistic expectations by making sure that you have accurate information. It's important that you be able to talk openly and honestly with your health care team. Let them know your fears and concerns and how they can best help you.

Family and friends also can provide support by helping to reduce the amount of stress in your life. The love and emotional support of those closest to you are invaluable. Logistically, the people around you can be of great help with everyday tasks such as getting you to and from your treatment sessions and buying groceries for the week.

To effectively manage stress and anxiety, you have to be willing to accept help and delegate tasks. Depending on others doesn't come easy for some women, especially if you're at the center of the family and all of its activities. But sometimes you need to let others help you.

When the worry is too much
Usually, feelings of anxiety tend to dissipate as you adjust to the changes you're going through. If your anxiety persists for more than a few weeks or it remains intense, it can affect your quality of life and interfere with your ability to function. In such a case, your anxiety may be part of a more specific disorder (see "Adjustment Disorder" on page 308), which needs medical attention.

You don't need to live with symptoms of persistent anxiety. The condition is treatable, and addressing it promptly can enhance your well-being and make your cancer treatment less worrisome.

Signs and symptoms that may indicate your anxiety exceeds a reasonable threshold and should be evaluated by a doctor include:

- Intense fear or worry
- Restlessness or irritability
- Trouble sleeping or waking up feeling wired
- Fatigue
- Difficulty concentrating or making decisions
- A rapid pulse
- Shortness of breath
- Sweating or chills
- Trembling
- Indigestion or diarrhea
- A feeling of detachment from yourself or others
- An inability to carry on with work or social functions

Your doctor can refer you to a licensed therapist, licensed counselor or other mental health specialist. Treatment for severe anxiety may include medications, counseling from a licensed mental health professional or both.

Dealing with sadness

Feelings of sadness, grief and loss are natural among people with cancer. A diagnosis of breast cancer can disrupt or even shatter your life plans and may make you feel discouraged and pessimistic about your future. Although these feelings take time to work through, they usually become more manageable over a period of weeks to months.

Among some women, though, these feelings linger and deepen. Grief and discour-

Adjustment Disorder

Adjustment disorder is the term used to describe a variety of emotional responses that may develop when a person encounters a major life stressor. Many people with cancer experience certain signs and symptoms of depression or anxiety. While perfectly normal, sometimes these signs and symptoms may reach the point where they interfere with daily living. However, they're not severe enough to be classified as an anxiety disorder or clinical depression. This in-between stage is called an adjustment disorder.

Adjusting to the fact that you have cancer doesn't occur as a single event. It usually consists of multiple responses and steps that occur throughout the course of the disease as you progress through diagnosis, treatment, follow-up and survivorship.

Adjustment to these events involves the ability to minimize their disruption to your life, regulate your emotional distress and remain actively involved in meaningful aspects of your life. In other words, even though you have fears, concerns and other difficult emotions, you are coping with your cancer and you still find meaning, joy and importance in your life.

If your feelings begin to cause significant impairment to your ability to function on a daily basis, whether at work, at home or in social settings, you may have an adjustment disorder. Doctors typically use these criteria in diagnosing an adjustment disorder:

agement can evolve into major depression, characterized by persistent sadness, loss of interest in life, feelings of hopelessness or worthlessness and continuous negative thinking. Uncontrolled pain, metabolic abnormalities and some medications also can contribute to depression.

It's not always easy to know if what you're feeling is just a natural response to having cancer or if it's major depression. If you're worried about what you're feeling and how you're reacting to your situation, discuss these concerns with your doctor or a member of your health care team. If you're having thoughts of suicide, seek help immediately.

Similar to anxiety, depression is highly treatable. Treating depression is vital to your quality of life. If you're in the midst of active cancer treatment, eliminating depression can help you better cope with your cancer therapy and any side effects it may have. You'll also feel more motivated to take part in rehabilitation activities to promote healing. Getting help for depression may also be worthwhile in terms of your relationships with your co-workers, partner, children, other family members and friends.

After treatment is over

Once the hustle and bustle of treatment is over, you might feel relieved that it's behind you. No more surgery, no more radiation or chemotherapy treatments, no more hair loss. But it's also not unusual to feel a bit lost and even scared.

- The individual's emotional or behavioral symptoms are in response to an identifiable event, such as a diagnosis of cancer or a cancer recurrence, that occurred within the last three months.
- The individual's response to the event is interfering with life. It's not that you cried for two hours when you were first diagnosed — it's that you keep crying and can't get things done.
- The individual is experiencing significant difficulty in social or work settings. You can't enjoy time with friends or accomplish tasks at work because you keep worrying about your cancer.

The person with cancer isn't the only one vulnerable to adjustment disorders. Sometimes, family members can experience an adjustment disorder as well, including children.

Age can play a role in the type of adjustment disorder people experience. Adults typically become depressed or anxious. Adolescents tend to act out their problems. This may include skipping school or doing some other type of uncharacteristic behavior.

Treatment usually consists of short-term counseling or psychotherapy, which involves talking about fears and concerns, dealing with thoughts and emotions, and changing behaviors. You and your doctor may consider use of medications.

An adjustment disorder is not a sign of emotional weakness. Some events in life are simply too great for people to manage without help. Professionals can speed the time it takes to adjust so that you can feel like yourself sooner.

As your medical appointments become fewer and farther between, contact with your health care team is reduced and friends and family members may expect you to rapidly return to your old self again. Meanwhile, you may be wondering how? How do you adjust to life after it's been upended on you? What if your previous ideas of how to feel and act just don't seem to apply anymore? And can you ignore the possibility of a recurrence or does life simply become a matter of sitting on a ticking clock, waiting for the cancer to come back? How do you find balance between living life and monitoring for recurrent symptoms?

Searching for meaning

Breast cancer not only affects your physical and emotional well-being, but also brings to mind questions about the meaning and purpose of life. What is it that makes life good and worthwhile and fulfilling? How do you live with a heightened sense of your own mortality? The part of you that reflects on these kinds of questions is often labeled as your spiritual side.

Paul Rousseau, a doctor who wrote about spirituality and illness, described spirituality like this: "Spirituality is characterized by the capacity to seek purpose and meaning, to have faith, to love and forgive, to worship, and to see beyond present circumstances, and enables a person to rise above or transcend suffering."

Possessing spiritual strength and resilience can be a great help in times of crisis. It can lead to hope and a sense of life's bigger picture. It can make you feel connected — to yourself, to others, to a higher order that takes you beyond your daily struggles. This kind of connection de-emphasizes fear and empowers you to be fully engaged in life's experiences.

Many women express their spirituality and resilience through religion, engaging regularly in prayer, meditation and religious worship. Others express their spirituality in a less formal manner. They may become re-energized by natural beauty, experiencing refuge in solitude and enjoying nature. Relationships with family and friends also can provide a sense of spirituality.

Strengthening your spirituality

A person's spirituality is always evolving. It matures with life experiences and is shaped by your upbringing, personality and life circumstances. A crisis such as cancer can affect your awareness of spiritual matters and highlight your spiritual needs. In essence, spirituality is linked with self-discovery and your sense of inner worth. Therefore, it's valuable to remember and share experiences that have moved you deeply or that have influenced your understanding of yourself. Ask yourself:

- What are my important relationships?
- Where have I found comfort and support in previous tough times?
- What are the things I enjoy most in life?
- What gives me hope?
- Was there a time or instance when I felt comfortable and felt all was right with the world?
- Was there a time when my life was filled with a sense of meaning or when I was filled with a sense of awe?

For many women, writing in a journal or diary helps them process their thoughts and feelings. Joining a support group or visiting with a cancer survivor who has traveled down a similar path can provide

Myth: **A positive attitude is all you need to beat cancer.**

Fact: Although many popular books on cancer talk about fighters and optimists, there's no scientific proof that a positive attitude gives you an advantage in cancer treatment or improves your chance of being cured.

What a positive attitude can do is improve the quality of your life during cancer treatment and beyond. You may be more likely to stay active, maintain ties to family members and friends, and continue social activities. In turn, this may enhance your sense of well-being and help you find strength. A positive attitude may also help you become a more informed and active partner with your doctor during cancer treatment.

At the same time, it's perfectly normal to feel sadness, anger or fear after a cancer diagnosis. It's a matter of degree. If you feel that negative emotions are taking up too much of your time, talk with a member of your health care team. Falsely putting on a happy face can increase your sense of isolation and hamper your ability to cope.

great comfort and help you feel less alone in your own journey. In addition, many clinics and hospitals have chaplains or mental health professionals on staff to help people who are struggling with spiritual distress.

Each woman's breast cancer journey is unique, and there are many people along the way to help you navigate yours, including members of your health care team. Going through a serious illness can be a positive journey of exploration and self-discovery. When you need help, don't be afraid to ask for it.

Tips for the Trip

As you learn to cope with and adapt to all of the changes in your life, eventually things will become more manageable. Many people are surprised to discover reserves of strength they never thought they had. But even years later, you may have times when you struggle to conquer feelings of fear, anxiety or discouragement related to your cancer. This is normal. Everyone has distressing times.

Self-help strategies

As you make your way on your cancer journey — through its ups and downs and occasional plateaus — here are some strategies that may help you along the way. If these strategies aren't helpful, ask for help.

Educate yourself
Knowledge is power. Learn as much as you can about your cancer and the treatment plan you and your doctor have set forth. When you know what to expect from your treatments, and why you're

receiving the treatments that you are, your fear decreases — you aren't dealing with fear of the unknown.

It can be difficult to absorb all the information that your health care team provides you at the beginning. Keep your notes and any educational materials you receive for future reference. Consider organizing your information in a folder or on your computer so that you can easily refer back to it if you need to. Many women keep personal journals as a way to track their journey. It can be a helpful way to remember your thoughts and ideas.

Keeping a journal can also help you track any side effects — which medications bothered you the most and how long after receiving them did you feel the worst. This information can help you prepare for future treatments and better manage your schedule.

Express your feelings

Share your feelings, good and bad, with the trusted members of your team. They want to help you and can best help you if they know how you truly feel. Tell them about the bad stuff — the side effects, how tired you feel and how much you long to have your old life back. Tell them the funny things, too — how your dog looked the first time he saw you taking his spot on the couch in the middle of the day, and about the grocery store clerk who loved your new look (you were wearing a wig). You're not alone and sharing how you feel can help to lighten the load.

If talking to others is stressful or awkward for you, consider writing your feelings in a journal. Writing gives you an outlet to express your anger, worries and

fears. Writing may help you identify matters that bother you most, sort out your priorities and put things in perspective. Perhaps the best thing about writing is that you can do it anytime you feel the need to express your feelings.

Learn from others

Talking to other cancer survivors can be an invaluable experience. They've been on much the same journey as you, and they can tell you a lot about the twists and turns ahead by sharing their own stories. But remember, everyone's experience is somewhat different. Take advantage of the expertise of others whenever you can. You can learn more about support groups made up of cancer survivors, and how these groups may help you, in Chapter 22.

Take care of yourself

You didn't have any control over the fact that you got breast cancer, but you can control how you take care of yourself. As you try to get and feel healthy again, do good things for your body. This is an opportune time to make better food choices, engage in regular exercise, and add fun or relaxing activities to your daily schedule.

Many women find that relaxation therapies such as meditation, yoga, massage, music therapy and other mind-body activities add a measure of support and comfort to their daily routine (see Chapter 21 for more on these therapies). The better you feel physically, the better you'll be able to cope mentally.

Exercise

During treatment, the last thing you may feel like doing is exercising, but it's

It Helps to Laugh

You may think there's nothing funny about your situation, but humor can help you cope. In fact, some studies have shown that being able to laugh in the face of adversity may not only help you cope but also ease pain.

The first studies on the effect of humor on the body were conducted in the United States in the 1930s. But it wasn't until 1979 that humor research got a real boost. That's when *Saturday Review* editor Norman Cousins countered a diagnosis of ankylosing spondylitis, a painful and potentially crippling arthritis, with a combination of mainstream medicine and daily doses of humor.

To get his humor fix, Cousins watched Marx Brothers and Three Stooges movies and videos of *Candid Camera*. Although his doctors had given him little chance of recovery, within eight days his pain began to subside, and he returned to work.

Cousins' experience spawned a wealth of humor research. Studies have indicated that laughter relaxes the skeletal muscles of your arms and legs, exercises your heart by raising your heart rate, releases pent-up feelings like frustration and anger, lessens pain, and, for some, makes breathing more comfortable. It doesn't, however, cure disease. Laughter may help relieve your symptoms, but it won't cure your cancer.

In one small study, women with breast cancer identified humor as an important coping skill. They said laughing helped them to relax, and it kept them from giving up and taking their situations too seriously. They reported feeling a strong need to laugh to survive low moments. The women also reported forming deeper, more-trusting relationships with health care professionals who used humor with them.

No one knows why laughter has the effects it does, but one theory is that it boosts the release of endorphins, brain chemicals that create a feeling of well-being. Whatever the reason, laughter helps. So look for something to laugh about, whether it's watching comedies or finding something humorous in each day.

important for you to keep moving to the best of your ability. Exercise can help build muscle, boost your energy level and counter fatigue. It can also lessen depression and anxiety, relieve stress and help you feel better about yourself. In addition, if you don't have much of an appetite, exercise may help stimulate it.

Your ability to exercise depends on the treatment you're receiving, its side effects and your general health and physical condition. If you exercised regularly before your cancer diagnosis, you may find you can still take part in the same types of activities, but perhaps at a lower intensity level. If you didn't get much exercise before your cancer, it's important to start off slowly. It's also a good idea to talk with your doctor or a member of your health care team about the best type of activities to begin with. For many women, walking is a good way to get exercise. You can walk almost anywhere and all you need is a pair of supportive shoes.

Diet

Cancer treatment can cause changes to your appetite and sense of taste. In addition, nausea and other side effects associated with treatment may make you not want to eat as much.

It's important, however, to get adequate nutrition so that you can maintain your strength and energy. Eat when you're hungry and eat what appeals to you. If you can, try to eat healthy, nonprocessed foods such as fruits and vegetables and whole grains. You may also find that eating several smaller meals throughout the day works better for you than the traditional three large meals.

For more information on what foods to eat and how to handle nausea from your treatment, see Chapter 20.

Stay connected

Unfortunately, some women isolate themselves during their treatment — they may feel embarrassed about their hair loss or not feel up to being out and about. But staying connected to the important people in your life provides much-needed support along the way.

Involvement with others — even if it means just sending an email or making a quick phone call — can help you take your mind off your troubles and restore a sense of normalcy to your life. More

likely than not, if you tell your family or friends that all you really want is to laugh a little (or a lot) and talk about "normal" things for a while, they'll be delighted to comply. It's also OK to set boundaries. If you're tired and you've had enough socializing, they'll understand if you ask for some time alone to rest.

Work when you can

Having breast cancer doesn't mean that you have to quit your job. If you're able to, continue to work. For many women, work is a meaningful part of life. It provides a sense of purpose and builds self-esteem, and it keeps you from focusing on your cancer. In addition, co-workers often provide ongoing support.

Going to work also creates some normalcy in your life. With so many changes around you, having a somewhat structured routine can help you find balance between cancer treatments and "real" life.

You might even consider talking with other women who've gone through similar treatment to get an idea of how it may, or may not, affect your ability to work and maintain your usual schedule.

Before you meet with your supervisor, make a list of what might be helpful to you. Would it help to have shorter or more flexible work hours, if possible? Would it be possible for you to work from home on occasion? If your workstation is near the break room, could you move to a different spot for a while to avoid cooking smells that may make you nauseated?

Try to schedule your treatments for days and times that interfere with your work as little as possible and leave you time to recuperate — perhaps later in the day or right before the weekend.

Treating the Whole Person

Cancer treatment often occurs in a setting of high-tech medicine and heavy-duty drugs. Medical staff is often so focused on treating the cancer that staff sometimes forgets about other needs that the person with cancer might have. Symptoms of stress, anxiety and depression, though deserving of care, may go unnoticed.

Doctors and nurses are becoming increasingly aware that just treating the cancer isn't quite enough. More care providers are recognizing the need to treat the whole person — the mind and spirit as well as the body.

A new approach to cancer care, called integrative oncology, seeks to combine the best of today's high-tech, cutting-edge cancer treatment with evidence-based nontraditional techniques and products that address the emotional and spiritual needs of people with cancer. Chapter 21 focuses on complementary therapies that can help you achieve a more holistic healing — therapies that can complement surgery, radiation, chemotherapy and other forms of standard care. You can also visit the Society for Integrative Oncology's website (see page 414).

Consider cleaning out your 'closet'

Cancer is a life-changing event. In facing it, you may feel a need to re-evaluate certain elements in your life, such as your priorities and your relationships. The new job or the promotion you worked so hard to achieve may not prove to be as important as you once thought. You may also find that there are people in your life who make you feel badly about yourself, or certain relationships that tend to drain your energy.

Cancer has a way of revealing life's clutter — the things or people who don't add value or richness to your life. Clearing them away or minimizing their effect on your life can offer a fresh perspective. In fact, you may be surprised by the silver linings behind an experience with cancer, if you're willing to be open to them.

Examine yourself

As you examine your relationships with others, examine your relationship with yourself. If there is something you regret, let it go. It saps your energy to hold on to old hurts and sorrows. If you feel you must right a wrong, do so but let go of lingering guilt.

Believe in yourself. Believe you have the strength and courage to complete the task ahead of you. Now is the time to concentrate on yourself and not on others.

Communicating With Family

When you learn that you have breast cancer, your entire family is affected. The challenges you face involve not only sharing the initial, often shocking news, but also helping your family adjust to the changes ahead.

In some families, cancer has a way of drawing people together. Previous arguments, disagreements and pet peeves seem to fade away in the face of the illness. Family members often learn to treasure their moments with one another. Eventually, the funny side of things starts to show up, and laughter and humor around the house sometimes increase. In essence, life becomes more real and precious than ever before. In time, family members adjust and move on to deal with the challenges at hand.

But illness doesn't always draw families together. In families where communication is already difficult, a crisis such as a cancer diagnosis may not improve the situation. Sometimes, it can make communication even more difficult and past conflicts even more problematic.

When cancer becomes a barrier

Even in the strongest of families, cancer can be a barrier to communication. Having to face this kind of illness can place tremendous stress on the family's foundations. If family relationships were strained before cancer entered the picture, they may become even more strained now. Family members may find it difficult to come to grips with the cancer and they may not be able to talk about important issues.

A family's responses to cancer are often very similar to those of the person diagnosed. In addition, feelings of helplessness and frustration at being powerless to solve the problem are a common response

among family members. Adjustment can be difficult for all involved.

Changing roles within the family also can exert pressure on relationships. For example, you may need to give up some of your responsibilities around the house or as an income provider in order to deal with treatment. In turn, your spouse or partner may need to pick up added responsibilities, such as making dinner, taking care of the children or working an extra job. The success of this transition often depends on how the family has functioned in the past. If household and child care responsibilities were shared before, the transition will likely be smoother. But if this wasn't the case, your spouse or partner may feel frustrated, inadequate or angry about having to take on additional responsibilities.

Teenagers also may need to shoulder chores and duties around the house. If these responsibilities were an expectation in the past, this will help things go smoother. If not, this sudden upheaval can increase tension in the family. Young children, meanwhile, may revert to more infantile behavior in an attempt to cope with the changes.

As in all difficult situations, communication is key. Have a clear understanding from your health care team about what side effects to expect from your treatments and how this will affect you on a day-to-day basis. Once you know what might be coming, you'll be able to explain your treatment to your family and help them understand when you may need their help the most.

Be prepared that if there's already tension and discord in your family, your cancer may lead to increased stress and frustration. Feelings of anger and resentment at the situation are not uncommon and sometimes they're inappropriately directed toward the person with cancer. Some family members who are frightened by your cancer may cope with it in unhealthy ways, such as inappropriate alcohol use.

Seek help

Coping with cancer may require skills that you, your family and friends don't use on a daily basis. It's not only appropriate but often wise to seek help in the form of counseling.

A chaplain or licensed mental health professional can provide you and your family an outlet for discussing fears and other feelings that may not otherwise be expressed. He or she may also offer coping skills to help strengthen your relationships. Many people with cancer also turn to support groups for help in coping with their disease.

Try to find a licensed counselor or adviser who works with people with cancer. Talk to your doctor or other members of your health care team if you need help. Meet with the individual to determine if you feel comfortable with him or her and to get a sense of whether you think you'll benefit from his or her help. If you're not comfortable, look for another person.

Communicating With Children

A woman with children still at home often finds the prospect of telling her children about her cancer especially daunting. Besides wanting to protect them from hurt and pain, she frequently doesn't know how to begin explaining the illness. It helps to come to grips with the diagnosis yourself before communicating it to your children, but at some point they must be told. Remember that children, particularly younger children, may not understand cancer in the same way that adults do. The response from your children may be very different from that of other family and friends. A child's response will also vary with his or her age and ability to grasp the concept of cancer.

Some helpful tips

Following are some suggestions from experts that may help you as you talk to your children. You know your children best. Try to recall how they may have dealt with problems in the past — they'll likely respond in much the same way now. Respect their resilience, but remember they need you now as much as ever.

Maximize their support system

Allow your children to carry on as normal of a schedule as possible, and assure them that it's OK to do so. Encourage your children's relationships with other trusted adults. By letting other adults help out with events and activities, your children will see that such relationships are OK and that they're not being disloyal to you. Alert adults close to your children, such as teachers, coaches, counselors and parents of friends, of what's going on.

The goal is to maintain as much stability as possible in your child's life. If you and your partner are having disagreements or difficulty communicating, it may help to rely on family members to bridge the gap for your children. Don't hesitate to seek professional help if needed.

Provide appropriate information

It's important to be open with your children and to talk with them in a way that's appropriate for their ages. Open communication with your children reassures them that they're valued members of the family, that they aren't being left out of important family matters, and that the family will pull through this together. Sometimes, just spending extra time holding and talking with your children can be valuable.

Children of different ages will have different levels of understanding. Preschoolers tend to think the world revolves around them, and they may see themselves as the cause of the illness. They may exhibit their distress through anxious behavior or angry, defiant outbursts. Find ways to reassure them that nothing they did or thought caused your cancer and that they'll continue to be loved and cared for no matter what happens. Older children may feel torn between being with you and going out with their friends and living their lives as usual. Encourage them to keep up their friendships and to maintain as much normalcy as possible.

Keeping Everyone Informed

As your treatment gets under way, you may feel overwhelmed at times by the number of questions you receive from friends on how you're feeling, how your family is coping and what they can do to help. It can be very challenging to keep up with everyone's communication needs. Some friends would like daily updates, others less often. It can take a lot of time and energy to meet everyone's expectations for information.

To stay in control of what information is shared and with whom, some women choose a family member or trusted friend to manage the role of communicator. Setting up an electronic communication plan, such as a blog or website, is a fast way to reach the most people with the least amount of effort. For example, CaringBridge is a non-profit organization that offers personalized websites at no cost to people facing a serious illness or hospitalization. A website such as this allows you to post updates as often as you like, and others can visit your page at any time to find out the latest news, send responses, and offer their comfort and support.

Be realistic about how often you want to send messages out and don't hesitate to ask for help in maintaining your communication lines. Older friends and family members may need to receive updates through a more traditional communication method. The bottom line is efficient communication can provide you and your family more time and energy to cope with the multiple changes affecting your lives.

Do your best to create a safe and open communication setting, allowing and encouraging your children to express whatever thoughts come to mind. As they ask questions you'll get a better idea of how much they understand and what they're worried about. Children may overhear conversations, read emails, blogs, websites and other communication, and they may misunderstand or become frightened by what they find. Checking in with them often encourages them to share their thoughts and worries with you.

Address common questions

It's important to be honest with your children about your diagnosis, what you're going through, and what they can expect at each stage of your disease and treatment. Although you may prefer to use words like *bad cells*, *lump* or *boo-boo* instead of *cancer*, these terms are often too vague, even for children. They may begin to think that every bump or lump is serious, leading to confusion and anxiety.

Encourage your children to ask questions and express their fears. Talking with them allows you to dispel misconceptions and ease the burden of legitimate worries. For example, some children think that cancer is contagious and that they might get it.

If you're worried about how much to share in terms of your illness, remember that overhearing information is worse than being told it directly. Inevitably, children tend to overhear the discussions of their parents. This can lead to misunderstanding and fear. If you and your husband need to talk about issues you're not ready to discuss with your children, you may wish to do it away from the home or while the children are gone. Otherwise,

make sure your children are in the family circle of information.

Questions regarding death may be especially hard for both the parents and the children. Tell them that there are different types of cancer and that some people with cancer are more sick than others. Acknowledge that cancer can be life-threatening but that you and your doctors are doing your best to fight it. Or assure them that you plan on living as long as possible and that you want them to continue to be as busy and active as before.

Some kids don't want to talk about the illness. If this is the case, don't force the issue. Feel free to share medical updates, but don't try to prolong the discussion if your child isn't ready to hear it.

Help them adjust to medical settings

If your children want to visit you while you're in the hospital and you're in a condition to receive them, encourage them to do so. Before they come to the hospital, have your partner or another adult prepare them for the visit by describing what they'll see, such as what you may look like and items that may be attached to you — intravenous tubes, a monitor, oxygen. Let the children stay as long or as little as they want.

If your child would rather not come to the hospital, don't force him or her. Other means of communication may be more appropriate, such as a card, email or phone call. Different children, even within the same family, communicate in different ways.

Following the visit, someone should follow up with the children and answer any questions or see if they wish to discuss anything that surprised them. This

Jeanne's Story

Jeanne Greenfield has heard the popular adage many times — the one about how people fear speaking in front of a crowd more than they fear dying. She's experienced both. "Not even close!" she responds.

More than 20 years ago, Jeanne was diagnosed with advanced cervical cancer — stage IVB, about as bad as it can get. At the time of her diagnosis, she was told the survival rate for women with this type and stage of cancer was zero. Zero.

When her doctors told her she had only a short time to live, the 38-year-old single mother of three fell apart. She cried uncontrollably, beat her pillow with her fists and refused to talk with people. She was angry, she was bitter, she was scared — and she was determined. Instead of going home and getting her affairs in order, Jeanne pleaded with her doctors to try something. "I refused to believe I was going to die."

Jeanne was placed on a clinical trial of chemotherapy medications, a combination of drugs she equates to ingesting drain cleaner. The drug regimen was eventually found to have too many severe side effects. For Jeanne, though, the chemotherapy worked very well. Next came radiation. She received 30 radiation treatments.

During her cancer treatment and the months that followed, Jeanne lived from week to week and checkup to checkup. "People would come and see me and they

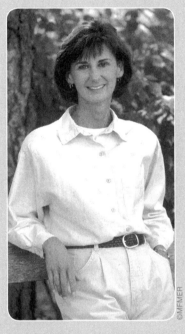

would say, 'I'll see you next week,' and that gave me hope. OK. I'm going to live another week then. I would go and see my doctor for a checkup and my doctor would say, 'I'll see you in two months.' That gave me hope. I'm going to live two more months."

Doctors were hopeful that Jeanne's treatment would buy her some time, maybe even enough time to see her oldest son graduate from high school. But they expected the cancer to return. A few months passed, then a few more. Still, no cancer. Soon a year had gone by, which gradually turned into two and three years and kept going. The cancer never came back. Jeanne has seen all three sons graduate from high school, she has watched her children get married, she has remarried, and she has celebrated the births of grandchildren.

So what happened? How did Jeanne survive when all odds appeared against her? The chemotherapy and long stretch of radiation treatments were undoubtedly key factors. But Jeanne, and even her doctors, feel other forces were also at play. Jeanne credits her strong faith, her unwillingness to give up and, aside from the cancer, her good physical health. Even when she was going through treatment, Jeanne would run or walk every day that she was able to. She also believes timing played a role. Jeanne began her treatment immediately upon diagnosis, at a time she believes the cancer was spreading rapidly.

Although Jeanne beat the cancer, recovery hasn't been easy. In a booklet that she wrote called *What I Learned from Having Cancer*, she writes, "The cancer did not kill me, but the cure has certainly tried to!" Jeanne has experienced shingles, blood poisoning and inflammation of the lining of her lungs. The femoral arteries in her legs closed up due to radiation damage, twice requiring bypass surgery. The same happened to the tubes leading from her kidneys to her bladder (ureters). She still experiences swelling in her lower torso, and she lives with chronic diarrhea. "Life isn't the same, but I wouldn't go back for anything. ... I've learned to appreciate life and all that I have."

Once very shy, Jeanne has become more bold and outgoing. She does mission work at her church. She acts in plays and speaks in front of groups. A speaking engagement at a cancer survivor seminar is what prompted her booklet, a lighthearted recollection of some of her experiences during treatment. Here are some excerpts:

If you wear your best outfit and get your hair done (that is, if you have any), and polish your nails and your tennis shoes and go to the tanning booth, your doctor might still give you bad news.

You might be in the hospital deathly ill with tubes coming out of every orifice of your body, but there's a good chance your teenager will call you up and say, "I need the car, Mom, I have a date tonight."

My mother went with me to my local doctor each week where I was given my interim drugs. When I got there the nurse always weighed me and took my blood pressure. Each week my mother asked them to weigh her and also asked them to take her blood pressure. What I learned from having cancer is that if your mother volunteers to go to the doctor's office with you, it might be so that she can get a free check-up.

Today, Jeanne spends a lot of time visiting with women who have recently learned that they have cancer. She knows their fears, worries, frustrations and joys — she has experienced them all. Jeanne says it's easy to be bitter and angry, but you have to let the bitterness and anger go or they'll get the best of you. Fear, she says, is the worst pain of all. To this day, she still experiences moments of fear and anxiety, but she has learned how to deal with them and how to move on. In her booklet, Jeanne offers words of advice for women struggling to find some sort of balance during a difficult time:

Life is simple. Don't complicate it. I think most everyone has asked themselves at one time or another, "Is this all there is to life?" My answer is a resounding, "Yes, yes!" This is all there is to life. That's this life. Now the more important question: What am I going to do with that information? What am I going to do with the life that has been given me? And, in my case and maybe yours, the life that has been given back to me.

person might also ask them if they want to talk about what was hard or enjoyable about the visit.

Make sure they know they're loved
Your children will take their cues from you and other adults in their lives. They don't carry all the anxiety and worry that tends to plague adults, so they process information based on what they see, hear and feel. Consistently affirming your love for them is critical to helping them adjust to changes in the family routine.

Communicating With Friends

Your friends want to help you. They may offer to bring meals to your home or ask if they can help with cleaning, grocery shopping and driving your children to school. Some may offer to hold fundraising events to help with your medical costs. Often friendships deepen during times such as these.

But sometimes friendships are lost, too. Some friends may be frightened by having someone so close to them develop a life-threatening illness. They're scared, and because they don't know what to say or how to handle the situation and they don't want to upset you, they may respond by distancing themselves. Reactions such as these can be difficult to accept, but they're usually driven by fear and there may be little that you can do to change them. With time, however, the relationship may improve.

People with cancer usually discover soon enough those friends whose energy is helpful and supportive. Your mind and your body aren't separate. The better you feel emotionally, the better you can physically cope with your illness. Surrounding yourself with positive, caring people helps boost your spirits and gives you confidence. Sometimes, you even make new friends, perhaps individuals who have been through some of the same experiences as you have.

Learning to accept relationship changes and leaning on friendships that are true is important. These steps can help minimize some of the stress that comes with cancer and with sharing the news with others.

Feel free to set your boundaries as to how much information you want to share with your friends. And don't feel that you have to be with your friends all of the time, or accept all of their offers of support. You know when requests to help out are good, and when they become too much.

Keep in mind that the most important thing at the moment is to focus on your needs and those of your loved ones.

Chapter 20:

Life After a Cancer Diagnosis

Treatment Side Effects

Fatigue	323
Causes of fatigue	324
Accepting your limits	324
Self-help strategies	325

Nausea and Appetite Problems	325
Nausea medications	325
Self-help strategies	326
Appetite and weight changes	327

| Hair Loss | 329 |
| Self-help strategies | 329 |

| Decreased Arm and Shoulder Mobility | 330 |

Lymphedema	333
Reducing your risk	334
Treating lymphedema	335

Sudden Menopause	336
Relief for hot flashes	337
Relief for night sweats and sleep disturbances	339
Relief for vaginal dryness	339

Sexual Changes	341
Painful intercourse	341
Difficulty reaching orgasm	342
Decreased interest in sex	342

| Osteoporosis | 344 |
| Prevention and treatment | 344 |

| Neuropathy | 345 |

| Joint Aches and Pains | 346 |

| Weight Gain | 347 |
| Reducing your risk | 347 |

| Cognitive Changes | 347 |

Cancer treatment can save or extend lives. But being treated for cancer also presents a number of challenges — from side effects such as fatigue and nausea, to the ongoing stress of doing battle with a life-threatening disease, to changes in home or work responsibilities.

In this chapter, we look at some of the physical challenges you may face during your treatment, and the emotional stress that often accompanies them. We also discuss ways to help you cope with common treatment side effects. The chapter begins with those challenges most often associated with the treatment of relatively early-stage breast cancer. Later on, you'll find information on some of the physical challenges associated with more advanced cancer.

Fatigue

When most people think of cancer treatment, often the first things that come to mind are nausea and hair loss. Fatigue, though, is probably the most common side effect of cancer treatment — not just of treatment but of cancer itself. In part, fatigue is a reaction to the physical and emotional toll that cancer takes. It can be one of the most debilitating side effects, interfering with everyday activities, including working and spending time with family and friends.

For individuals who haven't experienced cancer-related fatigue, it can be difficult to grasp what it's like. Everyone knows what it feels like to run out of steam after a hectic day, but a little rest usually helps you bounce back. Cancer-related fatigue is more encompassing, and rest may not make it better.

How people with cancer experience of fatigue can be different. Descriptions include feeling exhausted, being worn out, running on empty, feeling weak, having heavy limbs or having absolutely no energy.

Causes of fatigue

No one knows all of the causes of cancer-related fatigue, but we do know that certain conditions can contribute to it. Cancer specialists from the National Comprehensive Cancer Network have identified the following conditions as having a significant effect on fatigue:

- Chronic pain
- Emotional distress
- Depression or an anxiety disorder
- Reduced oxygen to the body due to a lack of hemoglobin in the blood (anemia)
- Sleep disturbances
- Low thyroid gland function (hypothyroidism)

If you're experiencing cancer-related fatigue, talk with a member of your health care team. You should be evaluated for anemia and possibly low thyroid func-

tion. If you're anemic, treatment may include taking iron supplements. For severe symptoms, you may need a blood transfusion. Injections of the synthetic hormone erythropoietin, given to stimulate the production of red blood cells, are no longer used because they may increase your risk of blood clots and stimulate cancer growth.

Low thyroid function isn't a common side effect from cancer treatment unless you received radiation therapy to your neck. However, it's a fairly common condition, caused by a number of diseases. Standard treatment for an underactive thyroid involves taking a synthetic thyroid hormone on a daily basis. This oral medication restores hormone levels to normal, easing fatigue.

Other factors that may contribute to your fatigue include medications you may be taking, such as pain relievers or antidepressants, other medical problems, poor nutrition, and inactivity. Be sure your health care team knows of any prescription or over-the-counter medications you're taking. If poor nutrition is a problem, your doctor may refer you to a registered dietitian, who can help you understand your nutritional needs. For fatigue caused by inactivity, simply getting out and walking — even for just a few minutes — can help.

Accepting your limits

Ignoring your fatigue and pushing yourself too hard may make your fatigue worse. Many people highly value their independence, and needing to ask others for help is a new and unwanted experience. But it's important to accept that you can't do it all. Call on friends and family to help with chores and errands.

In a few instances, fatigue may last for years. During the first year after cancer treatment, fatigue is one of the most common complaints.

Self-help strategies

Resting or sleeping more doesn't "cure" fatigue resulting from cancer treatment, but you can do things to help minimize it:

- Plan your activities for times when you usually have the most energy.
- Look for ways to conserve energy. For example, sit on a stool to chop vegetables or wash the dishes.
- Pace yourself. Take short naps or rest breaks when you need them.
- Work with your medical team to establish an exercise program to help lessen your fatigue. Moderate exercise after cancer treatment is strongly recommended.
- Try relaxation techniques, such as guided imagery or meditation (see Chapter 21 for more information).
- Reduce stress in your life whenever you can. Don't try to do everything. Learn to say no to some things.
- Ask your doctor if any of your medications could be contributing to your fatigue.
- Eat a good breakfast each morning to prepare your body for the day's demands. Then refuel every three or four hours. Limit high-fat and high-sugar foods. They tend to make you feel sluggish later.
- Make sure you're drinking enough fluids. Dehydration can contribute to fatigue.

If fatigue remains a problem, ask your doctor about other therapies that may help you. Over the years, doctors have explored the use of medications to reduce cancer-related fatigue. Most of the drugs studied have been psychostimulant medications. To date, the drugs haven't been found to reduce fatigue by a measurable amount and they carry side effects.

Some herbal medications may reduce fatigue by a small amount without the side effects of prescription medications (see Chapter 21).

Nausea and Appetite Problems

Eating healthy foods while undergoing cancer treatment is good for you. They can help you feel better and maintain your strength. But eating well can sometimes be difficult because cancer treatment can cause nausea, vomiting and changes in how food tastes, which may affect your appetite. There are ways to avoid or reduce these problems.

Nausea medications

Much progress has been made in development of medications that prevent and control the nausea and vomiting that accompany cancer treatment. Anti-nausea medications (anti-emetics) are routinely given before your chemotherapy treatment begins, as a preventive measure.

Chemotherapy drugs typically are rated on a scale of how likely they are to cause nausea. For drugs that tend to cause little nausea, you may not need anti-nausea

What to Eat

During chemotherapy treatment, it's best to avoid foods that are overly sweet, fried, spicy or fatty because they're more likely to trigger nausea. Foods that are cool or at room temperature may be more appealing because they produce less of an odor than do hot foods.

You may want to cook and freeze meals before your treatment or have someone else prepare your food when you're not around to smell the cooking odors. Easily digested foods include crackers, dry toast, broth and broth-based soups (such as chicken noodle), hard candy, frozen fruit bars, and flavored gelatin. If you tolerate those, try other mild-flavored, low-fat foods, such as cereals, rice, plain noodles, baked potatoes, lean meats, fish, chicken, cottage cheese, fruits and vegetables.

medicines, or your doctor may recommend a drug such as prochlorperazine, commonly used to treat nausea resulting from a number of causes.

If your chemotherapy treatment involves medications that are more likely to cause significant nausea and vomiting, your doctor may prescribe a corticosteroid medication and one of the newer anti-nausea drugs, such as ondansetron (Zofran), granisetron, dolasetron (Anzemet) or palonosetron (Aloxi). You may takes these with another medication to control nausea and vomiting called aprepitant (Emend).

You take these medications before chemotherapy and sometimes after your treatment, as well. To boost their effectiveness, these medications may be prescribed with other anti-nausea drugs. Side effects of some anti-nausea drugs include drowsiness and constipation.

If you're taking an anti-nausea drug and still experiencing nausea, talk to your doctor. Together you can try to find a combination of medications to better control your symptoms.

Self-help strategies

In addition to medications, some self-help strategies may help:

- **Eat lightly and frequently.** Eat small amounts throughout the day rather than three large meals. A light snack a few hours before treatment may help.
- **Eat and drink slowly.** Be aware of how quickly you're eating. Pace yourself. Put your fork down between bites. During your meal, pause to visit with others at the table or to reflect.
- **Eat moderate proportions.** Stop eating when you feel comfortably satisfied. Don't overeat.
- **Eat what you like.** Avoid foods that you find displeasing because of their smell or texture. Aim for variety, but choose foods you find easiest to eat and digest. During cancer treatment, your food preferences may change. Foods you once enjoyed may no longer appeal to you. And foods you didn't care for may seem appetizing now.
- **Drink plenty of fluids.** Sip on cool beverages such as water, unsweetened fruit

juice, tea and flat ginger ale. It may help to drink small amounts throughout the day rather than large amounts at one time. Limit liquids at mealtimes so that you have more room for food.

- **Make yourself comfortable after eating.** Rest after eating, but don't lie flat because doing so can hamper digestion. Wear comfortable, loosefitting clothes and do something to help keep your mind occupied.
- **Try relaxation techniques.** Relaxation techniques such as progressive muscle relaxation, guided visualization, deep breathing and meditation may help calm your nausea. A simple form of meditation involves sitting comfortably in a straight-backed chair. You close your eyes and breathe in and out naturally. If it helps, count from one to four as you breathe. For more on relaxation techniques, see Chapter 21.

Appetite and weight changes

Cancer treatment can have two effects on your appetite and weight. It may make you lose your appetite, and thereby lose weight, at a time in your life when getting the proper nutrients may be more important than ever. Alternatively, chemotherapy can cause unwanted weight gain in some women.

Weight loss

Once you begin treatment, you may find that food may not taste the way it did before your treatments. You also may have difficulty chewing or swallowing, or your mouth may be dry. Distress, anxiety or depression also can cause you to lose your appetite.

Anticipatory Nausea and Vomiting

After one or more chemotherapy treatments, some people develop a reaction by which they get nauseated and vomit before chemotherapy treatment. The nausea is triggered by something connected to the treatment, such as pulling into the hospital parking lot, walking into the chemotherapy suite or smelling an alcohol swab.

This is called anticipatory nausea, and up to half of all cancer patients who undergo chemotherapy may experience this.

Chances that you'll experience anticipatory nausea are greater if:
- You had severe nausea and vomiting after your previous chemotherapy
- You experienced weakness, dizziness, lightheadedness or sweating after your previous chemotherapy
- You have a lot of distress about your treatment
- You've experienced motion sickness

Unfortunately, standard anti-nausea drugs typically aren't very effective for anticipatory nausea and vomiting. Anti-anxiety medications, such as lorazepam (Ativan), may help a bit. Relaxation techniques and behavior modification techniques, which teach you to remain calm and relaxed when you encounter whatever triggers your nausea, also may help.

If you experience anticipatory nausea and vomiting, tell this to a member of your health care team.

If you're not hungry or interested in food, don't force yourself to eat, but do try to get enough nutrients. Here are some suggestions you can try to help make sure you're getting adequate nutrition:

- Think of eating a healthy diet as part of your treatment plan.
- Eat foods you like. Don't feel obligated to eat something you don't like just because someone went to the trouble of preparing it for you.
- Eat when you're hungry. Don't worry about traditional mealtimes.
- Eat small meals throughout the day.

If you're having trouble chewing or swallowing, try eating soft foods, such as scrambled eggs, milkshakes, applesauce and mashed potatoes. If you're choking on your food or coughing it back up during or after your meal, tell your doctor. If your mouth is dry, sip on water, unsweetened juice and other fluids throughout the day. Try eating soups, drinking milkshakes and consuming other foods that have a high liquid content.

Maintaining your weight can be a sign that you're eating enough. If you're losing weight and you need to increase the amount of calories you consume, try consuming more high-calorie foods and beverages, such as peanut butter, nuts, ice cream, malts, ice cream floats, milkshakes, nutritional drinks and eggnog. To increase protein and calories, add fortified dry milk to your beverages. Talk to your doctor if you've lost 5 or more pounds. He or she might recommend a medication to help stimulate your appetite.

Unwanted weight gain

A few decades back, it became apparent that many women tended to gain weight following a diagnosis of breast cancer, and that weight gain was more prevalent in women who received chemotherapy. There probably are multiple causes for this weight gain:

- Some women who are told that they might lose weight during treatment eat more to prevent weight loss.
- Some women who experience nausea tend to eat more hoping to decrease the nausea.
- Depression can lead some women to overeat.
- Some women don't exercise as much when they're going through cancer treatment.
- Chemotherapy might affect body metabolism in a way that causes increased weight.
- Chemotherapy may induce menopause, which can result in weight gain.

What can you do if you start to gain weight when you don't want to? In general, two common-sense steps can lead to weight loss: First, try to reduce your daily calories either by eating less or by reducing the amount of fat in your diet. Second, develop a routine exercise program to increase your level of physical activity.

If you're still having trouble losing weight, talk with your doctor about making an appointment with a dietitian or enrolling in a weight or exercise program.

On the upside, weight gain associated with chemotherapy is becoming less of a problem than it used to be. This is likely related to increased awareness of the potential for weight gain during treatment, better counseling by doctors and nurses, and shorter durations of chemotherapy medications.

Hair Loss

Many people who've been through cancer treatment will say that the most distressing part of their treatment was losing their hair (alopecia). In addition to the change in your physical appearance, hair loss is a very public banner that says, "I have cancer."

Hair loss is most often associated with chemotherapy treatment. The drugs work by destroying rapidly growing cancer cells in the body. But in addition to cancer cells, they attack other rapidly growing cells, such as those that make up your hair follicles. The result is hair loss.

Hair loss from chemotherapy medications depends on the type of drugs used, as well as an individual's response to the medications. Some women lose all of the hair on their heads in addition to their eyebrows and eyelashes. Others experience only hair thinning, and still others have no hair loss.

If you're going to lose your hair, it'll likely begin to shed 10 to 20 days after you begin chemotherapy treatment. Your hair may come out gradually or in clumps. Some women report scalp tenderness when their hair falls out. Keep in mind that your hair should grow back after treatment ends. In fact, it may grow back thicker than it was before you began chemotherapy. For some women, their hair starts to grow back before they finish treatment. It's not uncommon for the new hair to be different in color or texture.

Radiation therapy to the head also can cause hair loss. Unfortunately, if your hair loss is due to radiation, it may not grow back completely because the hair follicles may be permanently damaged.

Self-help strategies

Your doctor or another member of your health care team can tell you if the chemotherapy drugs you'll be taking are likely to cause hair loss, which gives you time to make some decisions beforehand. You may opt for a wig or plan to wear hats,

Cooling Your Scalp to Prevent Hair Loss

In the 1980s, researchers had an idea for preventing hair loss that involved placing ice caps on the scalp prior to and during chemotherapy treatment. Their thinking was that the ice would cause blood vessels in the scalp to constrict so that less chemotherapy could get to the scalp, resulting in less hair loss. The procedure, known as scalp cryotherapy, didn't work very well, and there was concern that it could potentially allow cancer cells in the scalp to grow.

In recent years, this procedure has made a comeback. Better means of applying cold to the scalp have been developed, and studies suggest the chance of cancer growing in the scalp is extremely low. Scalp cryotherapy is being used to varying degrees in various medical centers. It's still quite cumbersome and it can be uncomfortable. With time, better means of preventing hair loss will likely be developed.

turbans or scarves to cover your head. Or you may decide to leave your head bare. It's likely you'll choose different alternatives in different situations, such as when staying home or going to a social function. There's no right or wrong choice. Base your decision on what makes you feel most comfortable.

If you plan to wear a wig, consider getting it while you still have your own hair. That way, the wig maker can match it to the color and texture of your hair. Some shops specialize in creating wigs for women with cancer. To find out if such a shop is in your area, ask a member of your health care team, check the Yellow Pages or call your local American Cancer Society chapter. Many insurance companies will help pay for a wig if you have a prescription for one from your doctor.

When your hair begins to fall out, treat your remaining hair gently. Use a mild shampoo, brush it gently with a soft brush and set your blow-dryer on low heat. Don't color, perm or chemically relax your hair. Use a satin pillowcase when you sleep because it won't tug on your hair the way a cotton or synthetic pillowcase might.

Some women opt to shave their heads when their hair starts falling out. If you choose to do so, have someone help you and be careful not to nick your scalp, which could lead to an infection. Be sure to apply sunscreen or wear a hat to protect your head from the sun, and cover your head when it's cold outside to protect against loss of body heat.

Talking with your health care team about your distress over losing your hair may help you manage your feelings.

Decreased Arm and Shoulder Mobility

A common concern for women who've had surgery for breast cancer is regaining arm and shoulder mobility. Depending on the type of surgery you've had, the arm and shoulder adjacent to the breast

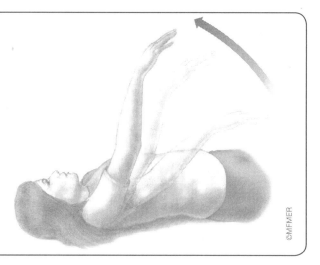

Arm raises

Lie on your back in bed with your arms at your sides. Slowly raise your affected arm straight above your head to stretch the muscles. Lower and repeat. If it would be helpful, fold your hands together and use your unaffected arm to help lift your affected arm.

©MFMER

Deep breathing

Sit in a straight-backed chair and breathe deeply in and out to expand your chest muscles.

Shoulder rotations

Sit in a straight-backed chair. Gently rotate your shoulders forward, down, back and around in a smooth, circular motion to loosen your chest, shoulders and upper back muscles.

Hand squeezes

Using an object such as a rubber ball or washcloth, make a fist and squeeze tightly. Repeat several times throughout the day to strengthen your arm.

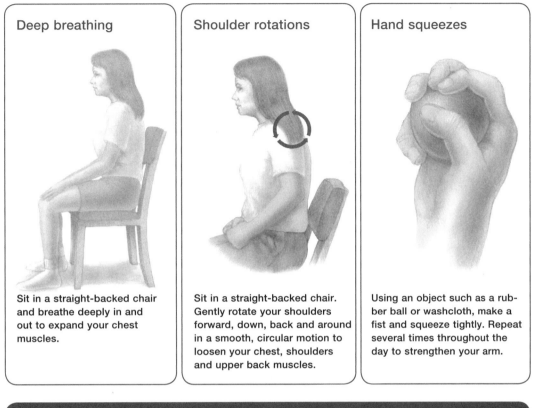

Note: The following exercises are a bit more strenuous. If you've had breast reconstruction, wait at least four weeks after surgery to do these.

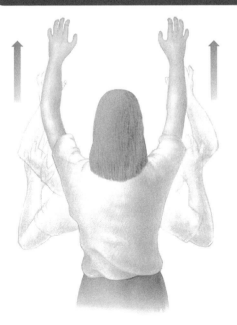

Wall climb

1. Stand facing a wall, with your toes as close to the wall as possible and your feet shoulder-width apart.

2. Bending your elbows slightly, place both your palms against the wall at shoulder level.

3. Using your fingers, work your hands up the wall — "walk up the wall" — until your arms are fully extended.

4. Work your hands back down to the starting point.

©MFMER

Arm swing

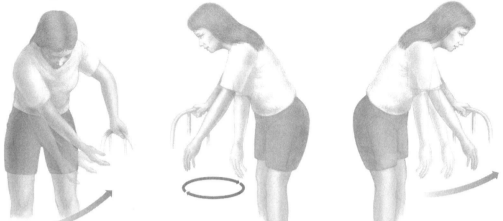

1. With your unaffected arm, hold onto the back of a sturdy chair.

2. Let your affected arm hang in a relaxed position.

3. Swing your affected arm from left to right. Be sure to move your arm from your shoulder, not your elbow.

4. Swing your affected arm in small circles, again making sure the movement comes from your shoulder. As your arm relaxes, the size of the circle will probably increase. Then circle in the opposite direction.

5. Swing your affected arm forward and backward from your shoulder, within your range of comfort.

Pulley

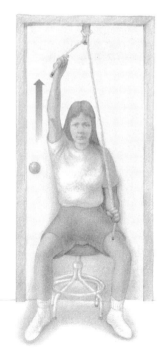

1. Obtain a rope-and-pulley system. These are usually available at medical supply stores and hardware stores. Fasten the system to an overhead beam. Over-the-door models also are available.

2. Sit or stand with the pulley overhead but slightly behind you.

3. Grasp one end of the rope with the hand of your affected arm, or let your hand rest in a loop tied at the end of the rope. Grasp the other end of the rope with the hand of your unaffected arm.

4. With the elbow of your affected arm slightly bent, slowly raise your affected arm forward and upward by gently pulling down on the rope with your other arm.

5. Stop the motion when you feel a pinch, but before you feel any pain in your shoulder.

6. Hold for 10 seconds. Then using the pulley, slowly lower your affected arm to your side.

©MFMER

that underwent surgery may be stiff and sore for a time. Limited movement of the arm and shoulder is most often associated with removal of lymph nodes from under the arm during surgery.

Because of the discomfort, you might be inclined to protect your arm by keeping it still and not using it. But that's not a good idea. Lack of movement can make your arm even weaker, and it can make your arm and shoulder less mobile.

Breast cancer surgery most often affects the type of arm and shoulder movement that you use when you reach upward (abduction), such as when you lift a brush to your hair. This type of movement is used in many everyday tasks, such as driving, retrieving an item from a shelf, and putting on a shirt or coat.

After breast cancer surgery, women typically are given instructions on exercises they can do at home to regain function of the affected arm and shoulder. If you haven't received such instructions, ask for them. Exercising is generally recommended once all surgical drains are removed.

Interestingly, one study found that women who participated in a physical therapy program to regain arm and shoulder mobility achieved better shoulder motion than did women who were just given an instructional booklet after surgery. You might ask your health care team about enrolling in a physical therapy program, and if you're able, find a physical therapist skilled at working with women recovering from breast cancer surgery.

Pages 330-332 contain some basic exercises that you can do yourself. The most important thing is to get your arm and shoulder moving.

Take it easy

Inactivity following surgery can cause your arm, shoulder and upper chest muscles to become stiff and weak. When you first begin your exercises, it's important to start slowly.

Gently stretching your arm and shoulder muscles will help lessen the stiffness and the feeling of weakness. This gentle movement is the key to maintaining arm and shoulder function.

The exercises shown provide the gentle stretching necessary to keep your arm and shoulder mobile.

Lymphedema

Surgery, radiation therapy or other cancer treatment that involves removal of or damage to your lymph nodes may cause you to retain lymph fluid in the area where the lymph nodes were damaged or removed. When this happens, your arms or legs can swell, a condition called lymphedema. *Edema* is a medical term that means "swollen."

Lymph nodes are small, bean-shaped structures found throughout your body, about 350 to 500 of them in total. They produce and store infection-fighting white blood cells, called lymphocytes. Lymphocytes are distributed through your body by way of your blood vessels and also through a network of vessels called lymphatic channels. These vessels carry a clear liquid known as lymph fluid from the tissues of your body to larger lymph vessels, which eventually empty into a large vein in your upper chest, just before the vein brings blood back to your heart.

Surgery or radiation therapy for cancer often results in removal of or damage to lymph nodes and lymph vessels. If your remaining lymph vessels can't maintain the proper flow of lymph fluid, excess fluid can back up and accumulate in the affected limb, causing swelling.

Signs and symptoms include:
- Fullness or heaviness in an arm
- Tightness of the skin
- Reduced movement or flexibility
- Clothing or rings that don't fit
- Visible pressure indentations in your affected skin, such as where you wear your watch

If you were treated for breast cancer and you had radiation therapy or had your underarm lymph nodes surgically removed or both, you're at risk of lymphedema in the arm on that side.

Sometimes, lymphedema occurs right after surgery and is mild and short-lived. At other times, it becomes a chronic problem. It might first occur months or years after treatment. The condition generally isn't painful, but it can be uncomfortable, due to the heavy feeling it causes in the affected limb.

Reducing your risk

There are no scientifically proven ways to prevent lymphedema, but most doctors believe you can do certain things to reduce your risk. Keep in mind, though, that the following suggestions need to be considered in the perspective of trying to live a full and active life.

Try to avoid infection
Your body responds to infection by making extra fluid to fight it. If your lym-
phatic system isn't operating to its full potential because of cancer treatment, this extra fluid can build up, triggering lymphedema. To avoid infection:
- Keep the skin on your arms clean and moisturized with a mild lotion.
- Keep your hands and cuticles soft with moisturizer, too. Don't cut your cuticles with scissors.
- Avoid having shots or blood tests done on an arm that might be at risk of lymphedema because of prior surgery, radiation or both. If you need a vaccination, suggest another location, such as your hip.
- Use an electric razor for shaving the underarm area of your affected arm. This type of razor is less likely to cause cuts than is a straight razor, and it's less harsh than hair removal cream.
- Be alert to early signs of infection. These include skin redness, blotchiness, tenderness, swelling or a feeling of warmth in an arm. Fever also is a sign of infection. If you suspect that you have an infection, contact your doctor.

Try to avoid burns
Like infections, burns can lead to excess fluid in women whose lymph nodes and vessels have been damaged or removed. To avoid burns:
- When you're going to be outside in the sun, use sunscreen. Try to avoid sun exposure during the hottest part of the day.
- Use oven mitts when taking dishes out of the oven or microwave.
- Don't test the temperature of cooked food or bath water with a finger of your affected limb.

QUESTION & ANSWER

Q: Can lymphedema be treated with medication?

A: In the early 1990s, researchers published a study in *The New England Journal of Medicine* reporting that a medication called coumarin (not related to coumadin, the drug used to treat blood clots) effectively reduced lymphedema in a variety of people. Most of the participants in the study had lymphedema for reasons other than cancer treatment.

To follow up, Mayo Clinic researchers developed a clinical trial to evaluate the use of coumarin in women with lymphedema resulting from breast cancer treatment.

Unfortunately, results of this study, which included 150 women, found no benefit in taking coumarin. In fact, a few women receiving the drug developed liver toxicity, a condition that may be life-threatening.

Presently, there isn't a medication known to effectively treat lymphedema.

• Use hot tubs and saunas with caution. The excess heat they produce may cause fluid buildup.

Other tips
You can also reduce your risk of lymphedema by:
• Not wearing clothes, gloves and jewelry that are too tight. Constriction can decrease the flow of fluid, which can lead to increased swelling.
• Eating healthy foods. Controlling your weight can help prevent fluid retention.
• Using your affected arm as normally as possible, but don't overuse it.
• Not having your blood pressure or a blood sample taken in your affected arm.

Treating lymphedema

Fortunately, lymphedema is less of a problem today than it was previously. Use of the sentinel node biopsy procedure (see page 166) has reduced the need for removal of the underarm (axillary) lymph nodes during breast cancer surgery.

Despite your best efforts to prevent it, lymphedema can still become a problem when lymph nodes are removed. If you do experience arm swelling, early intervention is key. It's easier to keep the swelling from getting worse than it is to reverse it once it has advanced.

The most common way of managing lymphedema is to wrap the affected arm or leg with elastic bandages and, once the swelling is reduced, to wear a compression sleeve or stocking, which is a special garment made of elastic material.

There's considerable debate about the best way to get fluid out of the limb. Some doctors prescribe various compression pumps to try to help the fluid flow out of the affected arm or leg. These pumps often put pressure on the furthermost part of the arm or leg and try to milk the fluid toward the heart. There's some concern that this might put too much pressure on already-compromised lymphatic vessels, making the problem worse.

Some doctors suggest massage as a better means of getting the fluid out of the limb. The massage begins at the hand, working the fluid out of this area, and then proceeds up the limb, helping to get the fluid out in a stepwise fashion. Some massage therapy treatments include extensive daily therapy over two weeks. Other times, the treatments are done periodically for an indefinite period of time.

If you're seeking treatment for lymphedema, your best bet is to visit a medical facility that has staff with extensive experience in treating the condition. The doctors and therapists there can help decrease the amount of lymphedema in your limb, teach you how to keep the fluid under control, and provide appropriately fitted elastic sleeves and stockings and ongoing therapeutic recommendations. Look for medical centers that have specialized lymphedema clinics.

To keep fluid from reaccumulating, exercise the affected arm regularly. Women who had axillary lymph node removal as part of breast cancer surgery were once told to avoid exercising the affected arm, due to concerns that the movement and stretching might lead to swelling. However, studies have found just the opposite — that use of arm muscles helps return excess fluid into circulation.

Sudden Menopause

Menopause occurs naturally in women at midlife. It begins when your ovaries start making less of the hormones estrogen and progesterone, which regulate your monthly ovulation and menstruation cycles. Eventually — when hormone production ceases — your ovaries don't release any more eggs, and your menstrual periods stop. Certain surgical or medical treatments for cancer can bring on menopause earlier than it would normally occur, which is generally about age 51.

A hysterectomy that removes your uterus but not your ovaries doesn't cause menopause. Although you no longer have periods, your ovaries still produce hormones. However, an operation that removes both your uterus and ovaries (total hysterectomy with bilateral oophorectomy) does cause menopause. If you're premenopausal, your periods stop immediately and you're likely to have hot flashes and other menopausal signs and symptoms. This is known as surgical menopause.

Chemotherapy and radiation therapy to the pelvis also may induce premature menopause. In addition, many of the hormone treatments for breast cancer can cause menopausal signs and symptoms. Premenopausal women receiving chemotherapy for breast cancer may experience a relatively abrupt decline in ovarian function.

The effects of sudden menopause are often more intense than are those of natural menopause. Unlike the more gradual hormonal changes of natural menopause, which usually occur over several years, hormone changes associated with surgical menopause are abrupt, often making the signs and symptoms more intense. Premature menopause also puts you at risk of other conditions, such as the bone-thinning disease osteoporosis.

Effects of sudden menopause

The signs and symptoms of menopause can range from mildly uncomfortable to severe. Some women experience several signs and symptoms, and others experience few, if any. The most common are hot flashes, sleep disturbances, night sweats, vaginal changes and emotional changes.

Hot flashes
Reduced estrogen in your bloodstream can cause abnormal regulation of your blood vessels, causing your skin temperature to rise. This can lead to a feeling of warmth that moves upward from your chest to your shoulders, neck and head. You may sweat, then feel chilled as the sweat evaporates. You may also feel slightly faint. Your face might look flushed, and red blotches may appear on your chest, neck and arms.

Sleep disturbances and night sweats
Hot flashes during the night can lead to night sweats. You may awaken from a sound sleep with your sleepwear and bed linens soaking wet, which may then cause you to feel chilled. In addition, you may have difficulty falling back to sleep, preventing you from achieving a deep, restful sleep.

Vaginal changes
Lack of estrogen can cause the tissues lining your vagina to become drier, thinner and less elastic. Decreased lubrication may cause burning or itching and may lead to increased infections of the vagina and urinary tract. These changes may make sexual intercourse uncomfortable or even painful.

Emotional changes
You may experience mood swings, be more irritable or be more prone to emotional upset. In the past, these symptoms were attributed to hormonal fluctuations. But the stress of having cancer and other life events understandably may contribute to changes in your mood, too.

Relief for hot flashes

If you're bothered by hot flashes, a combination of self-help strategies and medication often can reduce their severity.

Self-help strategies
Most hot flashes last from 30 seconds to several minutes, although they can last much longer. The frequency and duration of hot flashes vary from woman to woman. You may experience them once every hour, or you may be bothered by them only occasionally.

If you're experiencing hot flashes fairly regularly:
- **Dress in layers.** Wear cotton clothing that can be easily removed. Cotton promotes air circulation, and it helps absorb moisture.
- **Look for triggers.** Do certain foods or situations often lead to hot flashes? Some common triggers are smoking, hot beverages, spicy foods, alcohol, hot weather, a warm room and a stressful event.
- **Try to cool down.** Have a cold drink of water or juice and go somewhere cool when hot flashes start.

Medications
A variety of medications may reduce the effects of hot flashes. Discuss your options

Coming to Terms With Infertility

Loss of fertility is a possibility for some younger women who undergo cancer treatment that produces menopause. Infertility may be related to surgery, chemotherapy or radiation therapy.

If you were planning to have children, loss of fertility can be devastating. Some women experience grief and loss similar to that after the death of a loved one. When your friends and family members become pregnant, you may feel jealous and resentful — and then guilty for feeling that way. (See page 189 for information on ways to preserve your ability to have children before starting cancer treatment.)

Even women who weren't planning to have any more children may feel some grief at becoming infertile. They may feel they're less whole or less feminine.

To cope with infertility caused by cancer treatment:

- **Discuss your feelings.** Talk to someone you feel close to — your doctor, a counselor, your spiritual leader, a family member or a friend. Most importantly, share your feelings with your partner.
- **Allow yourself to feel the way you feel.** There is no right or wrong way to react.
- **Consider joining a support group.** You may find it helpful to talk with other women in the same situation. More information on support groups is available later in this chapter.

with your doctor, to determine what's right for you.

Hormone therapy

The most established treatment for hot flashes is the hormone estrogen, used in hormone replacement therapy (HRT). Estrogen reduces hot flashes by up to 90 percent. The hormone progesterone also can reduce hot flashes to a similar degree. However, because breast cancer and some gynecologic cancers are fueled by hormones, oncologists are often reluctant to prescribe HRT, and many women are reluctant to take hormones.

Vitamin E

Research suggests that taking 800 international units of vitamin E a day reduces

hot flashes a little bit more than does taking a placebo. What does that mean? In many clinical studies, women who took a sugar pill (placebo) daily reported about a 25 percent reduction in hot flashes after four weeks. Women receiving vitamin E reported about a 35 percent reduction in hot flashes four weeks later.

Clonidine

Clonidine (Catapres), a pill or patch developed to treat high blood pressure, also may help alleviate hot flashes to some degree. It does, however, have side effects, such as dry mouth, sleep disturbance, dizziness, drowsiness, lightheadedness and constipation, so doctors don't prescribe it as often as other remedies for hot flashes.

Antidepressants

Some antidepressant medications have demonstrated effectiveness in reducing hot flashes. Research indicates that a low dose of venlafaxine decreases hot flashes by about 40 percent. A slightly higher dose decreases hot flashes by about 60 percent. Venlafaxine is well tolerated by most women, although a few women taking it experience significant nausea or vomiting. For some women, the initial nausea goes away after a few days, despite continued drug use.

Venlafaxine has other side effects, such as mild dry mouth, decreased appetite and some constipation. If you have uncontrolled high blood pressure, your doctor may not recommend this drug because it may increase your blood pressure.

Other antidepressants also appear to relieve hot flashes. Medications such as paroxetine (Paxil) and citalopram (Celexa) appear to work as well as venlafaxine. Fluoxetine (Prozac) also may reduce hot flashes, but not as well as other antidepressants.

Anti-seizure medications such as gabapentin (Neurontin) and pregabalin (Lyrica) have been shown to reduce hot flashes. These medications can produce side effects such as lightheadedness and mild swelling, which some women find more bothersome than those associated with venlafaxine.

Relief for night sweats and sleep disturbances

Night sweats are usually the nighttime equivalent of hot flashes. You may awaken from a sound sleep soaked in sweat, followed by chills. You may have difficulty falling back to sleep or achieving a deep, restful sleep. Lack of sleep may affect your mood and overall health. If you experience night sweats or have trouble sleeping, try the following strategies:

- Use cotton sheets, wear cotton clothing to bed and keep an extra set handy. Cotton allows air to flow around your skin, and it effectively absorbs moisture.
- Keep your bedroom cool.
- Avoid drinking caffeinated beverages right before bedtime. These can cause trouble sleeping.
- Avoid exercising shortly before you go to bed because it can rev up your metabolism, which can make it difficult to fall asleep.
- Try relaxation techniques, such as deep breathing, yoga and progressive muscle relaxation. They can help quell sleep disturbances. See Chapter 21 for more information on relaxation exercises.
- Try to follow a consistent sleep schedule, and develop a routine before you go to sleep, such as reading or writing in a journal.

Relief for vaginal dryness

As your estrogen level declines, the tissues lining your vagina and the opening to your bladder (urethra) become drier, thinner and less elastic. With decreased lubrication, you may experience burning or itching, increased risk of vaginal or urinary tract infections, and discomfort during intercourse.

For vaginal dryness:
- **Use over-the-counter water-based vaginal lubricants or moisturizers.** Staying sexually active also may help minimize these problems because it increases

Concerns About Vaginal Estrogen

Over the years, there has been much debate about the use of vaginal estrogen therapy. Most doctors and cancer survivors opt against oral estrogen therapy because of concerns about increased estrogen in the bloodstream and associated breast cancer risk. With vaginal estrogen therapy, a small amount of estrogen is absorbed and enters the bloodstream. Theoretically, this could cause some concern. However, many oncologists and gynecologists believe that breast cancer risk associated with vaginal estrogen use is likely very small.

Vaginal estrogen therapy is a reasonable choice for controlling vaginal signs and symptoms associated with cancer treatment. If you're concerned about possible cancer risk from the therapy, it's OK not to use it.

blood flow to vaginal tissues, keeping them healthier.

- **Avoid use of douches.** They may irritate your vagina.

If these measures don't work, you might ask your doctor about vaginal estrogen replacement therapy. Because vaginal dryness results when your ovaries no longer produce estrogen, vaginal estrogen therapy can help relieve signs and symptoms. Vaginal therapy increases the amount of estrogen in the vagina, helping to relieve vaginal dryness.

Although doctors may be concerned about prescribing estrogen treatment in pill form to women with breast cancer, in some cases they may feel it's reasonable to use local estrogen treatment, such as a vaginal cream, to treat vaginal dryness (see "Concerns About Vaginal Estrogen").

Vaginal estrogen preparations

Vaginal estrogen cream (Premarin, Estrace, others) can help relieve vaginal dryness and itching. You insert the cream into your vagina with an applicator, daily for five to seven days. You can continue using it one to two times a week to control symptoms.

A vaginal estrogen ring (Estring) is a soft, plastic ring that you or your doctor insert into the upper part of your vagina. The ring slowly releases estrogen over a period of 90 days.

Vaginal estrogen also comes in the form of a tablet (Vagifem). You use a disposable applicator to regularly place a tablet in your vagina — every day for the first two weeks and then twice a week.

All of these methods increase the amount of estrogen in your vagina and should relieve vaginal dryness for as long as you use them.

Cautions

Virtually all vaginal estrogen preparations appear to get absorbed and travel to other parts of your body to some degree. One situation when it doesn't make sense to use a vaginal estrogen preparation is if a woman is taking an aromatase inhibitor. This type of medication is designed to decrease the body's estrogen to as low a level as possible. It's more reasonable to use vaginal estrogen treatment if you're receiving tamoxifen or if you have an estrogen receptor negative cancer.

Talk to your doctor about whether estrogen treatment is an option and, if so, which type might work best for you.

Sexual Changes

After treatment for cancer, your sex life may be affected in a number of ways. Studies have shown that about 25 to 35 percent of women diagnosed with breast cancer experience some type of sexual dysfunction.

Sexual changes that women may experience after cancer treatment include painful intercourse, difficulty reaching orgasm and decreased interest in sex.

Talk with your doctor or another member of your health care team if you're experiencing sexually related problems. Often, sexual problems can be treated.

Painful intercourse

Painful intercourse is a common sexual complaint after cancer treatment. The medical term for this problem is *dyspa-*

reunia. It's most often caused by estrogen loss that leads to vaginal dryness. Chemotherapy and hormone therapy can, in part, lead to sexual problems by decreasing estrogen.

Fortunately, there are things you can do to help make intercourse less painful:

- Use a water-based lubricant in and around your vagina before having intercourse. Several over-the-counter products are available. Experiment to find a product that you like. Avoid petroleum jelly and other oil-based lubricants. They may make you more prone to yeast infections.
- Make sure you're fully aroused before beginning intercourse. That's when your vagina is at its longest, widest and most lubricated.
- Choose a position for intercourse that allows you to control the pace and depth of the thrusts.
- Tell your partner if something is causing you pain, and suggest ways to touch you that aren't painful.
- Have your partner gently stretch your vagina with a lubricated finger before intercourse.

If your doctor recommends a vaginal dilator to stretch your vagina, use it as

---

QUESTION & ANSWER

Q: What is vaginismus?

A: Painful intercourse, whether caused by vaginal dryness, vaginal stenosis or a shortened vagina, can sometimes trigger a condition called vaginismus. The muscles around the vaginal opening become clenched in a spasm. With vaginismus, a woman's partner can't enter the vagina with his penis. The harder he pushes, the greater her pain becomes.

Kegel Exercises

Kegel exercises can help you learn how to tense and relax your pelvic floor muscles, which may help lessen discomfort during intercourse. To do Kegel exercises, contract the muscles you use to stop urine flow, hold for a count of three, and then relax. Repeat 10 to 20 times, a couple of times a day. If you're feeling pain during intercourse, stop and take a moment to relax your pelvic floor muscles.

directed. Vaginal dilators are latex, plastic or rubber cylinders that are made in a variety of sizes. They're lubricated and inserted into the vagina and left in place for about 10 to 15 minutes at a time, three times a week or every other day.

Difficulty reaching orgasm

Almost all women who are able to reach orgasm before cancer treatment continue to do so afterward. However, you may find that the steps necessary for you to become sexually aroused have changed. For instance, if a part of foreplay was stroking sensitive areas that have since been affected by cancer treatment, such as your breasts, you may need to find new areas that provoke sexual arousal when touched.

To help yourself reach orgasm, talk to your partner and make sure your partner knows which types of touch excite you. You might even have a sexual fantasy during lovemaking to distract you from negative thoughts.

Decreased interest in sex

Just as cancer treatment causes physical changes, it often packs an emotional wallop, too. You may experience several different feelings after cancer treatment or, perhaps, just a few.

A common problem following cancer treatment is loss of desire for sexual activity (libido). You may lose interest in sex for many reasons. It may be because of all the changes you're going through. You may be recovering from surgery, radiation therapy or chemotherapy, and perhaps you're tired or you don't feel well. Chemotherapy and other medications can disrupt your hormone balance, reducing your sex drive.

You may be fearful, anxious or depressed. These are common responses to a life-threatening illness. Many people find that their fears decrease with time and their libido improves. But for some, the emotional distress becomes overwhelming and medical intervention becomes necessary. Some medications used to treat depression and anxiety can interfere with your sex drive.

You may also have concerns about how your body has been altered by cancer treatment and whether your partner still finds you sexually desirable.

Women who have a mastectomy are particularly vulnerable to this problem. For both women and men, the breast represents a significant aspect of sexuality. Removing an entire breast (mastectomy) or changing its look and feel (lumpectomy) can alter a woman's perception of herself as a sexual being. According to some researchers, mastectomy leads to more post-cancer sexual problems than do many other treatments.

If you have a loss of interest in sex, and if it concerns you, try these suggestions:

Talk with your partner

One of the best ways to improve sexual intimacy is to open the lines of communication. For example, your partner may think you've lost interest. You may believe your partner isn't interested in you. A conversation about the issue can clear the air and restore emotional and physical intimacy. Begin by telling your partner how you feel about your sex life and what you would like to change. Explain why you think your sex life is the way it is and how it makes you feel. Avoid blame, and try to stay positive.

Set aside time for romance

When you're ready, make a date with your partner. Create a sensual mood using lighting, music and fragrance. Go slowly at first, focusing on foreplay. Slowly reacquaint yourself with your partner. Sometimes agreeing not to include intercourse can help you relax and focus on pleasurable activities.

Focus on new ways to make yourself feel sensual and attractive. Try a new haircut or color. Buy some beautiful new pajamas or a nightgown to help you feel more desirable.

Talk with your doctor

Sexual problems may not improve on their own. If you're having troubles and your doctor or another member of your health care team hasn't discussed sexual issues with you, take the lead. Your doctor can help determine if you need a referral to a specialist or, perhaps, suggest new ways to express sexual intimacy. If you're going to discuss your sex drive with your doctor, you might want your partner to attend the appointment, too. Having your partner with you will ensure that both of you receive the same information.

QUESTION & ANSWER

Q: I've heard that testosterone may increase a woman's libido. Is this true?

A: Evidence suggests that decreased sexual desire in women may be related to lowered concentrations of the hormone testosterone. Women's bodies do normally produce small concentrations of this male-associated hormone. After menopause, the levels are reduced. The administration of testosterone has been studied as a potential treatment for decreased libido. Some studies suggest it may be beneficial, especially when given to women who still have some estrogen in their bodies (premenopausal or taking estrogen replacement). However, most evidence suggests that it's not helpful for postmenopausal women with a history of breast cancer.

Osteoporosis

As more women survive cancer, the long-term effects of cancer treatment on bone health are becoming more apparent.

Osteoporosis is a condition in which your bones become brittle and weak, leading to an increased risk of fractures. Women who've been treated for cancer are at increased risk of osteoporosis for several reasons. Some breast cancer treatments inhibit bone formation. And medications used to control some of the side effects of chemotherapy, such as steroids, can lead to bone loss. In some cases, the cancer itself may cause bone loss.

Cancer treatment can also have indirect effects on bone loss. Aromatase inhibitor medications decrease estrogen concentrations in your blood, and this leads to bone loss. Surgical removal of the ovaries — sometimes a part of treatment for breast cancer — initiates immediate menopause. Chemotherapy and radiation therapy for cancer also may cause the ovaries to stop functioning. During the first few years after this occurs, you lose calcium from your bones at a much faster rate than normal, increasing your risk of osteoporosis.

Prevention and treatment

Several options are available for preventing and treating osteoporosis.

Calcium and vitamin D

Two of the most straightforward, highly recommended strategies are to get adequate calcium and vitamin D and to take part in weight-bearing exercises. Women at risk of osteoporosis should aim for 1,500 to 2,000 milligrams a day of calcium and 400 to 800 international units of vitamin D. The calcium and vitamin D can be from food sources or from supplements.

Exercise

Weight-bearing exercise can be as simple as walking and jogging. Non-weight-bearing activities, such as swimming, are helpful for general fitness, but they're not adequate for maintaining bone strength.

Estrogen

Estrogen therapy has been shown to be useful in preventing bone loss. However, given concerns about its use in women who've survived breast cancer, other options are more frequently recommended for these women.

Raloxifene

Raloxifene (Evista), a medication somewhat similar to the cancer drug tamoxifen, is taken to help maintain bone strength. It may also decrease breast cancer risk. However, there's some concern about prescribing raloxifene for women who've already taken tamoxifen for five years. Therefore, raloxifene generally isn't recommended for breast cancer survivors who've had tamoxifen. Raloxifene also may cause hot flashes.

Bisphosphonates

Medications known as bisphosphonates also can help preserve bone strength. These drugs appear to be as effective as estrogen in terms of promoting bone health. Bisphosphonates currently on the market include alendronate (Fosamax), risedronate (Actonel) and ibandronate (Boniva). You take these medications either once a day, once a week or once a month in a larger dose. Bisphosphonates should be taken first thing in the morning, on an empty stomach. Be sure to avoid lying down for at least 30 minutes afterward to avoid acid reflux into the esophagus.

Zoledronic acid (Zometa) is another form of bisphosphonate. It's different in that it's an intravenous medication, meaning it's administered by injecting the drug into a vein. Evidence suggests that receiving intravenous doses of this drug at six- or 12-month intervals may help maintain bone strength.

Denosumab
Denosumab (Prolia) is a newer type of osteoporosis drug. It's a type of antibody treatment that works in a different way but produces similar or better results, compared with bisphosphonates. Denosumab is delivered via a shot under the skin every six months. This same medication is also used to prevent bone complications from metastatic breast cancer. When used for cancer treatment, the medication is known as Xgeva.

Calcitonin
Calcitonin is an intranasal medication taken as an inhalant. It's another option for reducing bone loss in women with osteoporosis, but it's not as effective as bisphosphonates.

Neuropathy

Some chemotherapy medications can cause nerve damage (neuropathy), which can result in poorly defined pain throughout the body and in numbness and tin-

gling in the feet and hands. Taxane drugs, such as paclitaxel, used in the treatment of breast cancer are most commonly associated with neuropathy.

Some women who receive chemotherapy medications don't experience any problems with neuropathy. In others, it can become a substantial problem. New research suggests people affected by neuropathy may have a genetic makeup that predisposes them to these problems.

Acute pain syndrome

Taxane medications can cause a type of pain syndrome which peaks about three to four days after receiving the medication and then disappears a few days later. The pain is located throughout the body and it can be difficult to define — likely because most women have never had nerve pain like it before.

Women receiving lower, more frequent doses of taxane medications usually have less of a problem than do women who are given the drugs less often and in higher amounts. In recent years, the trend has been to administer taxane medications in smaller doses more often — weekly instead of every three weeks.

Peripheral neuropathy

Another side effect of some chemotherapy medications is peripheral neuropathy. It's a problem that affects the far (peripheral) extremities — the feet and hands. Often, the feet are affected more than the hands.

Peripheral neuropathy tends to become apparent the longer taxane medications are taken. Initially, symptoms include numbness and tingling in the hands and feet, which can make it difficult to button a button or manipulate small objects. Sometimes the symptoms will remain mild. Other times, they may worsen, and in addition to the numbness and tingling, sharp, shooting or burning pains may develop in the extremities. If the symptoms become too severe, the medication is generally stopped and replaced with a different type of chemotherapy drug.

Unlike acute pain syndrome, symptoms of peripheral neuropathy generally don't improve in between treatments, but they often get better once chemotherapy treatment is complete. Unfortunately, a few people experience symptoms for years after their treatment is complete.

There's no way to prevent chemotherapy-induced neuropathy other than to reduce or stop the medication. Sometimes prescription medications may be used to relieve pain associated with the condition.

Joint Aches and Pains

In addition to nerve pain, some medications taken to treat breast cancer can cause aches and pains in the joints.

Post-chemotherapy rheumatism

Some women who undergo chemotherapy as part of treatment for their cancers develop pain and stiffness in their muscles and joints, typically one to two months after completing treatment. This condition, which appears to be triggered by chemotherapy medications, is called post-chemotherapy rheumatism.

Doctors estimate the condition may affect up to 5 percent of women who receive a combination of chemotherapy medications.

The most common complaint of post-chemotherapy rheumatism is stiffness in the morning or after periods of inactivity. The hips and knees are most often affected. In most cases, symptoms of post-chemotherapy rheumatism go away without treatment, usually within six to 12 months. Researchers theorize that the condition may be a type of withdrawal from chemotherapy. Many questions about this condition remain unanswered.

Over-the-counter pain relievers haven't been found to provide much relief for this condition. But there are some things you can do that might help. If you're experiencing musculoskeletal pain after cancer treatment, avoid long periods of sitting. If you must sit for a long time, reposition yourself often to prevent or lessen stiffness. Turn your head at different angles, shift the position of your arms, and bend and stretch your legs. These slight movements may help prevent excessive stiffness. If you're able, get up and walk from time to time.

Aromatase inhibitor arthralgias

About half the women who take aromatase inhibitors experience joint aches and pains. The symptoms may be new or they may be a worsening of joint aches and pains that existed before your cancer was diagnosed. For mild symptoms, over-the-counter pain relievers may help. In severe cases, an aromatase inhibitor may have to be stopped. After a few weeks to a couple of months, your doctor may recommend that you try another aromatase inhibitor to see if the problem still persists.

Sometimes a different medication is more tolerable than the first one.

Weight Gain

As discussed earlier, some cancer survivors who've received chemotherapy drugs or are taking certain hormone medications have problems with weight gain. Unfortunately, in many cases, the extra weight stays on even when treatment ends.

Some studies suggest that weight gain is greater among premenopausal women treated for breast cancer than among women who've already gone through menopause. This could be because chemotherapy causes premature menopause in younger women, and menopause often is accompanied by weight gain. Women who were postmenopausal when treated for cancer may have already gained the weight associated with the onset of menopause.

Some women also report weight gain while taking the drug tamoxifen. However, about an equal number of women report experiencing weight loss. Again, weight gain associated with tamoxifen may have more to do with a woman's age than with the medication. Women tend to gain weight when going through menopause, and breast cancer — and the treatment that follows — is often diagnosed around the age when women start to experience menopausal symptoms.

Reducing your risk

Most doctors point to exercise as the best way to prevent or minimize weight gain after cancer treatment. In addition to helping you lose weight, exercise helps reduce fatigue, insomnia and anxiety, all of which can be consequences of cancer diagnosis and treatment.

If you've found that you've lost muscle and gained fatty tissue in your arms and shoulders during your treatment, you may find strength training exercises for your upper body to be helpful. Strength training exercises for your legs may be helpful, too.

Talk with your doctor about starting an exercise regimen that includes both aerobic exercise and strength training. And ask for a referral to a dietitian who can help you develop a healthy diet that won't add extra pounds.

Cognitive Changes

Some people treated for cancer report having problems with memory or concentration after receiving chemotherapy or radiation. Studies suggest that people who've been treated with chemotherapy are at greater risk of having such problems. Higher doses of chemotherapy seem to lead to greater problems. However, even people who receive standard doses can report memory or concentration difficulties. This problem is known as cognitive dysfunction and has been labeled by some as "chemo brain" or "cancer brain."

Most women who receive chemotherapy don't experience significant cognitive changes following their treatment, and they continue to effectively perform complex mental tasks.

The exact cause of cognitive changes and the degree to which they affect people aren't clear. Using radiologic imaging techniques, researchers have been able to visualize brain changes in women who received chemotherapy. They hope that within a few years — when more results of current research become available — they'll have a better understanding of the situation.

People who talk about the cognitive effects of cancer treatment tend to describe a blunting of their mental sharpness, fuzziness in dealing with numbers, trouble finding the right word and short-term memory lapses. Some people report changes in memory or concentration beginning sometime during cancer treatment. Others report symptoms sometime after their treatment ended.

At this time, there are no ways to prevent cognitive changes from chemotherapy. But there are some things you can do that can help you manage the situation:

- Keep yourself organized. Each day, make a quick note in a planner or on an electronic app about what you need to do or where you need to go.
- Use sticky notes to remind yourself of things at home.
- Check your math with a calculator.
- If you're having difficulty with a problem, run it by others for feedback.
- Learn relaxation skills (see Chapter 21) to control stress. Your memory and concentration may improve if you're less stressed.

If you're really bothered by your symptoms, talk to your doctor.

Shirley's Story

Shirley Ruedy has stared breast cancer in the face not once, but twice. The first time she was 43. The second time — 15 years to the day after her first diagnosis — she was 58. The first time was a terrible blow. The second diagnosis "felt like a comet hitting the earth." Instead of a cancer-free anniversary celebration, Shirley sat in her doctor's office coming to grips with a nightmare of every cancer survivor — another cancer.

Unlike the first cancer, which was caught early, the second one was more advanced. It had spread to a lymph node and her chest wall. Shirley underwent a second mastectomy, followed by six rounds of chemotherapy and 35 radiation treatments. It has now been about 17 years since her second breast cancer, and each day that Shirley wakes up, she knows that she's fortunate to be alive. She tries to live life to the fullest, not dwelling on the past or worrying about the future.

"I figure you do everything you absolutely can, and then you forget about it. I don't think that God has given you another chance at life to live it in misery. Worrying about it all the time is hellacious."

Shirley Ruedy knows cancer well — too well. She cared for her mother as her mother died a slow, agonizing death from colon cancer. She watched as her brother endured repeated treatments for breast cancer, until the cancer took his life. And she has stood by as good friends have received diagnoses similar to hers, and some haven't been as fortunate.

Shirley also knows cancer well because it became her life's work. Sometime after her first experience with breast cancer, Shirley returned to her writing career, accepting a job at the local newspaper in Cedar Rapids, Iowa. She proposed a regular column on cancer, feeling readers wanted, and could benefit from, more cancer information. For many years, until her recent retirement, Shirley wrote her award-winning "Cancer Update," a platform for anything to do with cancer. She shared the latest information on cancer screening and treatment. She encouraged readers to be proactive — to get second opinions, to challenge doctors if they felt it necessary, and to take steps to reduce their cancer risk. She also exposed the emotional side of cancer: common fears, feelings and frustrations.

Some of Shirley's most touching and popular columns were those in which she reflected on her own cancer battles and those of dear friends — putting into words the weighty surge of emotions in the power struggle between life and death.

Shirley Ruedy knows cancer well, but it's her sincere hope that future generations won't have to.

Here's one of Shirley's columns.

It's so good to feel good

By Shirley Ruedy
   Gazette columnist

It's been a year.

A very mottled year. In a way, it seems like a lifetime since I was told, one stunning Tuesday, that the breast cancer which had beat its drum so loudly in my life 15 years ago, dying to a dim sound in the distance, now beat violently once again.

It was back, they said. A brand new one. A new one to lick, to contend with, to watch its shadow, to sleep, it seemed, with one eye open.

And in another way, it's impossible to believe that a whole year has gone by. To think how innocently I tripped into last November, thinking of the holidays, thinking of finishing the work on our newly refurbished kitchen — certainly not thinking of another cancerous visit.

So busy was I that I forgot the follow-up appointment I had made with the oncologist for that funny "blip" on my rib. After a reminder call, I went blithely off; after all, the tests had been negative so far, right?

Ah, yes. So much for the "best laid plans of mice and men." Once again you are brought to your knees, made to recall that puny humankind has no firm grasp on the reins of life. What looks so leather-sturdy is as a dream, and you wake up holding only gossamer strands.

For that is, after all, all that life is: The most delicate thread (not the rope we fancy) tethering us to a final life — and we become so caught in our daily rushing about that we forget that at any given moment, the tether can reel us in to our eternal destination.

That is what I was abruptly reminded of last November. And I recalled that once there is the precedence of cancer cells in your body, in the family, one has to be forever the watchful sentinel.

REFLECTIONS: I did not have chemotherapy or radiation with my first mastectomy, as many readers know. So the "chemo" I began on Jan. 3, 1995, was a brand new world to me. My regimen, as I noted before, was not the most severe ever given, nor the lightest. I did what most of you would do: I endured, I prevailed, and I am here.

As I look back, what was most interesting, in light of the fear that so many people have worked up on the subject of chemotherapy, was simply, the chemotherapy suite.

It was, really, human nature at its best: Duty, love, compassion. The people — young, old, short, tall, fat, thin, rich, poor, men, women, white, black, brown, yellow

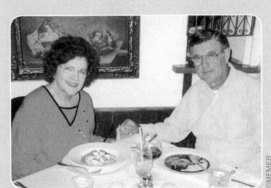

Shirley Ruedy and her husband, George, In Washington, D.C., for a national breast cancer awareness luncheon.

— showed up dutifully at their appointed times. They marched like soldiers to recliner chairs or beds (their choice), sitting or lying there quietly. They thought ... or read ... or talked with companions.

The patients were on the front line, but those steadfast companions were right at their sides — husbands, wives, parents, adult children or friends, loyally accompanying their beleaguered loved ones through the weeks and months of therapy. They never asked for credit, they never sought attention, they were just there: Love aflower, love abloom, love majestic.

Mostly, it was quiet in the rooms. Whatever fears, wishes or apologies that were tucked away in the corners of souls — well, they had already been talked about before going

there. Or, perhaps the thoughts would stay in their niches, never to come out. But everyone, patient and companion alike, knew why they were there. This was The Big Time. This was The Fight of Their Lives.

There was, of course, the silent drip-drip-drip of the IV — man trying anew to arrest one of the world's oldest diseases. The nurses went in and out, swiftly performing the mechanics of their trade, sometimes sensing a flagging spirit, sitting down to dispense some soft words of encouragement.

I learned that chemicals can teach you a lot about humans.

It's so good to feel good again, to see the hair on my head again. Do you want to hear something funny? It's curly! It's just a stitch! Little curls racing around my neckline. At times, I felt like the chemo was enough to curl my toes, but instead, it curled my hair.

Shirley Temple reincarnated! Wheeeee! Let a new year ring!

Reprinted with permission © 1995 The Gazette, Cedar Rapids, Iowa

Chapter 21:

Life After a Cancer Diagnosis

Complementary Therapies

Getting The Most of
Complementary Therapies 353
Discuss your options   353
Assess the risks vs. the benefits 354
Evaluate treatment providers   354
Consider the costs   354
Take a middle road   354

Types of Therapies   355
Mind-body techniques   355
Massage   357
Dietary supplements   358
Natural energy restoration   360

Finding
Reliable Information   362

There was a time that if you mentioned an interest in complementary or alternative therapies for your cancer, your doctor might look at you like you were a little crazy, and proceed to warn you about the dangers of such therapies. Even family and friends might have questioned your thinking.

But interest in therapies outside the range of standard medical treatments has increased substantially in recent years — not just among the general public but in the medical community as well. In a government-funded survey, almost 40 percent of adults interviewed reported using some form of complementary or alternative medicine, including natural and herbal products and therapies such as deep breathing, meditation, chiropractic care, yoga and massage, among others. Doctors and scientists also are taking a keener interest in studying the safety and potential benefits of nontraditional therapies and a number of rigorous research studies are underway.

Among women with breast cancer, the use of complementary or alternative medicine is even higher. Studies report that up to 80 percent of women with breast cancer use at least one type of complementary

Complementary, Alternative, Integrative: What's In a Name?

The terminology used for health care methods and practices that generally fall outside mainstream medicine has evolved quite a bit over the last several decades. It can be confusing to hear different people using different terms for what seem like the same things.

Once labeled as "unconventional" or "natural" medicine in the early 90s, dietary supplements and therapies such as yoga and hypnosis eventually came to be known as *complementary and alternative medicine* (CAM), an umbrella term that's still widely used today.

There's an important distinction, however, between complementary and alternative methods. Complementary therapies generally refer to treatments used in conjunction with conventional medicine, such as acupuncture for chemotherapy-induced nausea. In contrast, alternative medicine includes treatments used in place of traditional medicine. This might include seeing a homeopath or naturopath instead of your regular doctor. Among the general public, this distinction isn't always so clear. Many people use the term *alternative medicine* as a catchall phrase to refer to both — therapies used in addition to conventional care and those used in place of it.

Add to the picture another term. *Integrative medicine* is a fairly new concept that describes a growing movement in many health care institutions — integrating complementary therapies with conventional medicine in an effort to treat the whole person, not just the disease or condition. The treatments promoted through integrative medicine programs aren't substitutes for conventional medical care. They're used in concert with medical treatment to help alleviate stress, reduce pain and anxiety, manage symptoms, maintain strength and flexibility, and promote a sense of well-being.

It's the types of therapies being studied and practiced in a number of medical institutions, such as Mayo Clinic, that are discussed in this chapter.

or alternative therapy. People with cancer or chronic illness turn to complementary and alternative therapies for a host of reasons, including relieving physical distress, achieving emotional well-being and controlling symptoms such as pain. Surveys of women with breast cancer cite motivations such as:

- Boosting the immune system
- Alleviating side effects of treatment, such as nausea and fatigue
- Improving quality of life
- Preventing a cancer recurrence
- Providing feelings of empowerment and control
- Aiding conventional medical treatment

After learning that you have cancer or that you're at high-risk, your natural response is to want to do everything that you can to heal yourself and to live well. That may include use of complementary and alternative healing approaches.

Keep in mind, though, that no alternative or complementary therapy is known to cure cancer. If a claim for a type of therapy sounds too good to be true, chances are it is. You also don't want to pass up conventional medical treatment, such as surgery or chemotherapy, that's has been shown to help treat cancer or prolong survival, in favor of an unproven alternative approach. The best use of complementary and alternative medicine is to "complement" standard medical care.

This chapter focuses primarily on therapies that might complement your prescribed cancer treatment. These therapies are known to be generally safe and they may help improve the quality of your life by relieving symptoms, reducing stress or anxiety, or minimizing the side effects of conventional treatment.

The best approach is to learn all that you can about your options and the potential benefits and risks of each therapy that you're considering. It's also important that you talk to members of your medical team about the complementary approaches you feel may help you. Team members can assist you in making sure that you're pursuing the best therapies for your particular situation.

In the Additional Resources section of this book, located on pages 413-416, you'll find a listing of reliable institutions and organizations to help you in your quest.

Getting The Most of Complementary Therapies

One of the key differences between complementary therapies and conventional medicine is that conventional medicine, particularly in the United States, generally results from clinical trials that rigorously test medicines and other therapies on many people. A medicine or therapy is approved by the U.S. Food and Drug Administration, when it has been found to be safe and effective for people who meet the criteria for taking it and who take it as instructed.

Complementary therapies, on the other hand, have been used and practiced for much longer than conventional medicines, but they didn't originate in a lab or a study, and many lack good research. Thus, scientists today are playing catch-up in the sense that they are just now testing many unconventional therapies on a large scale to make sure that they truly are safe and effective.

Since not all of the evidence is there to tell you what works and what doesn't, it's important to use common sense when considering a therapy that you think might complement your cancer treatment or help you manage treatment side effects.

Discuss your options

Talk with your doctor or another member of your health care team about the therapy you're considering. Many people who use unconventional therapies don't discuss them with their doctors. They assume their doctors will either be indifferent or opposed to their use of such therapies. But not sharing information with your doctor about all of the therapies you're using could prove dangerous. For instance, some dietary supplements and herbs can interfere with conventional medications (see the chart on page 360).

When considering a complementary or alternative therapy, talk with your doctor first. He or she may be able to provide resources to help you evaluate your options or show you studies indicating potential risks or benefits.

Whether or not your doctor agrees with your decision, it's important that he or she knows what you're doing so that you receive the best possible care and avoid dangerous interactions.

Assess the risks vs. the benefits

Some therapies pose little risk while offering some obvious benefits. For example, meditation is unlikely to cause you harm, is easy to learn, is accessible at any time, and can help you relax and reduce stress.

To the contrary, buying an herbal supplement marketed online as a cancer cure could pose multiple risks. You don't know exactly where it came from or even exactly what's in it. Recent FDA regulations are improving the quality of most dietary supplements sold in the United States, but online products may be of suspect quality and purity. You also don't know how it will affect you personally. It may interact with your conventional treatment and, depending on the supplement, it may even increase your cancer risk. So, as you research unconventional therapies, use reputable sources and providers.

Evaluate treatment providers

If you decide on a particular treatment that requires a provider, such as acupuncture or massage, find a qualified and experienced practitioner who offers it. Ask for a referral from your doctor or another trusted health care professional. A number of teaching hospitals now have integrative health programs that offer a holistic, evidence-based approach to health care.

If you're given a referral from a friend, do your homework first before making an appointment. You can check your state government listings for agencies that regulate and license health care providers. Contact professional organizations, such as the American Academy of Medical Acupuncture, for the names of certified practitioners in your area. Keep in mind, though, that for many unconventional therapies, there are no licensure or certification standards.

Consider the costs

Your health insurance may not cover the complementary treatment that you're considering. Check with your insurance company. If you have to pay for the treatment out of pocket, find out how much it will cost. If possible, get the cost estimate in writing before you start your treatment.

Take a middle road

Regard complementary therapies with an open but objective mind. Stay open to possibilities, but fully evaluate any treatment you're considering.

Types of Therapies

Many different forms of complementary medicine are available, each designed to work in a different way to improve your health and quality of life. In this section we discuss some commonly used therapies that seem to have the most support from conventional practitioners.

Mind-body techniques

People have long believed that your state of mind influences your physical body. And there is, in fact, a substantial amount of scientific evidence that sustained stress can have a negative impact on your overall health. Stress can affect your emotions, your behaviors and even some of your physiologic responses.

Therefore, decreasing stress is widely thought to be beneficial. This is why mind-body techniques typically top the list of complementary therapies that doctors think are helpful.

The techniques discussed here can help reduce your vulnerability to stress and its harmful effects. They can help lessen the impact of treatment side effects, help you sleep better and feel better, lessen your sensitive to pain and contribute to your overall sense of well-being.

You can learn to do most of these techniques yourself, and many of them are inexpensive or free. To get the full benefit, though, you need to practice mind-body therapies regularly.

Meditation
Meditation techniques, which have been around for thousands of years and practiced by people of varied backgrounds, help you enter a deep, restful state that reduces your body's stress response.

Today, many people meditate for spiritual reasons, but meditation may have health benefits as well. Meditating regularly can help relax your breathing, slow your brain waves, and decrease muscle tension and your heart rate. You can teach yourself the art of meditation. Learn the steps on page 357.

Some people prefer moving meditation to sitting meditation. Walking meditation, yoga and tai chi, a Chinese martial arts form that combines gentle movement with deep breathing, are examples of moving meditation.

Yoga
Yoga involves moving through a series of body postures while practicing controlled breathing exercises. It's an excellent way to counteract stress and anxiety. Its quiet, precise movements focus your mind less on your stressors and more on the moment as you move your body through poses that required balance and concentration.

Practicing yoga regularly can improve posture, flexibility, strength and range of motion. Recent evidence also indicates that yoga can improve vigor and lessen persistent fatigue in women who've gone through breast cancer treatment. The women involved in one of the larger studies took a 90-minute yoga class twice a week for 12 weeks. Not only did they feel less fatigued, they also felt more confident in their ability to manage their fatigue and lessen its impact on their lives.

Yoga is an activity that you can do alone or in a group and it doesn't require a big investment to get started. You might begin by taking a class and then after you become adept at the postures and breathing continue the practice at home on your own.

Progressive relaxation

This is a method by which you learn to relax your body a little bit at a time. For instance, you might start by tightening the muscles in your toes and releasing them, then working your way up your body to the top of your head, tightening and releasing muscles as you go. Progressive relaxation teaches you to identify muscle tension and release it. Practicing it can help ease anxiety and distress.

Hypnosis

Hypnosis induces a state of deep relaxation while allowing your mind to remain narrowly focused and open to suggestion. Studies indicate that hypnosis can help reduce pain, anxiety, phobias, nausea and vomiting.

The success of hypnosis depends on the expertise of the practitioner and your willingness to try it. Some people eventually can be taught to hypnotize themselves. Contrary to ideas about hypnosis made popular by the film industry, while hypnotized you can't be made to do something against your will.

Biofeedback

During a biofeedback session, a trained therapist applies electrodes and sensors to various parts of your body to help you identify how your body responds to certain stimuli. Using this information, you can learn how to control certain body responses, such as decreasing muscle tension and lowering your heart rate and

skin temperature, all signs of relaxation. You can receive biofeedback treatments at physical therapy clinics, medical centers and hospitals. Computer-assisted biofeedback programs can be used at home.

Guided imagery

During guided imagery, you relax by following instructions — either from a recorded voice or by someone leading you — to create a pleasant mental picture. In your mind's eye, for example, you might see yourself lying on a beach on a warm summer day listening to gentle, rhythmic waves lapping against the shore. Sometimes, guided imagery is used with progressive relaxation, to increase the relaxation effect.

Music therapy

Music has been used to supplement healing for centuries, and it's still used today to improve quality of life for people with cancer. Listening to or playing music has many potential benefits. Music therapy may help reduce pain and, with the help of anti-nausea drugs, ease the symptoms of nausea and vomiting. It can also promote awareness and communication of your emotions and help you better manage your stress. More research is needed on the potential benefits of music therapy, but there's certainly no downside to its use.

More than just listening to soothing music, music therapy may involve working with a music therapist, who designs a program involving vocal or instrumental music, based on your needs.

To learn more about music therapy or to find a certified music therapist, ask a member of your health care team or check with the American Music Therapy

How to Meditate

One of the best things about meditation, other than its value as a stress reducer, is that anyone can do it. Here's how:

1. Find a quiet place. Experienced meditators may be able to tune out distractions, but if you're a beginner, the fewer distractions the better. So find a place where you're not likely to be disturbed. Turn off the phone; don't answer the door.

2. Get comfortable. Find a comfortable position, whether it's sitting on a straight-backed chair, sitting cross-legged on a cushion or kneeling on a meditation bench. Keep your back straight so that you're less likely to fall asleep, which is why lying down isn't a good idea. Close your eyes to shut out visual stimulation.

3. Breathe. If you're a beginner, start with this technique. Simply pay attention to your breathing. Focus on how it feels when air enters or leaves your nostrils or how your chest and abdomen move in and out as you breathe. If it helps you focus your attention, count your breaths, from one to four (in, out, in, out) and then start over. Or, you might pick a word or phrase to repeat over and over with every out breath. The word can be one that has a meaning for you, or it can just be a sound you find soothing. If your attention wanders — and it will — gently return your focus to your breathing, your counting, or your word or phrase. Practice for short periods — 5 to 10 minutes — and gradually increase the time. For optimal benefit, you should meditate 20 to 30 minutes daily.

Association (see page 413 for more information).

Massage

From birth, the warm touch of other human beings provides comfort and pleasure. So it seems reasonable to assume that massage and other therapies like it can contribute to improved quality of life for women with cancer.

Benefits of massage therapy include relaxation and decreased muscle tension. Studies indicate that massage therapy can help improve symptoms such as anxiety, pain, fatigue and distress. Types of massage therapy common in cancer care include Swedish massage, aromatherapy massage, foot or hand massage (reflexology) and application of light pressure at specific points on the body (acupressure). One type of massage, called manual lymph drainage, uses precise light rhythmic motions to reduce swelling of the arm after a mastectomy. This therapy has become a standard part of physical therapy after mastectomy.

Massage therapy, when provided by a massage therapist who's received additional training in massage techniques for people with cancer, has very few risks. If your cancer has spread to your bones, too much pressure applied during massage could lead to fracture. Vigorous massage may cause further harm to tissue that has already been damaged by surgery or radiation therapy if it's not applied carefully. Concerns about the possibility of massage increasing the risk of cancer spread appear unwarranted. Still, it's recommended massage not be applied directly to a tumor or enlarged lymph nodes.

If you have a massage, make sure the massage therapist uses care in areas of your body undergoing cancer treatment or that previously received treatment. Talk with your doctor about whether massage is safe for you and what areas of your body, if any, the massage therapist should avoid. Be sure your massage therapist graduated from an accredited program and meets state licensure requirements.

Dietary supplements

People with cancer will sometimes turn to dietary supplements, including vitamins and herbal preparations, to aid in their care. According to the American Cancer Society, about 40 percent of people with cancer report using vitamins or a nutritional supplement. Other surveys report even higher numbers. Breast cancer survivors report the highest use of any vitamin or mineral use, more than 80 percent in some surveys.

Although dietary supplements are popular among people with cancer, these therapies also have the least amount of evidence to indicate they aid cancer treatment or reduce side effects. Studies of botanicals and other biologically based products tend to be promising when performed in test tubes and in animals, but they fail to meet expectations when studied in humans. Herbs are composed of hundreds of different components and the key ingredients can be difficult to iso-late, making it hard to create a standardized, one-size-fits-all supplement. In some cases, it may be the synergy between multiple parts of an herb that make it effective.

In addition, people tend to think of products derived from plants and herbs as "natural" and, therefore, safe. Unfortunately, that's not necessarily true. Some dietary supplements may be harmful. In addition, they aren't regulated the way medications are and generally aren't put through rigorous testing procedures. The good news is the FDA now requires all herbs and dietary supplements sold in the United States to meet Good Manufacturing Practices. This means manufacturers are required to ensure what's on the label matches what's in the bottle.

Still, research, for the most part, hasn't established the effectiveness of most dietary supplements, or established guidelines concerning side effects or how much of a preparation is necessary to meet a specific claim.

A major problem with dietary supplements concerns their potential interactions with medications. For example, St. John's wort, an herbal preparation used to combat mild depression, can alter the action of a number of drugs, which is a serious concern if you're receiving anticancer medications. High doses of vitamins can pose risks, as well. So do your homework if you're considering taking a dietary supplement. Find out all that you can about any preparation you want to try, and discuss the information with your doctor before trying anything. The chart on page 360 lists supplements that may interact with chemotherapy drugs and cause harm.

Still, researchers continue to study certain plants, herbs and other biologically based substances to see if they might have beneficial properties, particularly for managing the side effects of breast cancer and its treatment. Following are some of the more popular dietary supplements taken by women who have or are at risk of breast cancer, as well as some of the more promising supplements being studied.

Green tea
Drinking green tea is one of the most common ways that women with breast cancer try to enhance their health. Although evidence for its usefulness is mixed when it comes to protecting against cancer, drinking a cup of green tea a day is unlikely to hurt you. However, be cautious about drinking large quantities of green tea if you're taking chemotherapy medications. The interaction may have harmful effects.

Vitamin C
Many people with cancer take high-dose vitamin C as a supplemental therapy in the belief that the antioxidant will enhance their body's ability to get rid of toxic free radicals. Unfortunately, there's little evidence that vitamin C helps prevent cancer. Large doses of the vitamin aren't necessarily dangerous because the excess is flushed away in your urine, but some research has raised concerns that vitamin C could interfere with the effectiveness of certain chemotherapy drugs.

Flax seed
Studies in mice have shown that components of flax seed and flax seed oil may

inhibit the growth of breast tumors and enhance the effects of the anticancer drug tamoxifen. But more research is needed in humans to see if this holds true for women with breast cancer.

Vitamin E
Research is ongoing regarding vitamin E's role in preventing breast cancer. As of yet, there's not enough evidence to recommend it as a supplementary therapy for breast cancer. And, as with other antioxidants, high doses might interfere with the effectiveness of chemotherapy.

Ginseng
The root of the American ginseng plant is being studied for its potential effects in improving cancer-related fatigue. A persistent feeling of tiredness is one of the most common unmanaged symptoms in people with cancer. Studies of ginseng support that it helps relieve some fatigue. A water-based extracted product is recommended instead of an alcohol-based one, which can produce unwanted estrogen-like effects.

Black cohosh
Hot flashes can be a bothersome side effect of menopause. Scientists are investigating whether black cohosh, an herb that has effects similar to the female hormone estrogen, might help alleviate hot flashes. Most studies, to date, haven't found the herb beneficial.

Vitamin D
Vitamin D supplementation is often recommended to improve or maintain bone health and prevent osteoporosis. Preliminary evidence also suggests that vitamin D may have protective effects

against breast cancer. Studies to define vitamin D's role in reducing breast cancer risk or recurrence are ongoing.

In the meantime, experts recommend women with breast cancer get at least enough vitamin D to optimize their bone health. The current recommended daily intake is 600 IU for women under 70 years of age and 800 IU for those over age 70. The upper limit is 4,000 IU daily.

Natural energy restoration

The theory of natural energy centers on the traditional Chinese belief that humans contain a vital life energy, called qi, which runs along pathways within the body. Illness results when there's a blockage or disturbance of the free flow of energy along these pathways. According to this theory, restoring natural energy flow restores health.

Acupuncture falls into this category. Although not every acupuncture practitioner ascribes to the energy theory,

the method is a proven treatment for many forms of pain, including cancer-related pain. Acupuncture is also noted for its potential to relieve nausea and vomiting associated with chemotherapy treatment.

Other energy therapies such as therapeutic touch and reiki are also known to be safe, although the evidence as to their effectiveness is limited. Research suggests that these practices primarily have a calming, relaxing effect, but they may also help relieve pain.

Acupuncture

Acupuncture is one of the most researched and accepted forms of unconventional medicine. It involves inserting from one to 20 or more hair-thin needles into the skin. The needles usually are left in place for 15 to 30 minutes. The practitioner may move the needles by hand or stimulate them with an electrical current.

It's possible that acupuncture may work, in part, because inserting needles

Herbal Products That Don't Mix

Available evidence indicates that the following herbal preparations may interfere with the strength or effectiveness of some chemotherapy or hormone therapy medications if the herbs are taken at the same time as the medications. Some of these products could possibly even work to stimulate tumor growth. The bottom line is that before taking any herbal preparation it's best to talk to your doctor.

Garlic	Ginkgo	Echinacea
Soy	Ginseng (alcohol-extracted)	St. John's wort
Valerian	Kava	Grape seed

Alternative Systems

Some health care practices are very different from conventional medicine. These include practices such as homeopathy, ayurveda and naturopathy. There's no evidence that any of these practices can cure cancer, and they may be harmful if they prevent an individual from receiving conventional medical treatment. However, the healthy lifestyle components of some of these practices may be beneficial if used in conjunction with conventional treatment.

Homeopathy
Homeopathy is based on two beliefs — the law of similars and the law of infinitesimals. The law of similars: A substance that causes certain symptoms in a healthy person can, when taken in tiny doses, cure someone with similar symptoms who is ill. The law of infinitesimals: The more dilute the substance, the more potent the medicine. Because this concept runs counter to most of conventional medicine, many doctors are skeptical of this therapy. Substances are prepared by a series of shakings, called succession, and are made from tiny amounts of plant, mineral or animal products or chemicals diluted in water or alcohol solutions. Although some of these ingredients are toxic, the amount used is typically too small to present any danger. There's no scientific evidence that homeopathic remedies are effective in treating cancer.

Ayurveda
Possibly the oldest system of medicine still practiced today, ayurveda begins with the premise that people differ from one another physically and psychologically, so treatments must take those differences into account. According to ayurveda, people are made up of three types of energy (doshas) — fire, water and air. In most people, one dosha is dominant, and different combinations cause different metabolic types. Disease is caused by energy imbalances and disharmony with nature. The system uses a variety of therapies, including healthy eating, herbs, exercise, intestinal cleansing, meditation, massage, and breathing exercises to promote health and cure disease. Although most of the techniques promote a healthy lifestyle, some of them, such as intestinal cleansing preparations, might be harmful.

Naturopathy
Based on the healing power of nature and the body, this holistic system uses a combination of approaches, including nutrition, herbs, acupuncture and massage. Practitioners also incorporate techniques from homeopathy, ayurveda, Chinese medicine and conventional medicine. Although some of the techniques may be harmful to someone with cancer, including certain herbal preparations and excessive dietary restrictions, most of the techniques are geared to promoting a healthy lifestyle.

into a person's skin releases endorphins, the body's natural painkillers, and other central nervous system chemicals. Other studies suggest that acupuncture may improve pain control by increasing the number of opioid receptors in the brain.

Acupuncture may provide relief of chronic pain associated with cancer or its treatments, as well as reduced nausea and vomiting that can accompany chemotherapy. Acupuncture has also been shown to improve dry mouth resulting from some forms of radiation treatment.

You should feel little or no pain from the insertion of the needles. Significant pain is a sign that the procedure isn't being performed properly. Adverse side effects are rare, but they do occur, usually as a result of a practitioner's lack of medical knowledge or inadequate training. Concerns about the risk of infection from acupuncture have largely disappeared as use of disposable needles has become a standard practice.

If you undergo acupuncture, you'll probably have several sessions. If you don't get relief after six or eight sessions, the procedure may not work for you.

Therapeutic touch

Proponents of therapeutic touch believe that the human body has an energy field and that blockages or disturbances in that field can be "fixed" with energy provided by a therapeutic touch practitioner.

During therapeutic touch, also known as healing touch, the practitioner moves his or her hands two to four inches above your body to survey your body's energy field, looking for areas of congestion. If a spot is found, the practitioner will use light touch or sweeping hand motions above your skin to assess and balance the energy in and around your body. A typical session lasts approximately 20 to 30 minutes.

Therapeutic touch hasn't been rigorously studied, but evidence so far indicates that it may promote a deep relaxation response, reduction of pain and anxiety, and faster wound healing. Some people have also found it helps to reduce certain side effects of cancer treatment, such as nausea and fatigue.

Reiki

Reiki practitioners channel healing energy by placing their hands just above or lightly on you when you're receiving treatment. The goal is to access your healing energy and use it to facilitate your own healing. During a reiki session, the practitioner uses a series of 12 to 15 different hand positions that are related to energy centers in your body. Each position is held for two to five minutes or until the practitioner feels the flow of energy slow or stop.

Similar to healing touch, the benefits from reiki may come from its ability to promote relaxation. It's not unusual to experience a relaxing tingling or warmness during the procedure. Reiki is most often used to restore a state of relaxation, balance and well-being.

Finding Reliable Information

Knowledge can be a powerful tool in your effort to treat your illness. There's no shortage of books, articles and websites that provide health information. But when it comes to alternative and complementary medicine, hype abounds. How do you know the information you're getting is accurate?

There may be no way to know for sure, but you can use certain safeguards. Here are some guidelines:

- Look for a reputable source, such as a well-known medical school or health care institution, government agency, professional medical association or familiar, disease-centered organization, such as the American Cancer Society.
- Be wary of any information that promises cures, makes claims that sound too good to be true or encourages you to give up conventional treatments.
- When using the Internet, look for a site with an editorial board or medical advisory board that reviews content.
- Check website dates. Outdated information can be wrong and potentially dangerous. Look for websites that review and update their information regularly. Avoid sites that don't date their material.
- Look for the Health on the Net (HON) Foundation Code of Conduct symbol. Only sites that adhere to the code are allowed to display its symbol. HON sites must provide clear information from a qualified professional, unless otherwise noted, and give contact addresses. The site must spell out advertising policies.

Sounds Too Good To Be True?

The Food and Drug Administration and the National Council Against Health Fraud recommend that you watch for the following claims or practices. These are often warning signs of potentially fraudulent dietary supplements or other so-called "natural" treatments that don't work.

- The advertisement or promotional materials include words such as *breakthrough*, *magical* or *new discovery*. If the product were, in fact, a cure, your doctor would recommend it.
- Promotional materials include pseudo-medical jargon such as *detoxify*, *purify* or *energize*. Such claims are difficult to define and measure.
- The manufacturer claims the product can treat a wide range of symptoms, or cure or prevent a number of diseases. No single product can do this.
- The product is supposedly backed by scientific studies but references aren't provided, are limited or are out of date.
- The product's promotional materials mention no negative side effects, only benefits.
- The manufacturer of the product accuses the government or medical profession of suppressing important information about the product's benefits. There is no reason for the government or medical profession to withhold information that could help people.

Even if you follow these guidelines, remember that there are no guarantees. Always verify the information you get, check more than one source, and talk with your doctor or other members of your health care team.

When it comes to use of unconventional practices, try to steer a middle course between uncritical acceptance and outright rejection. Learn to be open-minded and skeptical at the same time. Stay open to various treatments but evaluate them carefully. Also remember that the field is changing: What's unconventional today may well be accepted — or discredited — tomorrow.

Chapter 22:

Life After a Cancer Diagnosis

Survivorship

Moving Forward	366
Managing your fears	366
Reconnecting with old routines	368
Enjoying new and old relationships	370
Helping others	371

Taking Care of Your Health	372
Eat well	372
Stay physically active	372
Maintain a healthy weight	374
Get adequate sleep and rest	375
Continue with follow-up care	376

Support Groups	376
Is a support group right for you?	377
Choosing a support group	377

Public Events	378

Your treatment is over. "Celebrate," everyone says, "now you're back to normal!" Except … you're not really. Some of the side effects of your treatment may still linger. Your daily routine has changed in significant ways. Relationships have shifted and evolved. And you've gone through emotional and spiritual changes that have left indelible marks.

Making the transition from being a breast cancer "patient" to being a breast cancer "survivor" isn't always easy or smooth. During your treatment, you may have felt a sense of comfort in knowing that active steps were being taken to kill the cancer and that you were being checked frequently. But as your treatment ends and you return to your regular routine, you might be surprised by the uneasy feelings that can follow. You might feel like much of your support is gone. You may notice that, instead of celebrating, you're experiencing feelings of fear, loneliness and uncertainty.

Adjusting to a life that now includes a history of cancer means moving past or at least learning to manage some of these fears and uncertainties. But it also offers an opportunity for renewal, to once again take the reins of your life and move forward in a positive direction. This chapter will give you information, tips and practical strategies on re-engaging in life, taking good care of your body, getting the most out of follow-up care, rediscovering opportunities

What Does It Mean to Be a Survivor?

The National Cancer Institute estimates that there are over 11 million cancer survivors living in the United States today. This number is growing due to advances in early detection, diagnosis, treatment and care.

But what does being a survivor mean, exactly? The National Coalition for Cancer Survivorship (NCCS) was the first organization to introduce and define the term *cancer survivor* by stating that a person is considered a cancer survivor from the time of cancer diagnosis through the balance of his or her life. The Lance Armstrong Foundation, a nonprofit organization created to support people with cancer, defines cancer survivorship as a dynamic process of living with, through or beyond a diagnosis of cancer, regardless of the outcome. For practical purposes, this chapter focuses on the time period after your initial treatment is over.

For women with breast cancer, survivorship can mean different things based on the type of tumor they were diagnosed with and the treatment they received. For example, a lumpectomy and radiation therapy may not have as many late or long-term physical effects as a mastectomy combined with chemotherapy and radiation. Other factors that can affect a survivor's quality of life include the level of support she has in her family and community, her financial situation, her levels of stress or anxiety, and her emotional and spiritual state.

So survivorship can mean many different things to many different women. Some women are proud to be called breast cancer survivors, while others are not. They would rather emphasize different aspects of their identity. Whether you use the term or not, what's most important is you adapt and overcome, you live your life fully and richly — not overwhelmed by the illness, but in spite of it.

and maximizing your support network as you get started on this next phase of your journey.

Moving Forward

As you move on from cancer treatment, it will take time to develop a "new normal." Be patient with yourself. It's OK to feel a bit scared or apprehensive as you start a new phase of your life. There will likely be challenges ahead but there also may be great joys in store.

Managing your fears

One of the most common fears among cancer survivors is that the cancer will come back and that the next time there may not be a cure. This fear may become more tangible at certain times, such as when a doctor's appointment is approaching, when you feel various aches or pains, on anniversary dates of your diagnosis, or when a family member or friend becomes ill.

Although it's true that cancer can recur after treatment, it's also true that many women never experience a recurrence.

Thus, the challenge lies in living with uncertainty. In a world that emphasizes facts and knowledge, living with uncertainty can be particularly difficult.

Despite certain clues about the likely outcome of a particular cancer, it's impossible to be certain of the future. Therefore, you must learn to live with a degree of uncertainty.

Some anxiety about a cancer recurrence is healthy in the sense that it prompts you to respond to unusual signs and symptoms and take good care of your health. As time goes on, fear of recurrence generally tends to fade, although it may never go away entirely.

However, being continuously anxious about whether your cancer will come back isn't healthy. It can rob you of time that might be spent in a more worthwhile manner, such as focusing on your work or your family or simply enjoying life.

Pink Isn't Always My Favorite Color

The pink ribbon is recognized as the universal symbol of breast cancer awareness. It's worn with pride by many breast cancer survivors, their families and friends, and many other individuals and groups to increase awareness of the disease.

When you've been diagnosed with breast cancer, it may inspire friends and family to wear pink ribbons on their clothing to honor your courage in the face of the disease. You may receive gifts emblazoned with pink ribbons from well-meaning colleagues who want to show their support.

October is Breast Cancer Awareness Month and pink is widely used to demonstrate support for women diagnosed with breast cancer. There are pink athletic shoes for runners, the National Football League players wear pink on their uniforms, and even M&M's candy turns pink in October.

Many women with breast cancer appreciate the support and embrace the color with enthusiasm. But some women may want to distance themselves from breast cancer, at least temporarily.

As a breast cancer survivor, you may be asked to talk about your own diagnosis and treatment with other newly diagnosed women, perhaps by well-intentioned friends or co-workers. You may even feel an obligation to provide this support, especially if you've received it from other survivors. But it's OK to say no if you're not ready. Talking about your experience too soon may take you back to an emotionally difficult place and require additional time and energy to recover.

If pink is a painful reminder rather than a symbol of survival, be honest with your friends, family and co-workers. Cancer is a very personal journey and everyone has a unique perspective. Sharing your thoughts and feelings helps those who love and support you understand what does and does not make you feel better. It's OK if pink isn't always your favorite color.

Sharing your fears and concerns with a caring family member or friend is often an effective means of dispelling these fears. Seeking the help of a licensed therapist, counselor or professional support group also can be helpful in terms of learning to control your fears and put them in proper perspective.

One thing that many women discover as they learn to live with uncertainty is that their own feelings may be inconsistent or contradictory. For example, you may feel that you're a strong person but at the same time worry that you can't handle your cancer alone. One part of you is ready to fight, and another struggles to maintain hope.

Part of coping with uncertainty is learning to accept these paradoxes and letting go of preconceived notions of how things should be. One small, but perhaps enlightening, study focused on 10 women who had gone through treatment for cancer. Some had had early-stage cancer, others more advanced cancer. Learning to live with uncertainty was one of the major adjustment phases the women experienced. Letting go was a big part of entering this phase. To some, letting go meant giving up control over life and death. To others, letting go of their old selves helped them adjust to their new reality. Still others used humor to let go of emotional tension, to connect with others and to put the cancer into perspective.

Reconnecting with old routines

After treatment you may be dealing with the challenge of getting back to your regular work routine. Some people maintain a regular work schedule while going through treatment, while others may work fewer hours or in a less strenuous position. Or, maybe you needed to stop working during your treatment and are now thinking about returning to your job.

Perhaps returning to work is making you anxious. You may be concerned about fatigue, physical changes and performing your usual job responsibilities. Other concerns may include worry about future medical insurance coverage from your employer.

Meet with your supervisor or human resources representative before you return to your old routine to help alleviate some of your worries. If you decide to switch jobs, do your best to avoid a gap in insurance coverage. You may wish to consult a competent insurance adviser to help you work through the details.

With your co-workers, be honest and share what you feel comfortable talking about. You may find your co-workers are a great source of support and kindness. Your work family is important and can be an incredible source of strength.

Some women find that their cancer experience has given them a newfound desire to pursue a different career path. Instead of returning to their old job, they seek out a career they've always been interested in, but, for one reason or another, never pursued. As a result of their cancer, they now have a clearer vision of who they would like to be and what they would like to do.

It can be comforting to return to familiar routines. Work is just one example. Maybe it's meeting up with your coffee group, or getting back into gardening, jogging or other hobbies. Even your weekly trips to the grocery store can

Karen's Story

My name is Karen. I'm 65, and I'm a breast cancer survivor. I realize I'm not home free — it's possible there may still be cancer cells somewhere in my body. But that doesn't deter me. My plan is to survive cancer — and anything else life throws at me — for at least another 20 years.

My cancer story began with a routine mammogram that showed a very small mass, thought to be benign. I was advised to keep an eye on that breast and return in six months for another mammogram. Within those six months, the mass grew rapidly, and suddenly I was dealing with a 5-centimeter growth. Within days, my husband and I were at Mayo Clinic to start what would become an almost yearlong journey.

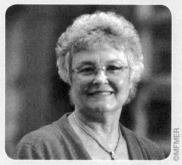

After several tests and a biopsy, I received the diagnosis: Stage III cancer, bordering on stage IV. Was I frightened? Yes! Was I determined to overcome this? Absolutely! My treatment began with a regimen of chemotherapy drugs to try and shrink the tumor. I was also asked if I would be willing to enter into various clinical trials. I agreed because of the possibility that I could be helped by the trials, and because I wanted my case to benefit future breast cancer patients. Fortunately, all of my treatments went well. After the chemotherapy, I had surgery to remove the tumor. My surgery was followed by radiation therapy.

Throughout my treatments, never did I look back. Survival was the order of the day! That's the universal part of my story. Survivorship. More women are surviving breast cancer. And many are overcoming incredible odds. An example is one of my doctors. She was diagnosed with breast cancer in her 30s, when she was starting her career and raising young children. Her sisters and her mother were diagnosed with breast cancer around the same time. Guess what? They're all surviving.

I wanted to survive for my husband, children, grandchildren and friends. I learned about survivorship almost as soon as my treatment started. At Mayo Clinic there is a group called Join the Journey. It's comprised of women who are breast cancer survivors, and they share their expertise and experiences with patients. They helped me, and their presence reminded me that people can survive breast cancer.

One piece of advice I have is to find survivors. Get as much information as you can, and stay positive. It's surprising what people can do when they have hope and determination. Another piece of advice is to trust your instincts. If you don't feel right or you think that something is wrong, don't wait. Get it checked out, and be aggressively vigilant. I'm here today because we moved quickly and because I had wonderful support — my doctors, my husband, my children, my friends. All of them are fabulous.

I was fortunate in that before I developed cancer, I understood how precious life is, and how important relationships are. It's surprising how many cancer survivors you meet in just everyday life. And when you discover that someone else survived breast cancer, you have an immediate bond with that person. You can talk to each other easily. You have much to share. And I think that's precious — that cancer, this terrible disease, has given me an amazing link to so many women, from many walks of life.

Making a Difference Within a Community

It started with a by-chance conversation in the grocery store one day. Effie was just completing treatment, and Patty was newly diagnosed. Effie realized that Patty was probably feeling the same way she did at the beginning of her treatment — overwhelmed and not sure what to expect — so Effie offered to provide Patty some support, including the use of her scarves and wigs that she no longer needed.

Little did Effie and Patty realize that this would be the beginning of a movement that would change the energy in their community. What started out as a basket of scarves being shared among friends soon turned into a local nonprofit organization in Rochester, Minn., called Join the Journey. Today, this group raises funds to support individuals newly diagnosed with breast cancer and it raises awareness in the local community about the disease.

Each year, Join the Journey launches a breast cancer survivors' dragon boat team, engaging in an ancient Chinese water sport that uses a long boat and a relatively large crew, usually about 20 paddlers. Together, the women form a floating support group that provides an opportunity for camaraderie, physical activity and fun. The team has inspired other dragon boat teams, as well.

Another offshoot of this group is the development of a mentorship program to provide newly diagnosed women with face to face emotional and informational support. The mentor, a survivor with a similar diagnosis, meets with the newly diagnosed woman within the health care setting to assist with emotional and physical changes. The success of the program is due both to the important connection between shared experiences and because of the willingness of these women to give back to others.

Join the Journey also makes it possible for women newly diagnosed with breast cancer to receive helpful educational information to help prepare them for issues they may confront or decisions they may have to make.

It was one small act of kindness — one woman helping another — that is now making a difference for hundreds of women each year.

make you feel normal again. Seeing familiar faces and getting on a familiar schedule often bring comfort. But, by the same token, don't be afraid to try something new, to mix things up a bit! Maybe you're tired of some of your routines and you'd like some new adventures. Now's a great time to think big and look for new opportunities.

Enjoying new and old relationships

Over the course of your diagnosis and treatment, your relationships with others — at home, at work and elsewhere — may have changed. Sometimes these changes can contribute to feelings of anger, sadness and loneliness. At the same time, many survivors find a new sense of appreciation and gratitude for those relationships that are the most meaningful to them.

Seeking out and developing positive connections to others are essential to thriving as a cancer survivor. Spend time with people you enjoy being around — people who make you happy and who make you feel good about yourself. These people may be old friends, they may be new friends, or they may be a combination of both. Feeling good about yourself, and about those around you, is important because it gives you strength and confidence.

This is also a time to redefine your relationship with yourself. Don't be too hard on yourself. Give yourself time to heal and to get accustomed to all of the changes in your life. Treat yourself to small things you enjoy and think about what it is that really makes you happy. Once you know the answer, make time to do those things that give you the most pleasure.

You will find that a key aspect of developing and maintaining relationships is good communication. Be honest with others and yourself. Talk with friends and family members about what you're thinking or feeling. Don't bottle up your emotions. Getting your thoughts and feelings out in the open can be a huge relief. By the same token, let them be honest with you, too. Try to develop relationships of honesty and trust.

Helping others

During your journey with cancer, you may have come in contact with a mentor or an advocate who provided you with support and encouragement. Oftentimes, these people are intimately familiar with cancer themselves. They've walked the same path, so they have a pretty good idea what you're going through.

As you heal and learn to live life as a cancer survivor, you might consider providing support and guidance to other women who are at the beginning of their cancer journey. For many cancer survivors, helping others or getting involved in a cancer awareness project makes them feel good. Giving back can be an empowering experience, and many women find they get back as much joy, love and support as they give out, or more. For the person receiving the support, it's inspiring to be with someone who knows exactly how they're feeling.

Your doctor or a member of your health care team can help you decide when might be a good time for you to consider becoming a mentor for another woman with breast cancer. In general, experts feel that there should be at least two years between the time you received your own diagnosis and when you go on to become a mentor. It's important that you have time to recover fully, both physically and emotionally, before exploring the role of mentor.

If mentoring is something you might be interested in, look for ways that you can help other women who would appreciate your experience and helpful insights.

Also keep in mind that helping others isn't limited to helping women with breast cancer. Maybe you would like to volunteer or mentor in different ways. Perhaps there's an organization in your community that interests you or volunteer activities where you worship.

Taking Care of Your Health

After going through breast cancer treatment, it's important to take good care of your body. Eating well, staying active, maintaining a healthy weight and getting adequate rest can make you feel better and more energized, ready to tackle the days ahead. It's also essential to keep up with your post-treatment care plan and to see your doctor regularly.

Practicing these healthy habits may even influence long-term outcomes, such as helping to decrease the chances of a breast cancer recurrence.

Eat well

Eating nutritious foods can help you regain your strength, rebuild healthy tissue and feel good. And because nutrient-rich foods are generally lower in calories than non-nutritious junk food, following a healthy diet can also help you achieve and maintain a healthy weight.

To date, there's no evidence that eating particular foods or taking specific nutritional supplements reduces the risk of breast cancer or of a cancer recurrence. However, an overall eating plan that's low in saturated fat and rich in fruits, vegetables and whole grains may be associated with longer life in breast cancer survivors, especially when combined with regular physical activity.

To give your body the right kinds of fuel for cancer survival, go for variety — no one food contains all the nutrients you need, so you want to eat from all of the food groups.

Foods to eat

As you plan your meals, consider these nutrition tips:
- Focus on plant-based foods
- Go for color with fruits and vegetables
- Emphasize whole grains and legumes, such as beans and lentils
- Go easy on fat, salt, sugar, alcohol, and smoked and pickled foods
- Choose low-fat dairy products and small portions of meat, fish and poultry
- Drink plenty of water

This combination of foods will ensure that you're eating plenty of the vitamins and nutrients you need to help make your body strong. While it may be tempting to supplement your diet with a host of vitamin and mineral supplements, resist that urge. Some cancer survivors think that if a small amount of vitamins is good, a large amount must be even better. But that isn't the case. In fact, large amounts of certain nutrients can hurt you. If you're concerned about getting all the vitamins you need, ask your doctor if taking a daily multivitamin is right for you.

Stay physically active

Regular physical activity is probably the closest to an elixir of life that humans will ever encounter. And it can be especially helpful for cancer survivors. It's an important and proven way to increase your overall well-being and speed your recovery after cancer treatment.

Being physically active can help:
- Increase your strength and endurance
- Increase bone density
- Minimize signs and symptoms of depression
- Lessen anxiety

- Reduce fatigue
- Improve your mood
- Increase your self-esteem

Regular aerobic activity and strength training can also help reduce swelling in your arms associated with lymphedema (see page 333). And it can help you lose weight, especially when combined with changes to your diet.

Mounting evidence also suggests that regular exercise after a cancer diagnosis — including breast, colorectal, prostate and ovarian cancers — may reduce the risk of cancer recurrence and improve overall survival. A critical analysis of six studies involving more than 12,000 breast cancer survivors suggested that being physically active after diagnosis was linked to a 24 percent lower rate of breast cancer recurrence, a 34 percent lower rate of death due to breast cancer and a 41 percent lower rate of death due to any cause.

While the evidence that exercise may reduce your risk of dying of cancer is still preliminary, the evidence regarding the benefits of exercise in relation to your heart, lungs and other body systems is not — it's proved.

Exercising with cancer

Regular exercise is highly recommended both during and after treatment for breast cancer, but there are certain situations that require some caution. The American Cancer Society offers these guidelines:

Treatment effect	Precaution
Severe anemia	Delay exercise, other than normal daily activities, until the anemia improves.
Compromised immune system	Avoid public gyms and pools until your white blood cell counts return to safe levels.
Severe fatigue	Aim for 10 minutes of light exercise every day.
Skin affected by radiation	Avoid chlorine exposure from swimming pools.
Indwelling catheters or feeding tubes	To prevent infection, avoid potential sources of germ exposures such as pools, lakes and oceans. Also avoid strength training muscles around the catheter (so it doesn't get dislodged).
Existence of other chronic illnesses, such as high blood pressure or arthritis	Talk to your doctor about how best to structure your exercise routine.
Numbness or pain in your extremities (peripheral neuropathy), muscle weakness, or difficulty coordinating your movements	Avoid activities that require significant balance and coordination, such as walking or jogging. Instead choose a stationary reclining bicycle or swimming, if possible.

Adding physical activity to your daily routine doesn't take a lot of extra work. Focus on small steps to make your life more active. Take the stairs more often or park farther from your destination and walk the rest of the way. Check with your doctor before you begin any exercise program.

With your doctor's approval, start slowly and work your way up. If you're dealing with side effects from your treatment, talk with your doctor about precautions you should take (see the table on page 373).

The American Cancer Society and the American College of Sports Medicine recommend that cancer survivors aim for at least 150 minutes of moderate physical activity a week — that's 30 minutes per day five days out of the week. Moderate activities include walking briskly, dancing, biking, canoeing, gardening — any activity where you're working hard but you can talk while you perform the exercise. You should also try to include at least two days a week of strength training. As you recover and adjust, you might find that more exercise makes you feel even better.

There may be days you won't feel like exercising, and that's OK. Don't feel guilty if lingering treatment side effects, such as fatigue, keep you sidelined. When you feel up to it, take a walk around the block. Do what you can, and remember that rest also is important to your recovery.

Maintain a healthy weight

An important lifestyle choice you can make as a breast cancer survivor is to achieve and maintain a healthy weight. A number of studies conducted over several decades have shown a link between extra weight and an increased risk of breast cancer recurrence.

What this means is that if you're overweight, you may be able to improve your odds for a successful outcome by losing some weight. In addition, evidence already exists that intentional weight loss can improve your hormonal status, physical abilities and quality of life after breast cancer treatment. It can also help head off other chronic diseases, such as high blood pressure and diabetes.

This doesn't mean that you need to embark on a crash diet or begin starving yourself. In fact, going on a diet after just completing cancer treatment might not sound very appealing at all. Don't think of what you're doing as "dieting." Think of it as developing a plan to eat better. Achieving and maintaining a healthy weight has a lot to do with changing the way you think about eating. It's about making gradual, healthy changes in your diet and exercise habits, which can eventually become engrained.

The American Cancer Society recommends these common-sense strategies for achieving and maintaining a healthy weight:

- Limit high-calorie foods.
- Drink fewer beverages with added sugar that are high in calories.
- Focus on low-calorie foods such as fruits and vegetables.
- Add more physical activity to your day.

If you need to gain weight
Maybe losing weight isn't your problem — perhaps you need to gain weight. If

your treatment has caused you to lose weight, achieving a healthy weight is just as important. Additional weight loss may delay healing and increase your risk of complications.

To gain weight, you'll want to increase your calorie consumption to achieve a positive energy balance. Try to consume more high-calorie foods and beverages, such as peanut butter, nuts, avocados, cheese, nutritional drinks and lean meats. You might also try eating more frequent meals.

If you're trying to gain weight, it's still important that you get regular physical activity because exercise provides so many health benefits. Seek out activities that increase your strength, such as yoga or resistance exercises, but don't use up too many calories.

Talk to your doctor or a dietitian if you're having trouble gaining weight. He or she can help you come up with a plan to help you consume the calories you need to reach a healthy weight.

Get adequate sleep and rest

Sleep is an important issue as a cancer survivor. Many people find that they feel tired and fatigued for months after they complete their cancer treatment. Although fatigue can sometimes be difficult to cope with, it is manageable. However, what works for one person may not work well for another, so it may take a little trial and error to find those practices that work best for you.

Sleep tips
Here are some simple strategies to help you sleep better:

- **Rest early.** Find time earlier in the day for short periods of rest, as opposed to late afternoon. This will help you sleep better at night.
- **Exercise.** Mild to moderate exercise helps to reduce fatigue. Yoga in particular may be helpful in treating cancer-related fatigue. You might also try walking or leisurely swimming.
- **Balance rest, sleep and activity.** While sleep and rest are important, don't overdo it. Too much rest can actually decrease your energy level.
- **Eat a balanced diet and drink plenty of liquids.** Your body needs protein, carbohydrates, vitamins, minerals and water to work efficiently. A dietitian can help to develop the best eating plan for you.
- **Reduce stress.** Stress steals precious energy. Try using relaxation methods or creative outlets to reduce stress. Some relaxation techniques include yoga, deep breathing, guided imagery, meditation, listening to music or creating art. See Chapter 21 for more information.
- **Maintain your social life.** Many people eliminate social activities altogether when they're feeling tired. To replenish your spirit, include activities in your life that are satisfying to you. These activities can also boost your energy level.
- **Develop good sleep habits.** To sleep well at night, try these suggestions: Create a pleasant, comfortable place to sleep, such as a dark, cool, quiet room. Avoid heavy meals before bedtime. Avoid, or limit, caffeine in the afternoon and evenings. Take part in relaxing activities before bed, such as reading, taking a warm bath or listening to quiet music.

Continue with follow-up care

After your treatment is complete, you probably won't see your medical care team as often as you once did, but you will need regular follow-up care. The purpose of follow-up care is to keep track of your overall physical and emotional health, identify and treat complications from your treatment, and watch for indications that your cancer may have returned.

You'll most likely continue to see your oncologist. If you transfer to another doctor's care after your initial treatment, such as your primary care doctor, you'll want a summary of your diagnosis, treatment and follow-up recommendations to take with you. Be an active participant in your care.

Initially, follow-up care visits may take place every four to six months, and then become less frequent as time goes by. During these visits, your doctor will want to know about any late or lingering side effects of treatment, do a physical exam, and possibly order some tests. You can read more about follow-up care and surveillance in Chapter 14.

Follow-up visits are also a good time to talk to your doctor about any concerns you may be having or to let him or her know if you're feeling down and unable to pick up with your life again. Sometimes, just talking with a professional can be reassuring. If you need additional help, your doctor may recommend a counselor or therapist to help you work through feelings of stress or anxiety.

In between visits, you can institute your own surveillance and prevention program with these simple habits:

- Be aware of changes in your body. Pay attention to new or unusual symptoms including skin changes, swollen lymph nodes, unusual bleeding, pain or excessive fatigue.
- Don't use tobacco.
- Protect your skin from sun exposure.
- Limit alcohol consumption.
- Get regular exercise.
- Eat healthy foods.

Support Groups

Once their treatment is over, some women feel isolated and lonely. They miss the emotional support they received from their health care team. Sure, friends and family can help fill the void, but sometimes only medical professionals and fellow cancer survivors can provide what's needed at this point.

Cancer support groups bring together people who've had cancer. Participants talk about their own experiences, feelings and concerns, they listen to the concerns of others, and they exchange practical information about how to deal with the challenges of life after cancer.

Cancer support groups can offer a variety of benefits. Simply by meeting others who've faced cancer, you may feel less isolated and gain a sense of belonging. Frank discussions can foster openness and better understanding. Shared problem-solving may help you find solutions to what may be bothering you or help you develop coping skills. Compassion and empathy from others in the group can help see you through a crisis. In addition, you may feel better about yourself by offering support and help to others.

Is a support group right for you?

It's certainly not mandatory that you join a support group. Not everyone wants or needs group support beyond their family and friends. Hearing other people's cancer stories makes some people more anxious. But others find it helpful to hear and learn from individuals outside of their immediate circle of family and friends.

If you're uncertain if a support group is for you, consider whether you like being part of a group and sharing life stories with others. Before joining a particular group, you might to want to find out some of the following information:

- How large is the group?
- Who attends (survivors, family members, types of cancer, age range)?
- How long are the meetings?
- How often does the group meet?
- How long has the group been together?
- Who leads the meetings — a professional or a survivor?
- What is the format of the meetings?
- Is the main purpose to share feelings, or do people also offer tips to solve common problems?
- Do you have to participate or can you just listen?

Choosing a support group

In general, cancer support groups fall into two main categories: Those led by a health professional, such as a nurse, social worker or psychologist, and those led by cancer survivors, often called peer groups or self-help groups. Some cancer support groups are for people with a specific type of cancer. Others are open to

anyone who has been treated for cancer. Still others are open to family members and friends of cancer survivors.

Some groups are designed to be more educational and structured. They may invite a doctor or another health professional to give a talk on a new cancer treatment. Other groups put more emphasis on emotional support and shared experiences.

The key is finding a group that matches your needs and personality. You may find that you prefer a structured, moderated group that provides organized discussions and educational information. A moderator or facilitator can help ensure that all of the participants have an equal opportunity to share if they wish to and that the discussions stay on track.

Or you may prefer a group with less structure. You may feel more comfortable meeting with a small group of people at someone's home, where emotional support is the focus.

In addition, there are online support communities that you can access virtually anywhere at any time. They can be a valuable source of emotional support, sometimes when you need it most. But be sure to double-check any health information you get from online support groups with your doctor. The information may be inaccurate or not applicable to your situation, and could be even potentially harmful.

If you decide to take part in a support group, try it out for a time. Keep in mind that it takes time to develop a "new normal," so try to be patient with yourself. If you don't find the group useful or comfortable, you don't have to continue attending.

Public Events

Some women on their cancer journey are reluctant to take part in cancer-related events. They're not sure what to expect or how they'll react. Other women embrace the events with excitement and enthusiasm. Your response may be somewhere in the middle.

Each year, hundreds of cancer events are held around the country to raise money for cancer research and education. Some events are strictly for breast cancer research, others support other forms of cancer, and still others raise money for cancer in general.

Think about taking part in a cancer event — a walk, bike trip or telethon — and see what you think. You may come away with an incredible sense of joy and hope. It's incredibly moving to see a group of people getting together to raise money or give support for the cancer cause. The whole idea has helped the country move from a time when cancer was a word rarely spoken, to the present, when support and awareness are free and open.

Cancer events provide a sense of doing something — moving forward with a real connection to others who have the same passion and drive to make a difference. Everyone is touched by cancer in some way in life, which is why it's so important to talk, walk and show support in every way possible.

Chapter 23:

Life After a Cancer Diagnosis

Making the Transition to Supportive Care

Accepting Your Situation   380

Maintaining Hope   381

When You and
Your Family Disagree   383

Managing
Signs and Symptoms   383
Pain   383
Shortness of breath   387
Appetite changes
and weight loss   387
Nausea and vomiting   389

Hospice Care   389
Services offered   390
Eligibility   393
Do-not-resuscitate status   393

When breast cancer reaches an advanced stage, there comes a point when many women realize the time has come to stop treating the cancer. Perhaps you're facing such a situation.

The decision to stop treatment aimed at killing the cancer (anti-cancer therapy) is generally considered after a woman and her doctor have discussed all of the remaining options, and they've determined that:

- No treatment will cure the cancer.
- There's little chance further surgery, chemotherapy or radiation therapy will change the course of the disease.
- There isn't good evidence that continuing treatment will prolong survival or improve quality of life.
- All evidence suggests that any positive response from continued treatment will be short-lived.

- The potential side effects from continuing anti-cancer treatment are significant.

If this is your situation, your decision to stop anti-cancer therapy is both a logical and an understandable one. Now, instead of trying to kill the cancer or slow its progression, the goals of your treatment are to:

- Reduce and manage the symptoms of the cancer as much as possible
- Experience the fewest medication side effects as possible
- Have the best quality of life
- Have the longest life

It's important to remember that just because you're stopping treatment aimed at fighting the cancer doesn't mean you're ending your medical care. You'll continue to receive regular care from your doctor.

Accepting Your Situation

In the beginning, right after receiving your diagnosis, the emphasis of treatment typically is on curing the cancer. If the cancer isn't curable, treatments are used to slow the growth of the tumor in an attempt to allow you to live longer. When efforts to slow cancer growth are no longer effective, the emphasis shifts primarily to alleviating discomfort and other symptoms. This is known as supportive (palliative) care (see page 388). Supportive care also includes addressing any of your psychological, social, spiritual and emotional needs, as well as providing support for your family.

'How Much Time Do I Have Left?'

Many people with a terminal illness want their doctors to tell them how much time they have left. This is a hard question for doctors to answer, and many may be reluctant to respond to it directly. For one thing, they can make only an educated guess. For another, answering the question requires a difficult balance between being realistic and hoping for the best.

Because doctors can't help becoming personally connected to their patients and their patients' families, they may overestimate prognosis in order to maintain hope. This could mean you may not have as much time as your doctor says you do.

Independent of trying to maintain hope, a doctor may simply be wrong in his or her estimate of the manner and speed in which the cancer will progress. Multiple studies have demonstrated that doctors tend to be overly optimistic regarding life expectancy in people with advanced cancer.

If your doctor does give you a time estimate, don't take it as gospel. Some people live longer than their doctors thought they would, others live less.

Having a time estimate may help you feel more in control, but no matter how much time you may have left, make the best of it. Live each day as fully as possible, doing the things you want to do.

How do you know when the time has come to stop fighting the cancer? It's a difficult decision to make. It's a personal decision that only you can make with advice from your health care team, family and friends. Some women find it difficult to end treatment aimed at destroying or controlling the cancer because it feels like they're giving up. But if the cancer has become resistant to anti-cancer therapies, such treatments may do more harm than good. For many women, the quality of their lives becomes paramount because they want to enjoy the time they have left.

The time when you may fare better without anti-cancer therapy arrives when the therapy stops working and the downsides of continuing it outweigh the potential benefits. For example, for many people with cancer, there eventually comes a time when the chances that chemotherapy will make them sick — and maybe cause potentially life-threatening side effects — may be far greater than the chances of it shrinking the cancer.

Deciding to stop anti-cancer treatment that's no longer helping you may be a way for you to take back control. You may feel as if your life has been out of control since you learned that you have cancer. Making the decision to stop cancer treatment and to be free of the side effects of treatment can be a powerful step in taking charge of your life.

Maintaining Hope

Even as you accept that your cancer isn't curable, you can still have hope. But your hopes might change as your circumstances change. For example, when you first received your diagnosis, you may have hoped that it was a mistake. Once you accepted the diagnosis, you undoubtedly hoped to beat the cancer. When you learned the cancer wasn't curable, you may have hoped that your treatment would work well enough to extend your life for several years.

So what do you hope for now that you realize further attempts at controlling the cancer likely won't work? That depends on your goals. This may be a time to reframe your hopes. They may include spending quality time with family, taking a trip, relieving your symptoms or living in comfort, without pain and suffering. Perhaps your hope centers on leaving a legacy for your children or grandchildren. This might involve putting your financial affairs in order, videotaping or writing family stories, or creating a document in which you write about your values, the lessons you've learned from life, and your love for family and friends.

Keep in mind, though, as you set your goals, that cancer's path can be difficult to predict. The course of your cancer can change abruptly, and it may not be possible for you to meet all the goals you've set. Some people think of it this way: Hope for the best while you plan for the worst. Make time to take care of responsibilities and essentials. Sign papers you need to sign, tell friends and loved ones what you want to say to them, and write down whatever thoughts you need to express in writing.

It's fine to have some longer term projects on your list of goals, but you may also want to be sure that you have a goal for each day, such as reaching out

Denying Impending Death

Some people with advanced cancer find it difficult, if not impossible, to accept that their treatments are no longer working and that their cancers are terminal. They may employ a defense mechanism known as denial.

Denial may be either harmful or beneficial. It's beneficial when it enables you to process information about your illness in your own time and in such a way that you can absorb it without being overwhelmed. But continued denial can cause you to insist on receiving anti-cancer treatments when it's clear they're no longer beneficial, and more importantly, it can keep you from getting your affairs in order, saying your goodbyes and, ultimately, dying a peaceful death.

In a study of people with advanced lung cancer, individuals who had difficulty accepting their eventual death and who continued to receive aggressive treatment didn't live any longer than those who stopped their anti-cancer therapy earlier.

Denial can be especially problematic if your family can't accept your illness and encourages or reinforces your denial. If you or family members are having a difficult time accepting that your cancer is terminal, it may help to talk with a counselor, chaplain, hospice worker or member of your health care team. An opportunity to express your fears, which can contribute to denial, may help you approach your illness more realistically so that you can make informed decisions regarding your future.

to friends and family or writing notes to people who have touched your life. On page 391, you can read the notes one mother wrote to her sons as she was in the later stages of her cancer.

Most people don't want to discuss dying. But rather than approach the subject with fear, why not treat this as a time to think about living and dying with the idea of compassion and kindness for yourself and your family. If you're interested in finding some peace for yourself, you might consider a couple of these ideas:

- Reflect on the positive aspects of your life; find strength in your deepest values.
- Keep in mind what's most important to you (in life and after you're gone).

- Write or tell stories of your fondest memories to your friends and family to reflect on now and later.
- Inquire early about hospice care (discussed later in the chapter). Receiving such care earlier, rather than later, can make a big difference. Palliative and hospice care provide a holistic approach that can assist you and your family members so that you can approach your last months and days in a positive manner.
- Talk about or write down what you want to happen after you're gone — this might include funeral planning, memorial ideas and any special requests related to the giving of meaningful personal items to others.

Keep in mind that some of your loved ones will feel a strong need to express their feelings at this time, and others won't feel capable of that. This can be a beautiful time of sharing, and you are the one with the most control over this opportunity. When you're ready, you and loved ones can share many simple but important words. These may include simple phrases such as: "I love you," "I forgive you," "I'm sorry," "Thank you" and — when the time is appropriate — "Goodbye."

When You and Your Family Disagree

Your illness affects your entire family. When you, along with your health care team, make the transition from anticancer treatment to supportive care, your family members may not understand. They may say that you're giving up. Maybe it's your spouse or your children or a relative who comes from out of town who hasn't been involved with your illness and treatment who wants you to "keep fighting."

Throughout your illness, you have experienced many losses. Although difficult, each loss may have caused you to establish new goals and to redefine hope. These losses, in some ways, prepare you for death. While your family members have experienced some degree of loss, too, it's different from your own. They may not be ready to let you go.

As you face the last phase of your illness, the support you receive from family and friends can influence how well you cope. If your goals are at odds with those of family members, arrange a meeting with them and members of your health care team. Ask someone from your health care team to explain your situation so that your family understands the basis for your decision and to answer questions family members may have.

Be firm in your resolve to do what's best for you. Don't be pressured to accept treatment just to keep the peace. That may do you more harm than good. Tell your loved ones that what's most important to you now is being able to enjoy high-quality time with them.

Managing Signs and Symptoms

It's natural for people with incurable cancer to fear pain and other symptoms the disease may cause. Once you stop treatment intended to kill or slow the cancer, that doesn't mean your care will end. Your health care team will still take care of you, helping you manage your symptoms and other conditions that may arise. The goal is to help you live as comfortably as possible. Many approaches can be used to manage symptoms and conditions that may develop. Depending on your situation, your primary care doctor or oncologist may enlist the help of an individual who specializes in supportive care.

Pain

Pain can be a major factor in your ability to enjoy life. It can affect your sleeping, eating and other day-to-day activities. For people with advanced cancer, pain is usually caused by the cancer spreading into organs, bone or soft tissue or by the cancer pressing on a nerve. Pain that involves an organ may be difficult to pinpoint and may be described as a dull, deep throbbing or aching or, occasionally, as sharp. Pain that involves skin, muscle or bone is usually limited to a specific area and may be described as sharp, aching, burning or throbbing. Pain that involves nerves (neuropathic pain) is often described as sharp, tingling, burning or shooting.

Pain may be severe but last a relatively short time (acute pain), or it may range from mild to severe and persist for a long time (chronic pain). Certain pain may also be associated with specific movements or activities and may be predictable (incident pain). There's also a type of pain known as breakthrough pain. It occurs when moderate to severe pain "breaks through" the medication that's controlling it. Breakthrough pain usually lasts a short time but may occur up to several times a day.

You will likely be asked to rate your pain on several occasions. This is so that your health care team can provide you with the right dosage of medication to keep on top of your pain — to control it adequately, but not provide you with so much medication that you have difficulty functioning.

For some people, rating their pain is a difficult thing to do. People's perception of pain is different, and what one person may consider mild another person may rate as severe. Still, your input is important. It's easier for your doctor to manage

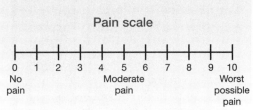

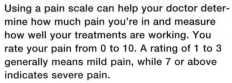

Using a pain scale can help your doctor determine how much pain you're in and measure how well your treatments are working. You rate your pain from 0 to 10. A rating of 1 to 3 generally means mild pain, while 7 or above indicates severe pain.

your pain with some input from you, than with none at all.

Seeing your doctor

Many medications can effectively manage pain, but your doctor needs to know the specifics of your pain to be able to treat it. To help your doctor assess your pain, provide him or her with as much information as possible, including the answers to the following questions:

• Where do you feel the pain?
• When did it start?
• What were you doing when it started?
• How does it feel — sharp, tingling, burning, aching, throbbing, shooting?
• Has it changed over time?
• On a scale of 0 to 10 — with 0 being no pain and 10 being worst possible pain — how bad is your pain?
• What, if anything, makes the pain better or worse?
• Have any of the medications you've taken had an effect on the pain?

It might help to keep a written record of your pain so that you can give your doctor an accurate report. Besides answering the questions above, keep track of your pain medication and the effect it has on your pain, and for how long. Let your doctor know if the medication is causing unwanted side effects, such as interfering with your activities or your ability to sleep or eat.

To assess your pain, your doctor will likely perform a physical examination and may request some tests, such as blood tests or X-rays, to determine the cause.

Treatment

The primary goal is to treat the source of the pain, if possible. This may include use of treatments such as radiation, surgery and targeted medication. With advanced cancer, though, it's not always possible to treat the specific cause. Then treatment typically involves use of analgesic pain medications, which range from

---

What About Addiction?

Studies have shown that many people with cancer are reluctant to take strong pain medications, such as opioids (narcotics), for two reasons. They're afraid of becoming addicted to the medications, and they're afraid that if they use strong medication too early in the course of their disease, it won't work for them later when their pain becomes more severe. These fears are understandable, but neither of them has a medical basis.

Addiction is a type of behavior where a person compulsively seeks drugs for the mental high they might provide. When opioid medications are used to treat cancer pain, addiction to these drugs is rare.

For people who take opioids for a long time, though, it's common for them to develop tolerance to a drug. With tolerance, the effects of the drug decrease with regular use, and the person taking the drug may need higher doses to achieve the same effect. Fortunately, doses of these drugs can be increased. There's no maximum

dose that can be given ("ceiling effect"). Therefore, if you become tolerant of a certain dose, your doctor can increase the dose until your pain is relieved or prescribe a different medication.

In addition, your body may become used to receiving the drug at regular intervals, a condition called physical dependence. If you stop taking it abruptly, you may experience withdrawal. Withdrawal can be avoided by slowly tapering off the drug if it's no longer needed. It's important to know that tolerance and physical dependence are not the same as addiction.

Tell your doctor about any problems with pain medication you've had in the past. Follow directions for taking your medication. And let your doctor know if it isn't providing enough relief.

Pain management is vital to maintaining a good quality of life. Cancer pain may require strong medications such as opiods. Work with your doctor to find the medication or combination of medications that works. Don't let fear of addiction keep you from getting relief from your pain. Ask your doctor to refer you to a pain specialist if needed.

simple pain relievers to opioids, also known as narcotics.

Simple pain relievers include acetaminophen (Tylenol, others), aspirin, and nonsteroidal anti-inflammatory drugs (NSAIDs), such as ibuprofen (Advil, Motrin IB, others) and naproxen (Aleve). Steroid medications also may be helpful in some situations. Opioids, the strongest pain-relieving medications, include codeine, oxycodone (OxyContin, Roxicodone, others), morphine, fentanyl (Duragesic) and hydromorphone (Dilaudid), among others. For severe pain, opioids are the best medications. Sometimes, regular doses of aspirin, acetaminophen or ibuprofen may be recommended in addition to an opioid medication to boost pain relief.

Opioids can be either long-acting or short-acting, referring to the period of time that they remain active in your system. Generally speaking, short-acting medications take effect quickly — within 30 to 60 minutes — and provide relief for up to two to four hours. Long-acting opioids, on the other hand, may take several hours to reach peak effectiveness, but their effects generally continue for about 12 hours.

For some people on long-acting opioids, taking an intermittent short-acting opioid can help relieve breakthrough pain that arises between scheduled doses of the long-acting drug. If you're experiencing breakthrough pain, a rapid-onset, short-acting opioid in addition to your long-acting medication should give you relief. If you know from experience that a particular activity triggers the pain, taking a short-acting opioid beforehand may block or significantly diminish the pain.

If you have continued pain, it's best to keep the pain under control by taking your pain medication at regular intervals rather than intermittently or as needed. This is especially true for the strong opioids. Steady dosing may diminish the side effects of the medication. Taking your medications on a regular schedule also provides better and more even pain control, and you actually may end up needing less medication than if you take the drugs intermittently.

Opioid medications may be given orally, by way of patches placed on the skin, by rectal suppositories or by injection.

Another method of receiving medication is by way of a pain pump. A pain pump can be implanted under the skin of your lower abdomen with a small tube placed in the spinal canal next to the spinal cord, where pain signals get transmitted to your brain. Though delivered to your spinal cord, the medication may help eliminate pain elsewhere in your body. Your doctor may suggest this method if you have severe pain that isn't controlled with regular opioids or if you're experiencing excessive side effects from the medication that can't be controlled.

Opioid medications may cause side effects such as drowsiness, dizziness, nausea and confusion. Most of these side effects are easily managed and, with steady dosing, they often diminish after a few days. One of the most common side effects is constipation. This occurs in almost all individuals who take opioid medications on a regular basis. Generally, only with appropriate treatment, does the condition improve. Your doctor will likely start you on a regimen of stool softeners

Controlling Pain Through Relaxation

Stress and anxiety can make your pain worse by creating tension in your body. Techniques designed to help relieve anxiety and help you relax may also help control your pain. These include deep-breathing exercises, meditation and progressive relaxation. See Chapter 21 for more information on relaxation techniques.

In addition, try to get your mind off your pain by doing activities that you enjoy, such as listening to music or engaging in a hobby. If you're able, exercise may make you feel better and help you relax and sleep. Try to get some exercise daily, even if you only feel well enough to walk for a few minutes on the arm of a family member or friend.

or bowel stimulants or both, as soon as you begin taking an opioid. It may be easier to prevent constipation than to treat it.

Other medications may be useful for specific types of pain. Anti-seizure drugs or other related medications may be helpful in individuals who have nerve damage. Medications called bisphosphonates that are used to treat osteoporosis may be helpful if you're experiencing pain from bone damage due to the tumor. Your doctor also may suggest other means of pain control, such as nerve blocks by injections of chemicals or radiation therapy to a localized area of pain.

If you find the side effects of a drug intolerable, if your medication isn't working well enough or long enough, or if you have frequent breakthrough pain, you may need to try another medication or other pain control methods.

Shortness of breath

Another condition that can occur is shortness of breath (dyspnea). It has multiple causes, including cancer spreading to the lungs, heart problems, muscle weakness, anemia and generalized fatigue. At times, the underlying cause of shortness of breath is treatable. To determine the cause of this condition and how best to treat it, your doctor will likely perform a physical exam and request some tests, such as a chest X-ray, blood tests or heart tests.

If the cause can't be determined or if your doctor can't treat the underlying cause, he or she will try to relieve the discomfort of shortness of breath. Having oxygen or cool air blown across your face may be helpful. Opioid medications, such as morphine, also provide relief by blunting the sensation of being short of breath. An inhaler or nebulizer that delivers medication to your lungs may provide relief.

Appetite changes and weight loss

With advanced cancer, you may find your appetite diminishing and your weight dropping. Your loved ones may be disturbed by your inability to eat, perhaps because we tend to equate a hearty appetite with good health. There's

Palliative Care

Palliative care is a relatively new specialty that aims to reduce pain and improve quality of life for people who have advanced illnesses, as well as provide support for their families. Palliative care takes into account the emotional, physical and spiritual needs and goals of the person who's being treated and his or her family. Palliative care doesn't replace primary medical treatment. Instead, it's provided in conjunction with other medical treatment.

Palliative care grew out of the hospice movement, but it differs from hospice in that it's available at any time during a serious or life-threatening illness, while hospice care is available only during the final months of life — when curative or life-prolonging treatments have been stopped. You don't have to be in hospice to receive palliative care.

Who can benefit from palliative care?

Anyone who has a serious or life-threatening illness can benefit from palliative care, either to treat signs and symptoms of the disease or to ease the side effects of treatment. In addition, palliative care can help if you or a loved one needs help understanding more about an illness or coordinating medical care.

Palliative care is available whether you or your loved one is being treated as an outpatient, in a hospital or nursing home, or through hospice. Often, palliative care specialists work as part of a multidisciplinary team to coordinate care. The team may be comprised of various specialists, including doctors, nurses, social workers, psychologists, counselors, chaplains, registered dietitians and pharmacists.

A palliative care specialist works with your primary care doctor and other members of your medical team to create a care plan that eases symptoms, relieves pain, addresses spiritual and psychological concerns, and helps maintain dignity and comfort. Together, these steps can lead to an improved quality of life.

A palliative care specialist can also help you or your loved one communicate with doctors and family members and create a smooth transition between the hospital and home care. If necessary, a palliative care specialist can help coordinate financial and legal assistance.

Research shows palliative care has a number of benefits including less time in the hospital, more time at home among family and friends, better control of symptoms, increased satisfaction with medical care and a reduction in the cost of care. People who seek palliative care also have a higher likelihood of dying at a place of their own choosing, such as at home instead of in a hospital.

If you're interested in obtaining palliative care for yourself or for a loved one, ask for a referral to a palliative care specialist.

no evidence, however, that a person with advanced cancer will live any longer if he or she eats more. Pressuring someone to eat can cause stress and nausea, which is an unnecessary burden if he or she is already experiencing the effects of advanced cancer.

If you're bothered by your loss of appetite, try these methods to possibly stimulate appetite:

- Eat more in the morning than in the evening, because your appetite is likely to diminish as you get tired.
- Eat small meals more often, rather than three large meals a day.
- Avoid cooking smells, especially if you're nauseated.
- Try to eat foods that are cold or at room temperature because you may find them more appetizing and easier to eat than hot foods.
- Try nutrition supplements, such as the beverages Ensure, Boost and Carnation Instant Breakfast.

In addition to trying these self-help tips, you might want to talk with your doctor about a prescription appetite stimulant. Perhaps the most widely prescribed and best studied is megestrol acetate (Megace). This drug also has an anti-nausea effect.

Nausea and vomiting

Loss of appetite and weight may be related to nausea and vomiting. Nausea and vomiting can result from many causes, such as spread of the cancer to the liver, interference with normal digestive functioning due to cancer spread to the intestines, constipation, and use of pain medications. Eating only those foods that appeal to you and eating frequent, smaller meals instead of three large ones may help. Anti-nausea medications may help to some degree. Those commonly prescribed to stimulate appetite (megestrol acetate and corticosteroids) also may help to decrease nausea and vomiting. Some people find patches for motion sickness that contain the medication scopolamine to be helpful.

If you experienced nausea and vomiting while receiving chemotherapy, you may have gotten relief from drugs designed to treat chemotherapy-induced nausea and vomiting. These same drugs may also help when nausea and vomiting are caused by advanced cancer rather than chemotherapy.

Hospice Care

Hospice is the term used to describe special programs in which a group of individuals — the hospice team — works together to provide optimal supportive care for terminally ill individuals and their families. The hospice team usually includes doctors, nurses, pharmacists, social workers, therapists, chaplains, volunteers and others. Hospice programs strive to enhance quality of life, while neither delaying nor hastening the dying process.

For some people, hospice care means the end of hope. It's true that hospice care can begin only after hope of a cure is gone, but initiating hospice doesn't mean that all hope is lost. The goal of hospice is to help you live well during the time you have remaining and to help you die with peace and dignity.

The Beginnings of Hospice

In the United States, modern-day hospice care began in Connecticut in 1974. The Connecticut Hospice in New Haven was modeled after a concept developed by Dame Cicely Saunders, a social worker who in 1967 opened the renowned St. Christopher's Hospice in Sydenham, England. Dame Cicely was so committed to providing high-quality, compassionate care for people near the end of their lives that she became a doctor to realize her goal. Her model of palliative care has since been replicated many times over in England, the United States and throughout the world.

Although hospice services initially were designed primarily for people with cancer, today they're available to people with other terminal illnesses, too.

Most hospice care is provided at home, but it may be provided in nursing homes and other residential settings. A few hospice programs have their own hospital or clinic facilities. In a home setting, although nurses and other members of the hospice team make visits as needed, the program is designed so that the person who's dying receives much of his or her care from loved ones, who can get advice and support from the hospice team 24 hours a day, seven days a week, whenever they need it.

Services offered

Hospice programs are designed to give access to around-the-clock support to terminally ill people and their families. The hospice team works with you and your loved ones, adjusting the services provided according to your needs and those of your family. Physical, social, spiritual and emotional needs are addressed throughout the last stages of illness and during the period of bereavement that follows a death.

Hospice programs provide comprehensive services, including management of symptoms, emotional support for you and your family, and spiritual care. Emotional (psychosocial) support is intended to help you and your family members deal with issues or problems you or they may be facing, such as depression, anxiety and fear. The intent of spiritual care is to help you maintain hope and address any questions you may have, perhaps about the meaning of your life.

Depending on the individual, hospice services may include:
- Medical services provided by your own doctor or a doctor who's affiliated with the hospice program
- Regular visits by nurses and on-call nursing support
- Chaplain services
- Counseling services
- Housekeeping and cooking services
- Medical equipment and supplies
- Medications to relieve symptoms
- Physical, speech and occupational therapy

A Good Death

As a person faces the prospect of death, he or she is likely to experience a host of feelings, including fear, concern about those left behind and possibly anger. Some people don't understand the concept of a good death. The following true story may help.

Gayle's Story

Gayle was diagnosed with a large breast cancer that had spread beyond the breast at the time of her diagnosis. For the next two and a half years, she was treated with surgery, radiation therapy, chemotherapy and hormone therapy. At times, as part of her treatment, she needed to have catheters placed in the tubes that lead from the kidneys to the bladder (ureters).

Although the chemotherapy was hard on her, she continued to live her life, enjoying time with family and friends until her final moments. Throughout her treatment, she had open discussions with her oncologist regarding the pros and cons of various treatment approaches. She and her family were actively involved in her treatment decisions. Eventually, she reached the point where she was no longer responding to a number of anti-cancer treatments, such as hormone therapy and chemotherapy. She chose to spend her final days at home with her family, receiving hospice care.

Three weeks before her death, on the day she, her family and her doctor concluded that treatments aimed at slowing the cancer's growth were no longer working, Gayle attended a high school football game with her family. One week before her death, one of her sons and his wife invited many close friends and family members to their home for a celebration of life, to allow Gayle and her family and friends to reflect on the many good times they had shared. It was also an opportunity for words of thanks and heartfelt goodbyes.

Several days before her death, with her youngest son's encouragement, Gayle wrote to each of her three sons. Her inspiring words provide an excellent example of making sure that loved ones know what they mean to you at the end of your life. Her children, reading her words at her funeral, called it "a special gift from an incredibly special woman." This is some of what she wrote:

To Our Firstborn — Jeff

We've always loved you best because you were our first miracle — the fulfillment of young love, the promise of our infinity. You sustained us through the hamburger years, the first home — furnished in early poverty — the many monthly payments, trying to make ends meet.

You were new, had unused grandparents and more clothes than a Barbie doll. You were the "original model" for unsure parents trying to work the bugs out. You got the strained lamb, open pins, tiptoe treatment and three-hour naps. We have always expected a great deal from you, and you have not disappointed us. God has blessed us because you've been a fine example to your younger brothers — and we love you for it.

You were the beginning.

To Our Middle Child — Jim

We've always loved you best because you drew the dumb spot in the family, and it made you stronger. You cried less, had more patience, wore faded clothes and never did anything "first." With you, we realized you could kiss a dog or miss a nap and not get sick. You crossed the street before you went to kindergarten, and we didn't get an ulcer about your using a hammer.

You were the child of our busy, ambitious years. Without you, we never could have survived job changes and the house we couldn't afford. You've always endured the pressures of an older brother's achievements and a younger brother's gregariousness. And we've loved you for it.

You were the continuance.

To Our Baby — John

We've always loved you best because endings are generally sad, and you are such a joy. You readily accepted the milk-stained bibs and the secondhand toys, skates and bikes.

You are the one we hold on to so tightly. For, you see, you are the link with the past that gives reason to tomorrow. You quicken our steps, square our shoulders, restore our vision and give us humor that security and maturity can't give us. And we've loved you for it.

You are lucky to have two older brothers who have taught you so much and set fine examples for you. When you are older, even when your children tower over you, you will still be "the baby."

You were the culmination.

In the last week of her life, Gayle told her husband that she needed to plan her funeral. Using the excuse that he was older than she, he said they needed to plan his funeral first. So that day, they planned both of their funerals, first his, then hers.

On the day she died, she called her children and grandchildren to be with her that afternoon. They all said their goodbyes and shared some last moments with her. When her oncologist came to visit her, he found her resting comfortably, her home filled with three generations of her extended family.

Shortly after the oncologist's visit, Gayle's parish priest arrived. With Gayle's family present, the priest asked if she felt safe. He told her she was about to go to a better place and asked if she was ready to die. She replied to both questions with a smile and a nod of affirmation. She died peacefully six hours later.

- Relaxation therapy
- Dietary counseling
- Grief and bereavement counseling

The hospice staff generally provides bereavement services to family members for up to a year after a loved one's death.

Eligibility

You're eligible for hospice services when you stop treatment aimed at curing or controlling your cancer and your doctor indicates that — if your disease follows the expected course — you're expected to live six months or less, a criterion established by Medicare. As long as you continue to meet the criteria, you may continue to qualify for hospice care. This may be longer than six months for some individuals.

Although hospice care is widely acknowledged as being very worthwhile for people nearing the end of their lives, only 20 to 50 percent of people with cancer who are eligible for hospice services receive them. And for individuals who do enroll in hospice, the average time they receive hospice services is just a few days to a few weeks, too little time for them to receive the full benefit of the range of services hospice offers. This is partly because of some people's reluctance to call hospice or because of their family member's inability to accept that a loved one is dying.

In addition, some doctors are reluctant to refer people to hospice, not because they don't see it as worthwhile but because they're hesitant to give up on anti-cancer treatment, or they don't want to tell individuals that they're dying.

Do-not-resuscitate status

The best time to make decisions about emergency care is before you need it. An example is when to decide on do-not-resuscitate (DNR) status. If you stop breathing or if your heart stops beating, do you want doctors to use extreme measures to try to bring you back? Extreme measures include performing cardiopulmonary resuscitation (CPR), shocking your chest to try to restart your heart or putting you on a machine that breathes for you (ventilator).

If you decide that you don't want to be resuscitated, it's best to convey that information to your health care team as soon as you make that decision. Requesting DNR status doesn't mean that you or your doctor will give up on your care, or that you cannot receive care for unrelated or potentially reversible conditions. DNR means that you don't want extreme or heroic measures taken to extend your life, if you were to die.

Attempting resuscitation in people with advanced cancer usually isn't effective at helping them get stronger, live longer or get out of the hospital. Doing so may prolong the dying process and it may cause more pain and suffering. Even if a person is "successfully" resuscitated in the short term and placed on a breathing machine, he or she may not be able to breathe independently again. And the family may then be faced with the decision of when to take the individual off the ventilator.

Doctors are mandated to discuss DNR status with all people who enter a hospital. Otherwise, the subject might not come up unless you were to initiate it.

Some people hesitate to sign a DNR order because they're holding onto the hope that coming back to life will give them another chance at beating their disease. Unfortunately, this is very unlikely with advanced, incurable cancer. They also believe that if a DNR order is in place, they may not receive routine care or they'll be abandoned, both of which are not true.

If you have these concerns, talk with your doctor and your family members about DNR status and what it does and does not mean regarding your care.

Chapter 24:

Life After a Cancer Diagnosis

For Partners

> Note: **This chapter is written specifically for the partners of women with breast cancer.**

When the woman you love learns that she has cancer, it's an intensely emotional time for both of you. It can also be a vulnerable time, bringing out both positive and negative aspects of your personality and relationship.

As the two of you come to grips with the situation and try to get your emotions in sync, your relationship will be tested. You may need to make short-term and long-term adjustments in everything from your daily routines to your sex life. There will be good days, and there will be bad days.

How you both respond to your loved one's cancer diagnosis may be influenced by many factors, such as differences in temperament, family structure, communication styles and cultural expectations. Your past experiences in dealing with crises also may influence your response. You may feel additional pressure because you've been taught that you need to be strong and resilient. You may have grown up in a home where problems weren't openly discussed. You may have had relationship problems before the diagnosis.

Although each cancer situation is unique, many partners experience the same kinds of problems and

Dealing With Your Loved One's Diagnosis	396
Your emotions and feelings	396
Common concerns	396
What to expect from your loved one	397

How You Can Help	398
Learn as much as you can	402
Ways to provide emotional support	402
Ways to provide practical support	403

Talking to Each Other	403
Communication barriers	404
Communication tips	404

Maintaining Sexual Intimacy	405
Barriers to sexual intimacy	405
Creating a healthy sexual relationship	406

Caring for Yourself	407
Finding balance	407
Seeking inner strength	408

Dealing With Incurable Cancer	408
Hospice care	409
Grieving	409

| Resources | 410 |
| Support groups | 410 |

| A Time of Growth | 412 |

day-to-day challenges that you may be facing. You have a special role in your loved one's life during the entire process, from her cancer diagnosis to her treatment to her recovery. This is a time when she can benefit from your support, but at the same time you can't forget about your own needs. This chapter addresses some common concerns of partners and offers encouragement and guidance.

Dealing With Your Loved One's Diagnosis

A diagnosis of cancer can be overwhelming. The first few weeks after a diagnosis often can be the most emotional and difficult time for everyone. Moods can change from moment to moment, and emotions and feelings can be intense and unpredictable as you and your loved one attempt to cope with news that has changed both your lives. Usually, the intensity of emotions is temporary, and over time some of the anxiety lessens. This process varies with different individuals, and the two of you may come to terms with the diagnosis at different times.

Your emotions and feelings

It's understandable that the primary focus of everyone's attention is caring for your loved one, but your feelings and emotions also are important and valid. Even though you aren't the one with cancer, you may experience feelings and emotions similar to hers — helplessness, anger, anxiety, fear. In addition, you may

feel unappreciated if family and friends neglect to ask how you're doing.

Your role and position in your loved one's life is unique because the love and level of commitment you share is different compared with that of other family members or friends. You're the one who's expected to be by her side no matter what. It's normal to be unprepared for and overwhelmed by such an enormous responsibility. Don't be afraid to acknowledge your frustrations and fears so that you can find comfort, or at least learn how to persevere through this difficult time.

Common concerns

Each couple's experience is unique, but certain concerns and feelings may be universal. Three common concerns and challenges of partners of cancer patients are:
• Fearing cancer and its spread
• Knowing how to offer support
• Making adjustments to daily life

Fearing cancer and its spread
More than once, you may have found yourself asking or thinking: "Has the cancer spread?" "Will it continue to spread?" "What's the chance of it coming back?" "How many hours, months or years will she live?" Fear and worry are normal responses.

In addition to the status of the cancer, you may fear seeing your loved one in pain or watching her die. You might even worry about what would happen if you became ill, especially if you feel that everyone is depending on you. You may worry about your own death and then feel guilty for thinking about yourself.

Knowing how to offer support

Many partners worry that they aren't handling the situation correctly or aren't providing enough emotional support, love and understanding. Common questions include "How do I help?" "Am I really being helpful?" "Am I capable of being helpful and supportive?"

One of your greatest frustrations may be learning how to deal with your loved one's emotions, which may be unpredictable and, at times, intense. You may feel helpless and powerless because you desperately want to fix things or at least do what you can to make her feel better, but you don't know how. Or perhaps you've tried to talk with your loved one about her feelings and fears, but it hasn't gone well. You may question if your efforts are hurting the situation instead of helping it. This is a time to take stock of the strengths of your relationship. A diagnosis of cancer doesn't magically change a relationship. But you can build on its strengths even in difficult times.

Making adjustments to daily life

"Who's going to take care of the children?" "Who's going to cook dinner?" "What happens when my sick days and vacation days are used up?" Beyond the emotional turmoil is the day-to-day reality of living with someone who has cancer. And for some cancer patients and their families, there may be no end to the adjustments that need to be made because the situation may keep changing throughout the different stages of cancer.

Many aspects of life are affected in one way or another when a family member receives a diagnosis of cancer. You may need to take on added child care and household responsibilities, as well as become the caregiver for your loved one. For some partners, this may be especially challenging. Like many, you may not feel prepared for your new role as a caregiver. This can cause feelings of helplessness and frustration.

Perhaps you need to spend so much time at the hospital that no time is left for anything else. You might feel guilty for wanting to be free from the situation. If additional treatments are necessary, you may feel even more restricted.

What to expect from your loved one

After your loved one has learned that she has cancer, she may need some time before she's ready to share what she's feeling. She may distance herself from you both physically and emotionally. It's important to let her bring up the subject. If she confides in you, it's probably because she wants to share her concerns and anxieties with you. Let her know that you're available to listen to her when she's ready. There may be times when she prefers sharing her concerns with other women who've had similar experiences. This doesn't mean that your support is less important or less helpful.

Anger, fear, stress, anxiety, loneliness, depression and powerlessness are some of the emotions your loved one may experience. Her feelings may be unpredictable, changing from day to day and even hour to hour. You may be on the receiving end of emotional outbursts or mood swings. Remember, even though the outbursts may be directed at you, she's acting out toward the situation. These are some of the emotions you may see from your loved one:

- **Anger or hostility.** Expressing anger or hostility may help your loved one reduce feelings of stress and tension. It may be her way of asking, "Why me?" Unfortunately, you may have to withstand the worst of her anger. Try not to take it personally.
- **Fear.** Fear is a common response to a diagnosis of cancer. Your loved one may fear death, pain, an inability to work, physical changes, changes in personal relationships and uncertainty about the future. She may worry that she'll become a burden to the family.
- **Stress and anxiety.** Stress and anxiety can cause a wide range of physical symptoms, such as headaches, muscle pains and loss of appetite. Your loved one may experience these.
- **Loneliness.** Many cancer patients and their families may feel isolated and lonely. Friends who don't know how to deal with cancer, or simply can't deal with it, may start distancing themselves by staying away and not calling. Your loved one may be surrounded by caring people but still feel that no one else can understand what she's experiencing.
- **Withdrawal.** Some people need time and space, even from those they love the most. Sometimes withdrawing is the only way to regain some control, if only temporarily. Periods of withdrawal are not uncommon. If your loved one's withdrawal worries you or if your withdrawal from her worries her, talk about it.
- **Depression.** Your loved one may be overwhelmed by feelings of deep sadness and despair. If you notice that she's experiencing a strong sense of helplessness, sadness, grief and a feeling that life is meaningless, these could be signs of clinical depression. It's important that she share these feelings with her doctor.
- **Powerlessness.** Your loved one may feel like she's losing control. She may feel a loss of independence because she has to rely on others for many of her needs. It may be difficult for her to hand over control to you or to accept help from others, especially if she's accustomed to being in charge of certain responsibilities or handling things a certain way. In addition, while your loved one's body is trying to heal, it may not be functioning normally, and she may feel abandoned by her body.

How You Can Help

You're an essential part of your loved one's healing. She needs your support throughout the entire process, from diagnosis to treatment to recovery. On some days, she may need emotional support or someone to talk to. On other days, she may need help with daily tasks, such as going to the grocery store or cooking dinner.

Your long-term commitment to your relationship is especially important because with some cancers, treatment can last for years. Initially, she may have strong support from family and friends, but over time these people may become less involved. Your support and encouragement may be the only constant in your loved one's life.

It's important to try to focus on living as normal a life as possible. Many challenges lie ahead, and you'll probably say things or do things that you'll regret, so patience is important. One of your ongoing challenges may be finding a good balance between giving your loved one added support while, at the same time, allowing her to hold onto as much independence as she can. Encourage your loved one to tell you if your support is overwhelming her.

Communicating With the Team

Although doctors, nurses and other health care providers are a valuable source of information, they may assume that you understand everything they're communicating unless you ask them to explain things. Following are some ways you and your loved one can establish good communication with her doctor and other members of her health care team.

Keep in mind that only if your loved one gives permission can her doctor or other members of her health care team talk with you or other family members about her condition. If she chooses not to grant this permission, you need to honor her desires, even though it may be difficult. She may have her reasons for limiting your communication with her health care team. Talk with her about such things.

Preparing questions before appointments
Ask your loved one if she would like you to help write down questions to ask her doctor.

Taking notes and asking questions during appointments
Ask your loved one if she would like you to accompany her to her doctor's visits. You can help take notes and ask questions she may have forgotten to ask. This will also help you to become more knowledgeable about her situation.

It's important that both of you understand what's happening. Don't be afraid to ask the doctor to explain information you don't understand. Every question is important, and if an answer doesn't make sense to you, ask again. Make sure that you understand the available treatment options and the advantages and disadvantages of each. If your loved one needs time to think about her treatment options, let her doctor know.

Supporting a second opinion
If your loved one wants a second opinion, help her look for another doctor. A second opinion often confirms the options that have already been presented. However, sometimes a second opinion may bring to light a different treatment approach that your loved one may want to consider. Most insurance companies cover the cost of a second opinion, but you may want to check first.

Information Gathering Checklist

Throughout the course of your loved one's illness, the amount of information presented to you can be overwhelming. Keeping track of that information and learning as much as you can about the physical and emotional effects of treatment may help you support her. Here's a checklist to help you gather and organize information.

Care providers
❑ **Primary care doctor:**_____
   Phone number: _____
❑ **Oncologist:** _____
   Phone number: _____
❑ **Surgeon:**_____
   Phone number: _____
❑ **Nurse:**_____
   Phone number: _____
❑ **Pharmacist:** _____
   Phone number: _____
❑ **Social worker:**_____
   Phone number: _____
❑ **Chaplain:** _____
   Phone number: _____
❑ **Other:** _____
   Phone number: _____

Testing for cancer
❑ Type of diagnostic procedure: _____
❑ Purpose of the procedure: _____
❑ Date test results were discussed with us: _____
❑ Name of the person coordinating care:_____
❑ Current hopes and fears: _____
   _____
❑ What will help us cope while we wait? _____
   _____

Surgery
❑ Type of surgery: _____
❑ Date the pathology report was discussed with us: _____

❑ Length of time in hospital: _____

❑ Home-going instructions after discharge from the hospital: _____

_____

❑ Current hopes and fears: _____

_____

❑ What will our family need? _____

Treatment
❑ Type of treatment: _____
❑ Number of treatments: _____
❑ Possible side effects of treatment: _____
❑ Ways to minimize side effects: _____
❑ Current hopes and fears: _____
❑ What can I do for my loved one during this time? _____
❑ Support groups and other resources: _____

_____

After treatment
❑ Next follow-up appointment: _____
❑ Current hopes and fears: _____
❑ Ways to balance the needs of my loved one and family members: _____

_____

❑ Support groups and other resources: _____

Recurrence
❑ Type of treatment: _____
❑ Number of treatments: _____
❑ Ways to minimize side effects: _____
❑ Current hopes and fears: _____
❑ What can I do for my loved one during this time? _____

_____

❑ Support groups and other resources: _____

Adapted from Laurel L. Northouse and Holly Peters-Golden, Cancer and the Family: Strategies to Assist Spouses. *Seminars in Oncology Nursing,* 1993;9(2):74.

Learn as much as you can

Most people are afraid of what they don't know or understand. Knowing the facts about your loved one's cancer can help both of you cope with your worries and fears.

If you know ahead of time what your partner's treatment will involve, you'll be better prepared to cope and to plan for disruptions that may occur in your daily routine.

Gathering information may be a concrete way you and your loved one can regain control of the situation. It may also be an important part of the coping process as the two of you create feelings of confidence by making informed decisions together. You may gain valuable insights from each other. In addition, when visiting with her health care team, the two of you may feel more confident because the information you're hearing will sound familiar to you.

Health information is available in many places, such as community, hospital and medical school libraries, and major cancer research and treatment institutions. Many organizations offer their materials online. See pages 413-416 for a list of reliable and credible sources.

Offer to help your loved one search and sort through information about her cancer. Realize that she may be overwhelmed with the amount of information you find, so let her determine when or if she's ready to read it.

But be careful not to go overboard. Some women and their partners seek out several expert opinions, try to collect all the relevant materials they can, spend countless hours on the Internet, and then try to make appropriate medical decisions themselves. This can cause considerable angst. If you find yourself in this situation, it's important to find a cancer doctor you trust and allow him or her to help you make appropriate medical decisions.

Ways to provide emotional support

You can support your loved one in many ways, but often what's most important is your presence. You're in a unique position to attend to her with your heart, mind and soul. Your loved one needs your support to help her through a very emotional time.

- **Reaffirm your commitment.** Let her know that you intend to support her and stay by her side. She needs to know that you'll continue to love her, especially through the difficult times. It's important to remember to say, "I love you."
- **Spend quality time together.** Schedule time when the two of you can be alone without any distractions. Go on a date. If you're home, shut off the television or radio and let the answering machine answer your calls. Try to set aside at least 30 minutes every day when the two of you can simply talk. If you find that both of you are exhausted at the end of the day, try scheduling time in the morning.
- **Listen attentively.** While your loved one is sharing her frustrations and fears with you, you may not be giving her your full attention. Instead, you may be thinking about what you're going to say when it's your turn to talk. Rather than worrying about coming up with

solutions or providing the right answer, give her your complete attention. You may not feel like you're doing much by just sitting and listening, and it may be difficult to accept what you hear, but your presence and acceptance may be exactly what she needs at the moment.

While being a sounding board for your loved one's fears and frustrations, don't be afraid to express your own fears and frustrations — but within limits, of course. She may not be able to take on the added emotional task of comforting you.

- **Find out what her wishes are.** Ask your loved one to be honest about what she wants and needs from you and others.

Ways to provide practical support

In addition to emotional support, helping out on a day-to-day basis is important. Here are some suggestions:

- **Cook dinner and clean up afterward.** If life is really hectic, now and then buy prepared foods, dine out or order food to be delivered.
- **Drive her to doctor visits.** Doctor appointments can be nerve-racking, and if she's receiving treatment, such as chemotherapy or radiation therapy, she may not feel well afterward.
- **Help keep the house in order.** If you can afford it, consider hiring a housekeeper. Or, perhaps, family members or friends can help you keep the house in order.
- **Screen telephone calls and visitors.** Family and friends may have good intentions when they call or visit, but at times your loved one may not be feeling well and may not be up to seeing visitors or talking on the phone. Try to convey this to visitors in a caring way so as not to discourage them from visiting or calling in the future. You may suggest that they send a card, or you may suggest a better time to call or visit.
- **Give your loved one peace and quiet.** Your loved one may need some time alone to reflect, relax and emotionally recharge. Encourage her to do so.
- **Help out with the children.** If you previously weren't involved in packing lunches or chauffeuring the kids around, offer to help out now. It may take time for the children to adjust to relying less on mom, but it can be an opportunity for you to spend more quality time with your children. In addition, it may be time for your children to be a little more independent. Have them help with chores, too.
- **Help your loved one resume her regular activities.** Don't put your lives on hold. Continue to enjoy spending time with friends and family and, as much as possible, doing other things you've always liked to do, such as eating out or going to the movies. Your loved one may have less energy, so try to follow her cue.

Talking to Each Other

Communication is important in any relationship, but even more so during times of stress and uncertainty. Two things that can hinder communication are wrong assumptions and poor communication skills. Open and honest communication is important. In your discussions, it's OK to use the word *cancer*.

Don't Be Afraid to Seek Professional Help

If the cancer experience is causing problems in your relationship, it may be because you're experiencing a breakdown in communication. A trained professional may be able to help you resolve some misunderstandings and suggest ways that you can strengthen your relationship. You might consider seeking professional counseling, especially in the following circumstances:

- If you start distancing yourself from your loved one because you're uncomfortable talking about cancer
- If your discussions end up as arguments
- If you and your loved one are having difficulty maintaining sexual intimacy

Communication barriers

A common problem among couples is making assumptions. One person simply assumes the other knows his or her needs without actually discussing the problem or situation. Because cancer is likely a new experience for both of you, be careful to not make assumptions. You won't truly know what the other needs unless you talk about it.

If you or your loved one aren't the type to talk about difficult issues, the two of you may have trouble doing so now. A diagnosis of cancer may not instantly change the way the two of you communicate, but it's an opportunity to make an improvement in your relationship. Just because you haven't been entirely open with each other in the past doesn't mean that you can't start now. Big changes may not occur, but small steps are possible.

Communication tips

As your loved one attempts to open up to you — to share her feelings, worries, fears and hopes — keep these points in mind:

- **Respect her feelings.** Your loved one may want to talk about her cancer diagnosis one day and be silent about it the next. If she doesn't bring up the topic, you may be afraid to do so. The best thing to do is simply ask your loved one if she has anything she wants to talk about, and then respect her wishes.
- **Be a good listener.** If your loved one wants to talk, be attentive. Listen to what is said and how it's said. And listen without becoming defensive.
- **Be patient.** Be prepared for periods of silence and crying. Silence can be comforting because it allows your loved one time to reflect. Allow her to cry or sigh because these behaviors help release tension and anxiety.
- **Speak from your heart.** If your loved one asks you questions that you don't know how to respond to, be honest and say that you don't have an answer but that you'll try to find one. A simple touch, hug or smile is a sign of affection that shows you care.
- **Ask questions.** Your loved one may want you to simply ask questions or listen. Try asking, "What are you feeling?"

not just "How are you feeling?" It may be a refreshing break to change topics. Reminisce about a happy childhood memory or tell a joke. Laughter is great medicine.

• **Be prepared.** When your loved one is ready, don't be afraid to discuss important decisions regarding her treatment.

Maintaining Sexual Intimacy

Sexual intimacy is an important aspect of many relationships. It can be shared and expressed on many levels — physically, spiritually, psychologically and emotionally. A breast cancer diagnosis doesn't need to put an end to sexual intimacy, but you may need to make some adjustments.

Sexual drive, sexual function and sexual acts are different aspects of sexuality. Sexual drive (libido) is the natural desire for sexual activity. The desire can be an emotional or physical need. Sexual function is how your body responds to sexual stimulation, such as erection, vaginal lubrication or orgasm. Sexual activity is the action taken to satisfy the sex drive, such as kissing, touching, sexual stimulation or intercourse.

Difficulties with sexual issues may arise during and after cancer treatment. If this is an area with which you and your loved one are struggling, talk about it. Communication is one of the best ways to improve intimacy.

Although cancer treatment often affects sexual intimacy between partners in one way or another, often patients

and doctors don't discuss this aspect of treatment. It may be helpful to discuss potential problems with the doctor ahead of time so that you're better prepared to deal with them. Or if you're currently having problems, your loved one's doctor or a member of the health care team may offer some practical tips to overcome the barriers. You may also consider counseling from a trained specialist.

Barriers to sexual intimacy

To help the two of you deal with and overcome sexual barriers, it's important that you know what they are. The type of problems your loved one may experience will depend on the type of cancer she has and the treatment she's receiving. Sexual problems that can result include:

Lack of sexual desire
Side effects of treatments such as chemotherapy or radiation therapy may make your loved one tired, nauseated, anxious or depressed. All of these things lessen sexual desire. She may also experience less sexual desire due to stress.

Painful intercourse
Surgery, radiation therapy or other types of treatment that affect a woman's hormones may affect the vagina's shape and moistness. If her vagina stays tight or dry during intercourse, it becomes painful. Dryness may also result from difficulty becoming aroused.

Difficulty achieving orgasm
Your loved one may have difficulty achieving orgasm during this time. Given everything that she's going through physically

and emotionally, this is understandable. She may be anxious, distracted or fatigued from her diagnosis and treatment.

Menopausal symptoms

Menopause is a natural phase of life for women. Common symptoms include hot flashes, increased urinary tract and vaginal infections, vaginal dryness, and some loss of shape and flexibility of the vagina. When these changes are caused by surgical removal of the ovaries, the symptoms are often abrupt and can be very uncomfortable. Chemotherapy also can cause a fairly abrupt slowing of ovarian function.

Change in body image

Cancer treatments may result in the loss of hair, the loss of one or both breasts, or scarring — changes that affect your loved one's body image. If she has had one or both breasts removed, it can be a devastating experience for her. She may feel less attractive and less feminine, and she may worry that she'll no longer be sexually appealing to you.

Creating a healthy sexual relationship

The two of you will need to work together to overcome any barriers that may affect sexual intimacy. As with other aspects of your relationship, it may take some time and effort developing or maintaining your sexual relationship. Here are ways that may help you stay sexually healthy during and after cancer treatment:

Take a break

It may take some of the pressure and anxiety away if the two of you agree to abstain from sexual activity for a period of time. You can use this time to focus on building more emotional closeness and intimacy through hugging and snuggling.

Make a date

Set aside one night for an hour or two of intimate time and get reacquainted. This can be a time to strengthen your relationship. Even though the moment may not be spontaneous, this time together can be just as exciting.

Talk with her

You may be reluctant to initiate sexual activity because you're afraid or worried that your loved one may experience discomfort or pain. But she may view your reluctance as a sign that you're no longer attracted to her. The best approach simply is to ask her if she's ready for sexual intimacy and then follow her lead.

Acknowledge the loss

If a mastectomy or lumpectomy has been performed, it may help if you looked at the scar together. It's important that both of you are able to acknowledge the loss or alteration of a breast as soon as possible so that the grieving and healing process can begin. Acknowledge and discuss what has changed.

Many women who lose a breast miss the pleasure they felt from being stroked in that area during sex. During sexual activity, you might try stroking your partner's whole body. She may find new places to replace the pleasure she used to feel.

Let her be the guide

Because your loved one's body may be sore in some spots, let her guide your

QUESTION & ANSWER

Q: Do I need to worry when my partner and I are sexually intimate that I'll get her cancer?

A: One person's cancer cannot survive in another person's body. Thus, cancer is *not* contagious, and it can't be spread by kissing, hugging or having sexual intercourse.

touch. Ask her what areas of her body she would like you to kiss or touch. Most cancer treatments won't affect her ability to feel pleasure from touch or to reach orgasm. However, you may need to change the manner in which you give her pleasure or help her achieve orgasm.

Many couples find it helpful to take it slow once they're ready to resume sexual activity. You might begin simply with allover body touching. If you both feel relaxed during the first touching session, the next time include some touching of the genitals.

Experiment with different positions

If sexual activity is painful for your loved one, it won't allow her to reach orgasm. You might need to try different intercourse positions or different types of genital touching. If she has pain or stiffness in her arms and shoulders, especially if her surgery involved lymph node removal in an armpit, avoid positions that put weight on her shoulders and arms.

Caring for Yourself

When a loved one is diagnosed with cancer, it's easy to focus solely on that person's desires and needs and to ignore your own. Over time, this approach can be emotionally draining, making you moody and tired.

Balancing work, family needs and social life may have been a challenge before your loved one was diagnosed with cancer, so you may be concerned about how you'll keep everything in order with your added responsibilities. Perhaps you already feel overwhelmed and exhausted.

It's important that you take care of your personal needs in addition to your loved one's. Otherwise, you'll build resentment toward her — a situation that will be unhealthy for both of you. To be able to help your loved one, you need your emotional, mental and physical strength.

Be realistic about what you can and can't do. And accept that you'll probably make some mistakes, but learn from them and move on.

Finding balance

While caring for your loved one, don't forget to care for your own needs:
• **Live your life.** Don't feel guilty if you look forward to going to work because it gives you a break from the pressure and stress at home. Continue to spend time doing the things you enjoy, such as going to the gym or spending a night out with friends.

- **Take a break.** Mental and physical breaks are more important now than ever. For example, you might ask a family member or friend to stay with your loved one so that you can go on a weekend golfing or fishing trip with friends.
- **Ask for help.** You probably know many people who are willing to assist with household tasks, run errands or allow you some time away. You just need to ask. Let them know specifically what they can do. If someone offers to help, take them up on the offer. There's nothing wrong with admitting that you need help.
- **Take care of your body.** Crazy schedules, added responsibilities and stress can lead to some unhealthy habits — not eating right, not exercising, not getting enough rest or sleep. It's important that you pay attention to your physical needs because you need all the strength you've got.
- **Talk with a friend or counselor.** You may find it helpful to share your feelings with a friend or counselor. It's important to share any resentment you may be feeling. A formal support group is another place to vent your feelings and to find others who can relate to your experience.

Seeking inner strength

Serious illness or tragic events often remind us of our mortality and may cause us to think about the purpose and meaning of life and to become more aware of our spiritual self. Spirituality is the pursuit of the sacred, the search for meaning and purpose in life. Spirituality involves connecting with something larger than ourselves — beyond what we can see, hear, smell and touch.

Throughout the cancer experience, you and your loved one may find strength and comfort in your spiritual beliefs, whatever they may be. Even if your spiritual paths are different, you need to respect each other's beliefs. The strength you gain as individuals contributes to strengthening your relationship as a couple.

You may be encouraged by reading religious materials, praying or meditating. Another source of spiritual strength may be talking with spiritual advisers, who are often trained in and knowledgeable about counseling patients and families dealing with serious illness.

Dealing With Incurable Cancer

If your loved one has an incurable cancer and is nearing the end of her life, you're facing many additional worries and concerns. The knowledge that death may be nearing is extremely frightening. And you may be worried about whether you can cope, whether you can make it through a long and difficult process.

It's also a profound time for your loved one. She needs you close by, listening to her concerns and offering support with a smile or gentle touch. She may withdraw from life as she enters the dying process, but she still needs to know that you're present and available if she needs you.

If you don't know what to do, just simply touch her — hold her hand or rub

Keeping a Journal

Some people have difficulty expressing their feelings to others, and they tend to keep everything bottled up inside. If you happen to be such a person, you may find it therapeutic to write your thoughts in a journal.

A journal is a way to release your innermost thoughts, observations and experiences. You can be as honest as you want to be about your fears and frustrations. It's also a place where you can write about happy moments and your hopes for the future. You don't need a special notebook or to follow any special format. However, for future reference, it may be helpful to write down dates, times, your feelings at the time and other details.

You can share your writings with others if you like, but you don't have to do so. The main purpose of a journal is to release what you're feeling inside.

her back — and talk. If she feels up to it, encourage her to talk about her life — a life review. These can be the times when marvelous stories are told. Sometimes, when adult children are present, they're amazed to find out that they've never heard these stories.

Hospice care

Don't feel guilty if you can't do it alone. No one can. This is a time when you and your loved one will likely want to consider hospice care. Hospice organizations are meant to provide expert and compassionate care for people near the end of life.

Hospice care allows your partner to spend her last weeks or months in the comfortable surroundings of your home or in a homelike setting, while under the care of a team of professional and volunteer caregivers.

Oftentimes, your loved one's doctor coordinates the team, and a nurse handles the details of daily care. Chaplains and social workers can offer counseling and

support. Trained volunteers are available to assist with daily tasks, such as light housekeeping and cooking meals, and they offer companionship. For more information on hospice care, see Chapter 23.

Grieving

When people are keeping a vigil for a loved one who is dying, or after a loved one has died, they often say it feels like a bad dream. You may feel the same way. Feelings of grief, loss and sadness come in waves. Emotions can be overwhelming, making even simple tasks seem difficult for a time.

This is all normal. It doesn't mean you're going to be unable to function the rest of your life. It means that right now, most of what you can do is grieve. It's all part of being human and loving. Grief is a natural response to loving and feeling loss.

If you're concerned that you have spent too much time grieving and are unable to function or if others have expressed concern about you, consider seeing a counselor. Sometimes a loss is more than a person can handle, and depression occurs.

The line between profound grief and depression is blurry. But if you're still having trouble sleeping and concentrating months after your loved one's death, make an appointment to see a counselor.

Resources

You and your loved one don't have to face cancer alone. In addition to family and friends, a network of resources is available. Begin your search by contacting organizations that offer programs to assist cancer patients and their families or that can recommend other organizations.

Support groups

Some partners of women with cancer find support groups to be helpful. Although you may be reluctant to share your feelings with strangers, being in a support group has these advantages:

- You may find it beneficial to connect with others experiencing the same or similar cancer issues.
- You may learn something new or be encouraged by someone else's story.
- You may learn how other partners have adapted to changes and have coped.
- It may be a relief just to know that you're not alone.

As your loved one may seek the camaraderie of other women with cancer, you too may find it beneficial to connect with partners in a similar situation.

You can begin your search by contacting various cancer organizations. Many types of cancer support groups exist. They're designed to meet the different needs of individuals with cancer and their loved ones. It may take you some time to find the group that meets your needs and interests.

When Your Loved One Is in Denial

Denial can be an important coping mechanism. Some individuals deny that they're facing death because reality is too frightening. Denial is a form of natural protection that allows a person to let reality in bit by bit. It allows a person to continue living while he or she contemplates death.

Your loved one may be in denial for a variety of reasons: She doesn't want to say goodbye. She may be afraid of the pain that might be ahead. She may be afraid of losing her bodily functions. She doesn't want to lose control over her life. She may be afraid of becoming a burden to others.

One of the ways you can support her if she's in denial is to ask her to talk about her fears. Or you might encourage your loved one to visit with a member of her health care team. Sometimes, it's easier for a dying person to share what she is afraid of with someone other than a family member.

QUESTION & ANSWER

Q: Is it wrong to tell a loved one that it's OK to let go?

A: Sometimes, it appears as though a dying person is having difficulty letting go. Perhaps the experience isn't evolving as you thought it would. Perhaps it's taking longer than you expected. People die in their own time. Whether someone really holds on until the last family member is there, for example, medical experts have no way of proving, even if it seems that way. If you think your loved one is holding on for your sake, it's OK to tell her that you'll be all right and that she can let go.

Types

Not all support groups are the same. Following are several types of support groups for partners.

Peer support groups

Peer support groups make up the majority of support groups. Members of peer support groups help each other out by sharing similar experiences. Individuals leading the meetings may or may not have professional training.

Educational intervention groups

Educational intervention groups meet to learn about and discuss a specific topic related to cancer. The meetings often begin with a formal presentation, given by an expert. Some women with cancer and their partners find it empowering to learn more about cancer and its treatment.

Coping skill intervention groups

In this type of support group, participants learn concrete coping skills. During one class, participants might learn about relaxation techniques to help relieve stress. Another class might provide tips on mental health exercises to help keep a positive mental perspective. Coping skill intervention groups are usually led by mental health professionals with expertise leading these types of interventions.

Therapy groups

Therapy groups are led by mental health professionals trained in group therapy. These types of support groups usually focus on specific personal issues. Members are asked to share personal stories, as well as respond to others in the group. Each member is challenged to take action concerning a particular issue with which he or she needs help.

Online support groups

Online support groups allow members to communicate with others on the Internet in chat rooms and on message boards. If you participate in an online support group, be aware that chat rooms are not always reliable sources of health information.

Finding the right group

If you're searching for a support group, it may be helpful to think about what type of group would best meet your needs. Ask yourself the following questions:

Who's in the group?

Most support groups have two types of membership: open and closed. Open membership doesn't require the same level of commitment as closed membership. With open membership, you're generally not required to sign up ahead of time nor are you expected to attend all meetings. Closed membership usually requires preregistration.

Who's leading the group?

Meetings may be led by health professionals or group members, such as a partner of a person with cancer. Health professionals often are licensed and have some skill in leading groups. Although a partner may be able to empathize and share personal experiences, the discussion may not be as productive unless the facilitator has some leadership skills.

What's the format?

Some groups have a more structured program with different topics of discussion each week. Other groups have open discussions around topics members bring up.

A Time of Growth

Partners do have vital roles in the lives of women with cancer. While your experiences can be very stressful and difficult at times, they also can be rewarding. A cancer diagnosis can lead to positive growth in your relationship, as the two of you find strength in each other and as you re-explore your love for each other.

Additional Resources

This book is devoted to providing the answers you need to a wide range of health and medical questions, but no single volume can address all of the issues that may interest you and other readers. For more information about breast cancer and coping with cancer treatment, contact these organizations. Telephone numbers and Web addresses are subject to change.

Caregiving and Hospice

Family Caregiver Alliance
www.caregiver.org
800-445-8106

National Family Caregivers Association: Caregiving Resources
www.nfcacares.org/caregiving_resources
800-896-3650

National Hospice and Palliative Care Organization
www.nhpco.org
800-658-8898

Clinical Trial Information

Center Watch
www.centerwatch.com
866-219-3440

Coalition of Cancer Cooperative Groups
www.cancertrialshelp.org
877-227-8451

EmergingMed
www.emergingmed.com
877-601-8601

Mayo Clinic: Clinical Trials
clinicaltrials.mayo.edu

National Cancer Institute: Clinical Trials
www.cancer.gov/clinicaltrials
800-4-CANCER (800-422-6237)

Complementary and Alternative Medicine

American Music Therapy Association
www.musictherapy.org
301-589-3300

ConsumerLab.com
www.consumerlab.com

Food and Drug Administration: MedWatch
www.fda.gov/medwatch
888-INFO-FDA (888-463-6332)

Mayo Clinic: Complementary and Integrative Medicine Program
www.mayoclinic.org/general-internal-medicine-rst/cimc.html

MD Anderson Cancer Center: Complementary/Integrative Medicine Education Resources
www.mdanderson.org/departments/cimer

Memorial Sloan-Kettering Cancer Center: About Herbs, Botanicals & Other Products
www.mskcc.org/mskcc/html/11570.cfm

National Center for Complementary and Alternative Medicine
www.nccam.nih.gov
888-644-6226

Office of Dietary Supplements, National Institutes of Health
ods.od.nih.gov
301-435-2920

Society for Integrative Oncology
www.integrativeonc.org

Coping

Cancer Hope Network
www.cancerhopenetwork.org
800-552-4366

FORCE: Facing Our Risk of Cancer Empowered
www.facingourrisk.org
866-288-RISK (866-288-7475)

Español (Spanish)
Resources for Cancer Information

American Cancer Society: Informacíon de referencia sobre el cáncer
www.cancer.org/Espanol/index
800-227-2345

Cancer Care: En Espanol
www.cancercare.org/espanol
800-813-HOPE (800-813-4673)

Instituto Nacional del Cáncer
cancer.gov/espanol
800-4-CANCER (800-422-6237)

MedlinePlus: Institutos Nacionales de la Salud
www.salud.nih.gov

Y-ME Apoyo Contra el Cáncer de Mama
www.y-me.org/es
800-221-2141

Financial

Cancer Care
www.cancercare.org
800-813-HOPE (800-813-4673)

Corporate Angel Network
www.corpangelnetwork.org
866-328-1313

National Association of Hospital Hospitality Houses
www.nahhh.org
800-542-9730

National Patient Travel Center
www.patienttravel.org
800-296-1217

Pharmaceutical Research and Manufacturers of America
www.phrma.org/issues/access-affordability
202-835-3400

General Cancer Information

American Cancer Society
www.cancer.org
800-ACS-2345 (800-227-2345)

American Society of Plastic Surgeons
www.plasticsurgery.org
847-228-9900

Association of Cancer Online Resources (ACOR)
www2.acor.org
212-226-5525

Cancer Education
www.cancereducation.com

Cancer.Net (American Society of Clinical Oncology)
www.cancer.net

Centers for Disease Control and Prevention
www.cdc.gov/cancer
800-CDC-INFO (800-232-4636)

Mayo Clinic Cancer Center
cancercenter.mayo.edu

Mayo Clinic: Cancer Education
www.mayoclinic.org/cancer-education

Mayo Clinic: Health Information
www.mayoclinic.com

National Cancer Institute: Cancer Information Service
cancer.gov
800-4-CANCER (800-422-6237)

Research

American Institute for Cancer Research
www.aicr.org
800-843-8114

American Society of Clinical Oncology
www.asco.org
571-483-1300

Cancerpage: Cancer Information and Community
www.cancerpage.com

PubMed
www.ncbi.nlm.nih.gov/entrez/query.fcgi

MedlinePlus
www.nlm.nih.gov/medlineplus

Myriad Genetics
www.myriad.com
800-469-7423

National Library of Medicine
www.nlm.nih.gov
888-FIND-NLM (888-346-3656)

Specific Cancers

Breastcancer.org
www.breastcancer.org

Foundation For Women's Cancer
www.foundationforwomenscancer.org
800-444-4441

National Ovarian Cancer Coalition
www.ovarian.org
888-OVARIAN (888-682-7426)

Ovarian Cancer National Alliance
www.ovariancancer.org
866-399-6262

Susan G. Komen for the Cure
ww5.komen.org
800-GO-KOMEN (800-485-6636)

Women's Cancer Network
www.wcn.org
312-578-1439

Y-ME National Breast Cancer Organization
www.y-me.org
800-221-2141

Survivorship

American Cancer Society: Cancer Survivors Network
csn.cancer.org

Cancervive
www.cancervive.org

LiveStrong Lance Armstrong Foundation
www.livestrong.org
855-220-7777

Living Beyond Breast Cancer
www.lbbc.org
610-645-4567

Mayo Clinic: Living With Cancer Blog
www.mayoclinic.com/livingwithcancer/

National Coalition for Cancer Survivorship
www.canceradvocacy.org
877-NCCS-YES (877-622-7937)

Treatment

American Medical Association
www.ama-assn.org
800-621-8335

MyOncofertility
www.myoncofertility.org
866-708-FERT (800-708-3378)

RadiologyInfo
www.radiologyinfo.org

Resolve: The National Infertility Association
www.resolve.org
703-556-7172

Glossary

A

abdominal hysterectomy. An operation to remove the uterus that's performed by way of an incision in the abdomen.

absolute risk. The actual numeric chance of developing a condition, such as cancer, during a specified time.

adenocarcinoma. Cancer that starts in glandular tissue or cancer that forms glandular-like structures.

adjuvant therapy. Additional treatment that's given to a person with no visible evidence of any remaining (residual) cancer after completion of the first (primary) treatment.

advanced (metastatic) cancer. Cancer that has spread to distant parts of the body, such as the bones, lungs or liver.

angiogenesis. Development of new blood vessels, allowing cells to receive nutrients.

antibody. An immune system protein whose function it is to bind to and eliminate a foreign substance (antigen).

anti-cancer treatment. Therapy that focuses on shrinking and killing cancer cells.

anti-emetic. A medication given to prevent or lessen nausea and vomiting.

antigens. Foreign substances that elicit an immune system response.

antioxidants. Substances that protect the body's cells from the damaging effects of free radicals, highly reactive and potentially toxic oxygen molecules.

areola. The area of dark skin around a nipple.

aromatase inhibitors. Breast cancer medications that block the production of estrogen.

ascites. Accumulation of fluid in the abdomen.

axillary node dissection. Surgical removal of lymph nodes under the arm in an attempt to remove cancer cells that may have spread from a tumor in the adjacent breast.

axillary nodes. Lymph nodes located under the arm (in the axilla).

B

benign. Not cancerous.

benign tumor. A growth that doesn't invade surrounding tissue or spread to distant parts of the body.

bilateral. Affecting both sides. Bilateral breast cancer is breast cancer that occurs in both breasts at the same time. Bilateral oophorectomy is the removal of both ovaries.

biologic therapies. Nonchemotherapy approaches to treat cancer, such as immunotherapy and growth factor blockers. They target tumor cells through biologic pathways.

biopsy. Removal of a small sample of tissue for analysis in a pathology laboratory.

bone scan. A test to look for bone damage, possibly caused by spread of cancer to bone.

brachytherapy. *See* internal radiation (brachytherapy).

BRCA1 and BRCA2 genes. Genes that help govern a cell's response to DNA damage. When altered, they result in a marked predisposition to breast and ovarian cancers.

breast reconstruction. A surgical procedure designed to restore a relatively natural-shaped breast mound after breast tissue removal.

breast self-examination (BSE). Examination of your own breasts for lumps or changes.

C

calcifications. Calcium deposits in body tissues, including the breast. Depending on their size and clustering pattern, they may signal a benign or malignant process.

cancer. Growth of an abnormal population of cells that have acquired aggressive properties, including the ability to spread to new tissues in the body.

CA 125 blood test. A blood tumor marker test that measures the level of CA 125 in blood. CA 125 is a protein that's produced by most ovarian cancers.

carcinogen. A cancer-causing agent.

carcinoma. Cancer that originates in epithelial tissue, which covers or lines an organ or body structure.

carcinoma *in situ*. Cancer cells that are confined to the layer of cells in which they started to develop. Also known as noninvasive cancer.

cell proliferation. Cell multiplication by way of cell division.

cervix. The lower, neck-like portion of the uterus, which extends into the upper portion of the vagina.

chemoprevention. Use of medication to reduce the risk of cancer.

chemotherapy. Medications that can kill cancer cells.

chromosome. One of 46 (23 pairs) rod-shaped structures in the nucleus of human cells that carry genetic instructions for each cell.

clinical breast examination (CBE). Examination of the breasts for lumps or changes by a health care professional.

clinical trial. A research study in humans that tests new approaches for diagnosis, treatment or prevention of a condition, or for relief of symptoms.

complementary therapies. Treatments used in addition to mainstream medicine.

complete blood count (CBC). A test to count levels of white and red blood cells and platelets.

complete remission. After treatment, disappearance of all evidence of cancer by physical examination and medical tests.

computer-aided detection (CAD). A computer technique that gives radiologists an additional tool to help them detect questionable areas on a standard mammogram.

computerized tomography (CT) scan. An X-ray technique that produces more detailed images of the internal organs than do older X-ray studies.

contralateral. Referring to the opposite side of the body.

contralateral prophylactic mastectomy. A means of lowering the risk of a new breast cancer by removing the unaffected breast.

core needle biopsy. A type of biopsy in which a needle is used to withdraw a small core of tissue from a mass. A smaller needle is used for fine-needle aspiration.

corpus. The upper, larger portion of the uterus.

cyst. A fluid-filled sac that's benign.

cytokines. Immune system proteins, some of which either attack and kill cancerous cells directly or stimulate the body's immune system cells to help attack a cancer.

D

debulking (cytoreduction). Surgical removal of as much cancer as possible.

deoxyribonucleic acid (DNA). The chemical code of genes found in the nucleus of cells that carries hereditary information.

diagnostic mammogram. A breast X-ray used to investigate breast changes, evaluate abnormal findings on a screening mammogram or evaluate breasts with implants.

dilation and curettage (D&C). Opening (dilating) the cervix and scraping the lining of the uterus (endometrium) with an instrument called a curet.

disease-free interval. The time extending from the initial diagnosis of a cancer to the time when a recurrence becomes apparent.

distant cancer. Cancer that has spread from its original site to other parts of the body. Also called metastasis.

dosimetrist. An individual who calculates and measures radiation dosage and delivery.

doubling time. The time it takes for a tumor to become twice its size.

ductal carcinoma. Cancer that begins in the ductal cells of the breast.

ductal carcinoma *in situ* (DCIS). A noninvasive breast cancer in which the abnormal cells haven't spread through duct walls into the connective or fatty tissue of the breast.

ductal cells. Cells that line the milk ducts in the breast.

ductal lavage. Injecting saline into a breast duct through the nipple openings and then withdrawing the solution for analysis.

ductoscopy. Use of a very slender catheter with a microscopic video camera at its tip that's inserted into openings in the nipple of the breast to visualize the lining of the ducts of the breast and look for cellular changes.

ducts. Thin tubes within the breast that connect the milk-forming bulbs, lobules and lobes to the nipple.

dysplasia. A precancerous process in which normal cells begin to change in size, shape or structure.

E

endometrial hyperplasia. An increased number of cells in the lining of the uterus.

endometrium. The thick, blood-rich inner lining of the body (corpus) of the uterus.

epithelial cells. Cells that line or cover most organs.

epithelial hyperplasia. An overgrowth of epithelial cells.

epithelial ovarian cancer. Cancer that develops in the epithelial covering of the ovary, the most common type of ovarian cancer.

epithelium. The thin layer of cells that lines the outside and inside of most organs.

estrogen. A primary female hormone. It stimulates the growth of cancer cells in hormone receptor positive tumors.

estrogen receptor. A protein found in certain cells within certain tissues, such as breast and uterine tissues, to which estrogen binds.

excisional biopsy. Surgical removal of a mass.

external beam radiation. A form of radiation therapy in which doses of radiation from a large X-ray machine located outside the body are aimed at the tumor area.

external risk factors. Outside influences on the body, including lifestyle and environmental factors. Some can contribute to cancer development.

F

fallopian tubes. The passageways for eggs to travel from the ovaries to the uterus.

fibroadenoma. A solid, benign tumor that often occurs in the breasts of women during their reproductive years.

fibrocystic breasts. The presence of benign fibrous tissue in the breasts, with or without fluid-filled sacs (cysts).

fine-needle aspiration biopsy. A type of biopsy that uses a very fine needle and syringe to collect a sample of cells from a mass.

flap surgery. Reconstructive surgery in which a section of tissue taken from one part of the body, such as the abdominal wall, is used to fashion a new breast mound.

free radicals. Highly reactive and potentially toxic oxygen molecules within cells that are created as a byproduct of normal metabolism.

frozen section. A tissue sample that's quickly frozen, sliced and analyzed under a microscope so that a surgeon can receive information on the sample within minutes.

G

Gail model. A statistical tool that allows doctors to estimate the likelihood that a woman with certain risk factors will develop invasive breast cancer in the next five years and also during her lifetime.

gene. A defined segment of DNA within a chromosome. Genes are the blueprints for how the cells of the body function.

gene therapy. The process of supplying abnormal cells with healthy copies of missing or defective genes in an effort to treat, cure or possibly prevent disease.

genetic marker. An identifiable substance associated with a normal or abnormal gene.

genetics. The study of genes and the diseases caused by gene abnormalities.

genetic testing. Testing to determine whether an individual carries a specific gene mutation that puts her or him at increased risk of a certain condition.

genomics. The study of the human genome, the complete set of approximately 25,000 genes in a human being.

germ cells. Cells in an ovary or testicle that develop into eggs and sperm, respectively.

Gn-RH analogs. Drugs resembling hormones that control production of the hormones estrogen and progesterone. Gn-RH stands for gonadotropin-releasing hormone.

grade. A measure of how much cancer cells differ from normal cells when viewed under a microscope. The grade often reflects the aggressiveness of the cancer.

H

hereditary cancer. Cancer caused by mutations in a gene, which can be passed on to a child from a parent.

HER2. HER2 is an abbreviation for human epidermal growth factor receptor 2, a protein that stimulates cell growth and is overproduced in about 20 to 25 percent of breast cancers and some other cancers.

histology. The study of the microscopic appearance of tissue.

hormone receptor. A cell protein that can bind to its specific hormone or to hormone-look-alike drugs.

hormone therapy. Treatment of cancer by removing, blocking or adding hormones in an attempt to inhibit cancer growth.

hospice care. A program designed to provide palliative care to people with terminal illness and supportive services to their families and significant others.

hyperplasia. Increased cell growth.

hysterectomy. Surgical removal of the uterus.

I

immunotherapy. Using various means to stimulate a person's own immune system to kill cancer cells.

implant, breast. A breast-shaped device placed under the skin of the chest wall and held in place by the chest muscles. It's used for cosmetic surgery or breast reconstruction.

incidence. The number of new cases of a disease within a defined time frame.

inflammatory breast cancer. Cancer that's associated with redness, warmth and swelling of the skin of the breast.

internal radiation (brachytherapy). A form of radiation therapy in which radioactive substances are placed in the tumor or near where the cancer was removed.

internal risk factors. Influences within the body that may increase the likelihood of disease, including hormonal factors, inherited genetic mutations and immune conditions.

interstitial radiation. A type of internal radiation in which radioactive material is sealed in a container and placed into or near the cancer, but not in a body cavity.

intracavitary radiation. A type of internal radiation in which the radioactive material is placed in a body cavity, such as within the uterus.

intraductal hyperplasia. A condition in which too many cells line the wall of a milk duct in the breast.

intraductal hyperplasia with atypia. A form of intraductal hyperplasia in which the cells begin to take on an abnormal appearance.

intraoperative radiation therapy (IORT). Radiation treatment during surgery in which the radiation is aimed directly toward the site intended to receive the treatment.

invasive cancer. Cancer that has spread from its cell or cells of origin into adjacent connective tissue.

ipsilateral. Referring to the same side of the body.

L

laparoscopy. Use of lighted instruments and small cutting tools that are inserted through small incisions in the abdomen and pelvis to gather cell samples or perform surgery.

laparotomy. Surgery that involves opening up the abdominal cavity by way of an abdominal incision.

lifetime cancer risk. The chance that an individual will develop cancer during his or her lifetime.

lobes. Fifteen to 20 sections of the breast made up of milk-forming lobules.

lobular carcinoma. Cancer that originates in the lobules of the breast.

lobular carcinoma *in situ* (LCIS). A condition in which lobular cells of the breast are abnormal, but the abnormal cells are confined within the breast lobules.

lobules. Tiny milk-forming structures within the breast.

locally advanced breast cancer. Breast cancers with one or more of these features: larger than 5 centimeters, extensive involvement of the regional lymph nodes, or spread to breast skin or the chest wall.

local recurrence. Regrowth of cancer cells at or near the site of the original tumor.

local-regional therapy. Treatment, including surgery and radiation therapy, that's targeted directly at the tumor and nearby tissue.

lumpectomy. Removal of the portion of a breast that appears to contain cancer cells, but not the whole breast. Also known as breast-conserving surgery.

lymphadenectomy. Surgical removal of lymph nodes from a specific location.

lymphedema. Accumulation of fluid in an arm or leg from disruption of lymph vessels.

lymph node. A collection of lymphatic tissue found in many parts of the body.

lymphoma. A tumor that develops in lymphatic tissue.

lymph vessels. Vessels that carry lymph, a clear fluid that contains immune system cells and that drains waste products from tissues.

M

magnetic resonance imaging (MRI). An imaging technique that uses a magnetic field and radio waves to create a detailed, three-dimensional (3-D) representation of the body.

malignant. Cancerous.

malignant tumor. Abnormal growth and multiplication of cells, causing the cells to form a mass (tumor). The cells have acquired aggressive features, including the ability to spread into other tissues. Another term for a cancer.

mammography. A procedure in which X-rays are taken of the breasts to detect any abnormalities.

margin of resection. The edge of a sample of tissue (specimen) that's removed during surgery.

mastectomy. Surgery to remove a breast.

metaplasia. A change in tissue cells to a form that's not normal for that type of tissue, but not necessarily abnormal enough to be called cancer.

metastasis. The process by which cancer cells break away from the primary tumor and spread, usually through blood and lymph vessels, to other parts of the body.

microcalcifications. Tiny calcium deposits that can appear in the breast and often show up on a mammogram. Depending on their size and other features, they may suggest a noncancerous (benign) or cancerous (malignant) process.

mismatch repair genes. Genes that help repair damaged DNA. When these genes are defective or damaged, mutations are more likely to accumulate.

modified radical mastectomy. Surgery that removes breast tissue, the areola and nipple, and lymph nodes under the arm near the breast.

monoclonal antibodies. Antibodies are one branch of the body's immune response. Monoclonal antibodies attach themselves to one specific target (antigen) in the body.

multifocal cancer. Cancer that starts within multiple areas of an organ.

mutation. An alteration in a gene.

myometrium. A layer of smooth muscle that makes up the muscular wall of the uterus.

N

negative margins. Edges (margins) of a tissue sample that are cancer-free.

neoadjuvant therapy. Chemotherapy given before a planned surgery to remove the cancer.

neoplasia. A new growth that may be benign or malignant.

nipple-sparing mastectomy. Removal of the underlying breast tissue, while keeping most of the breast's exterior, including the breast skin and nipple and areola.

noninvasive cancer. *See* carcinoma *in situ*.

nuclear medicine imaging. Injection of tiny amounts of radioactive tracers into the body. The tracers concentrate in given tissues and are viewed by a special camera.

O

omentum. The fatty apron in the front of the abdomen where cancer cells can collect.

oncogenes. Genes that play a role in normal cell growth and differentiation. If mutated, they can result in uncontrolled cell growth.

oncologist. A doctor trained in diagnosing and treating cancer.

oncology. The study of cancers and their treatments.

oophorectomy. Surgery to remove the ovaries.

optimal debulking. Abdominal-pelvic surgery that leaves behind only minimal or no cancer deposits.

ovarian cysts. Benign fluid-filled pockets (sacs) within or on the surface of an ovary.

ovarian suppression (ablation). Shutdown of ovarian function by way of surgery, radiation or medication. It reduces the production of estrogen in premenopausal women.

ovary. The female reproductive organ that contains eggs and produces hormones.

P

Paget's disease of the breast. Scaling and inflammation of the nipple associated with an underlying breast cancer that may be invasive or noninvasive.

palliative care. Therapy aimed at controlling symptoms caused by a disease or treatment for a disease.

palpate. To examine a tissue or organ by feeling it.

Pap test. A screening test in which a doctor obtains a sample of cells from the cervix for examination by a pathologist.

paracentesis. A procedure by which excess fluid in the abdomen (ascites) is withdrawn with a needle.

partial remission. Reduction, but not elimination, of cancer as a result of treatment.

pathology. Study of the cause and nature of a disease, and especially its structural appearance.

pathology report. A detailed report that contains information about the pathological appearance of a tissue specimen.

peau d'orange. Swollen breast skin that resembles an orange peel, caused by blocked lymph vessels in breast skin.

pedigree. A structured diagram that shows a family tree.

pelvic exam. Examination of a woman's external and internal reproductive organs.

peritoneal implant. Tumor spread to the lining of the abdominal-pelvic cavity (peritoneum).

peritoneum. The lining of the abdominal-pelvic cavity.

phytoestrogens. Plant chemicals, such as those in soy, with similarities to estrogen.

placebo. A medically inactive substance that may be used as part of a clinical trial to determine if a new treatment works.

platelets. Small particles in the blood that aid in blood clotting.

pleural effusion. Accumulation of fluid within the pleural space around the lungs that may or may not be cancerous.

positive margins. Edges of a tissue sample (margins) that show signs of cancer.

positron emission tomography (PET). A nuclear medicine study in which a tracer is injected into the body that accumulates in malignant cells.

precancerous. Referring to a condition that may develop into cancer.

primary tumor. The initial site of origin of a cancer.

progesterone. A female hormone that rises in the second half of the menstrual cycle.

progestin. A synthetic form of the hormone progesterone, used in hormone therapy.

prognosis. The predicted outcome of a disease.

prophylactic mastectomy. Surgical removal of one or both breasts in a woman at high risk of breast cancer to reduce her cancer risk.

prophylactic oophorectomy. Surgical removal of the ovaries in a woman at high risk of ovarian cancer to reduce her risk of ovarian and peritoneal cancer. In a premenopausal woman, the surgery may also reduce breast cancer risk.

prosthesis, breast. A soft device that's shaped like a breast and worn outside the body.

proteomics. The study of the body's proteins.

punch biopsy. Use of a hole-punch-type instrument to remove a sample of skin tissue.

Q

quadrantectomy. Surgical removal of the quarter of the breast that contains cancer cells. Also called partial mastectomy.

R

radiation therapy. Use of high-energy X-rays to kill cancer cells or damage them to the point that they lose their ability to grow and divide.

radical mastectomy. Surgical removal of the breast, chest wall muscle below the breast and all of the lymph nodes under the arm.

radioisotope. A radioactive substance.

recurrent cancer. Cancer that comes back after initial treatment.

regional recurrence. Cancer that recurs in lymph nodes or other tissues located near the original tumor.

regression. A decrease in tumor size.

relapse. Redevelopment of cancer after a cancer-free time period.

relative risk. A numeric comparison between the number of cancers (or other conditions) in a group of people with a particular trait and the number of cancers (or other conditions) in a group of people without that trait but who are otherwise similar.

remission. Disappearance of the cancer as determined by clinical evaluation, resolution of symptoms or both.

residual disease. The amount of cancer that remains after surgery.

risk factor. A factor that increases the chance of developing a condition.

S

sarcoma. A cancer that originates in connective tissue such as bone, cartilage and muscle.

screening. Being tested for a disease in the absence of symptoms.

screening mammogram. An X-ray of the breast used to look for changes in women who have no signs or symptoms of breast cancer.

sentinel node biopsy. A dye or a radioactive solution is injected into the primary tumor area to determine which lymph nodes are the first to receive drainage from the cancer area (sentinel nodes). These lymph nodes are removed and examined for cancer cells.

serosa. The thin, fibrous, outermost layer of many organs.

simple hyperplasia. An excess of normal-appearing cells. This is the most common form of endometrial hyperplasia.

simple (total) mastectomy. Surgical removal of the breast tissue, skin, areola and nipple, but not any lymph nodes.

skin-sparing mastectomy. Removal of breast tissue while preserving as much of the breast skin as possible.

speculum. A device used to hold the vaginal walls apart during a pelvic exam.

squamous cells. Flat cells that cover the surface of the skin and the lining of some hollow organs of the body.

staging. Determination of the extent of the cancer or its spread. Cancer stage is generally based on a tumor's size and whether it has spread to lymph nodes and other areas of the body.

stroma. Tissue supporting the structures of an organ.

subcutaneous mastectomy. Removal of breast tissue, but not the nipple and areola.

supportive (palliative) care. Treatment designed to alleviate symptoms caused by cancer or anti-cancer therapy.

surgical biopsy. Surgical removal of a portion of a mass (incisional biopsy) or the whole mass (excisional biopsy) for pathological examination.

surgical menopause. Menopause that's caused by surgical removal of the ovaries.

systemic. Affecting the entire body.

systemic therapy. Treatment delivered to the entire body by way of the bloodstream, including chemotherapy and hormone therapy.

T

targeted therapies. Nonchemotherapy treatments that target a specific pathway that's driving a cancer.

total abdominal hysterectomy. Surgical removal of the entire uterus, including the cervix, through an incision in the abdomen.

transvaginal ultrasound. A procedure in which a transducer is inserted into the vagina to check for suspicious masses in the pelvic region.

tubal ligation. A surgical procedure to prevent pregnancy by cutting or sealing the fallopian tubes.

tumor. An abnormal mass of tissue that results from excessive cell growth and division, which may be benign or malignant. Also called a neoplasm.

tumor marker. A substance circulating in blood that's produced by a certain tumor. The level of the tumor marker may reflect the activity or extent of the tumor.

tumor suppressor genes. Genes normally responsible for restraining cell growth.

U

ultrasound. An imaging procedure that uses high-frequency sound waves to produce images of the inside of the human body, which are displayed on a computer screen.

uterine cancer. Cancer that starts within the uterine body (corpus).

uterine fibroids. Benign tumors that develop in the muscle wall of the uterus.

uterus. A hollow organ where a fetus grows and develops during pregnancy.

V

vagina. A muscular tube that connects the uterus with the outer genitals.

vaginal hysterectomy. A hysterectomy that's performed through a vaginal incision.

W

wide local excision. A procedure in which a doctor removes the tumor and some surrounding tissue.

wire localization. Use of fine wires to show the surgeon the location of a breast mass that can't be felt so that the mass can be removed.

Index

A

abdominal hysterectomy, 417
abortion, 51
absolute risk
  defined, 62, 417
  example, 62–63
  relative risk versus, 64–65
  in studies, 63
  See also risk(s)
acceptance, supportive care, 380–381
acupuncture, 360–362
acute pain syndrome, 345
addiction, 385
additional treatment
  decision factors, 183–184
  reasons for, 179
  who should consider, 179–184
  See also invasive breast cancer
adenocarcinoma, 417
adjustment disorder, 308–309
Adjuvant!, 184
adjuvant systemic therapy
  anti-HER2 therapy, 197–199
  chemotherapy, 185–188
  decision guide, 196
  decision tools, 195
  decision making, 186
  defined, 417
  elements of, 184–185
  hormone therapy, 189–195
advanced breast cancer
  bone marrow transplants and, 262
  bone metastases, 269
  central nervous system metastases, 269–270
  chemotherapy, 257–259
  clinical trials, 263
  defined, 247, 417
  disease extent, 249
  disease locations, 249
  disease-free interval, 248
  drug therapy decision, 261
  HER2 medications, 259–261
  HER2 status, 248–249
  hormone receptor status, 248
  hormone therapy, 250–257
  localized treatments, 262–270
  medications that prevent blood vessel growth, 261
  new therapies, 262
  personal and treatment factors, 249
  pleural effusions, 269
  prognosis factors, 248–249
  stories, 264–268
  treating, 247–270
  treatment goals, 250
  treatment monitoring, 262–263
  treatment options, 250–262
  when treatment stops working, 270
age
  in additional treatment decision, 183
  in advanced breast cancer prognosis factor, 249
  as breast cancer cause, 54
  in DCIS treatment, 155
  as risk factor, 25
  as uterine cancer risk factor, 289
Agnes's story, 159
alcohol consumption
  prevention and, 97
  as risk factor, 72
alkylating agents, 257
angiogenesis, 60, 417
antibodies, 417
anti-cancer treatment, 417
anticipatory nausea/vomiting, 327
antidepressants, 339
antigens, 417
anti-HER2 therapy
  chemotherapy, 199
  defined, 197
  lapatinib (Tykerb), 198
  trastuzumab (Herceptin), 198
  watchful waiting, 199
anti-metabolites, 257
antioxidants, 96–97, 417
anti-tumor antibiotics, 256
anxiety level, 307–308
appetite problems
  self-help strategies, 326–327
  supportive care, 387–389
  weight gain and, 328
  weight loss and, 327–328
  See also side effects
arm/shoulder mobility
  arm raises, 330
  arm swing, 332
  decreased, 330–333
  deep breathing, 331
  hand squeezes, 331
  inactivity and, 333

pulley, 332
shoulder rotations, 331
wall climb, 331
See also side effects
aromatase inhibitors
defined, 109, 193–194, 417
as postmenopausal metastatic breast cancer
treatment, 255–256
tamoxifen versus, 194
use after tamoxifen, 194
use of, 194
aromatase-inhibitor arthralgias, 346–347
Ashkenazi descent, 67, 76, 85-87, 274-275
atypical hyperplasia
defined, 34
illustrated, 151
as precancerous condition, 150
axillary node dissection, 418
axillary nodes, 418
ayurveda, 361

B
benign breast conditions, 44–45
benign breast disease
defined, 45
hyperplasia, 73
lobular carcinoma *in situ* (LCIS), 73–74
benign tumors, 418
bevacizumab (Avastin), 261
bilateral breast cancer, 216
biofeedback, 356
biopsy procedures, 132–139
core needle, 134–136
defined, 132–133, 418
fine-needle aspiration, 133–134
guiding with ultrasound, 132
surgical, 136–139
types of, 133
in uterine cancer diagnosis, 297, 298
See also breast cancer diagnosis
birth control pills, 276
bisphosphonates, 344–345
black cohosh, 359
blood tumor markers, 231–232
blood vessel growth inhibition medications,
261
blood vessels, 45
BOADICEA model, 67
bone marrow transplants, 262
bone metastases, 269

bone scans
defined, 418
metastatic recurrence, 246
staging with, 143–144
BRCA carriers, 214–215
BRCA genes
BRCA1, 77
BRCA2, 77
breast cancer risk, 81
defined, 77, 418
discovery of, 78
family example, 80
mutation, 79–80
mutation likelihood, 84, 85
ovarian cancer risk, 81, 275
role in hereditary breast cancer, 77–79
summary, 79
BRCAPRO model, 67
breast cancer
advanced, 58, 247–270
advancing science, 57–60
bilateral, 216
coping with, 317
defined, 45–47
detection advances, 43–44
ductal carcinoma *in situ* (DCIS), 48, 153–160
grouping estimation, 147–148
growth, 49
HER2-positive, 197, 198
hereditary, 50, 51–52, 75–90
inflammatory, 212–213, 424
invasive ductal carcinoma (IDC), 47–48
invasive lobular carcinoma (ILC), 48
lobular carcinoma *in situ* (LCIS), 48
locally advanced, 212–214
lumps, 128
in men, 222–224
metaplastic, 217–218
at molecular level, 48
nonhereditary, 76–77
overview, 43–60
Paget's disease, 48
pregnancy after, 222
pregnancy and breast-feeding, 220–222
preventing, 91–110
racial and ethnic differences in survival
rates, 57
rates, 54
spread, 49
stage I, 36

breast cancer continued
  stage II, 36
  stage III, 36
  stage IV, 37
  statistics, 11, 43, 55–57
  stress and, 52–53
  triple-negative, 199
  types of, 47–48
  as uterine cancer risk factor, 292
  See also invasive breast cancer
breast cancer causes
  aging, 54
  environmental factors, 53–54
  genetic factors, 50–52
  hormonal and reproductive factors, 51, 52
  identification of, 49–50
breast cancer diagnosis, 127–148
  absorbing, 306–307
  basics, 144
  biopsy procedures, 132–139
  DCIS, 154
  having children and, 189
  hereditary question, 76–79
  imaging tests, 130–132
  importance of, 128
  male breast cancer, 223
  medical history, 128–129
  pathology report, 139–143
  physical examination, 129
  process, 127
  repeating tests, 140
  signs and symptoms, 128
  staging, 143–148
  survival estimation, 147–148
breast cancer recurrence, 235–246
  cancer cells spreading and, 237–238
  DCIS, risk of, 157
  difficulty in dealing with, 235–236
  early detection and, 227
  local, 226, 236, 238–242
  metastatic, 227, 236, 244–246
  monitoring for, 225
  new cancer versus, 227
  prognostic and predictive tools, 184
  reconstructive surgery and, 184
  regional, 226–227, 236, 242–244
  signs and symptoms to watch for,
      228
  types of, 226–227, 236
  understanding, 226–227

breast lumps
  as breast cancer sign, 128
  evaluation of, 127
  as palpable mass, 128
breast lymphoma, 218
breast reconstruction. *See* reconstructive
      surgery
breast sarcoma, 218–219
breast self-exams
  defined, 116, 418
  dimpling, 118
  lumps, 118
  lying down, 119
  performing, 116–119
  possible cancer signs, 118
  standing in shower, 117–119
  thickening, 118
  visual exam, 117
breast-feeding, as risk factor, 69
breasts
  benign conditions, 44–45
  composition, 45
  density, 74
  fibrocystic, 104
  illustrated, 46
  with implants, evaluating, 132
  lobes, 46
  normal tissue, 47
  self-awareness, 116–119

C
CA 125 blood test, 278, 418
calcifications, 123, 418
calcitonin, 345
calcium deposits, 45
cancer
  advancing knowledge of, 26–32
  biology, 33
  causes, 24–26
  chromosomes, 21
  as curable, 18
  "cure" for, 16
  death rates, 17, 32
  defined, 18–21, 418
  development, 20
  diagnosis, responses to, 11
  external factors, 24
  as family affair, 16
  internal factors, 24
  invasive, 35, 47

noninvasive, 35, 47
occurrence of, 23–24
ovarian, 271–286
radiation exposure contribution to, 27
resources, 415–416
risk factors, 24–26
scientific discoveries, 17–18
statistics, 12, 17
understanding, 17–32
uterine, 287–302
See also breast cancer
cancer cells
    anti-growth signals and, 20–21
    blood supply, 21
    bone, 237
    characteristics of, 19–21
    in DCIS treatment, 155
    defined, 19
    growth, 20, 24
    life cycle and, 21
    liver, 237
    reproduction, 23–24
    spread of, 237–238
    stage IV, 37
cancer development
    as long process, 23–24
    visual guide, 34–35
cancer drugs, new, 29
cancer survivors, 366
carboplatin, 185–186
carcinogenesis, 34
carcinoma, 419
carcinoma *in situ*, 419
Carol's story, 264–266
Cathy's story, 158–159
cell membrane
    defined, 33, 40
    illustrated, 33
    medications acting on, 40
cell proliferation
    in additional treatment decision, 184
    defined, 419
cells
    abnormal, 34–35
    cancer, 19–21
    division, 22
    normal behavior, 18–19
    nucleus, 22
central nervous system metastases, 269–270
changed life, 15

chemotherapy
    in anti-HER2 therapy, 199
    carboplatin, 185–186
    combinations, 188, 258
    cyclophosphamide (Cytoxan), 185
    defined, 185, 419
    doxorubicin, 185
    duration, 185
    eating and, 326
    epirubicin (Ellence), 185
    fluorouracil, 186
    local recurrence after mastectomy, 242
    long-term side effects, 187–188
    pregnancy and breast cancer, 222
    short-term side effects, 186–187
    taxanes, 186
    See also adjuvant systemic therapy
chemotherapy for metastatic breast cancer,
        256–261
    alkylating agents, 257
    anti-metabolites, 257
    anti-tumor antibiotics, 256
    combination, 258
    drug classes, 256
    drug options, 259
    holidays, 259
    mitotic inhibitors, 256
    single-agent versus combination, 257–258
    vinca alkaloids, 257
    See also advanced breast cancer
chest X-rays, staging with, 143
children, communicating with
    addressing common questions, 319
    adjustment to medical settings, 319–322
    appropriate information, 318–319
    challenge of, 317
    knowing they're loved, 322
    tips for, 317–322
choices, 14
chromosomes, cancer, 21
Claus model, 67
clinical breast examination, 119, 419
clinical trials
    advanced breast cancer, 263
    defined, 28, 29, 419
    enrolling in, 30
    finding, 30
    importance of, 28
    invasive breast cancer, 199–202
    mammography, 112–113

clinical trials continued
    patient safety, 31
    phase I, 28–30
    phase II, 30
    phase III, 30–31
    prevention medications, 106
    proton therapy, 171
    resources, 413
    risk factors and, 66
    See also research
clonidine (Catapres), 338
cognitive changes, 347–348
Colleen's story, 181–182
combination chemotherapy, 258
communication
    with children, 317–322
    with family, 315–317
    with friends, 322
    with the team (partners), 399
communication (partners)
    barriers, 404
    importance of, 403
    sexual intimacy, 406
    with the team, 399
    tips, 404–405
complementary and alternative therapies,
        351–364
    acupuncture, 360–362
    alternative systems, 361
    ayurveda, 361
    biofeedback, 356
    costs of, 354
    defined, 351–352, 419
    dietary supplements, 358–360
    getting most out of, 353–354
    guided imagery, 356
    homeopathy, 361
    hypnosis, 356
    learning about, 353
    massage, 357–358
    meditation, 355, 357
    middle-road approach, 354
    mind-body techniques, 355–357
    music therapy, 356–357
    natural energy restoration, 360–362
    naturopathy, 361
    options, discussing, 353–354
    progressive relaxation, 356
    reiki, 362
    reliable information, finding, 362–364

    resources, 413–414
    risk versus benefits assessment, 354
    therapeutic touch, 362
    treatment provider evaluation, 354
    types of, 355–362
    use of, 351–352
    yoga, 355–356
computerized tomography (CT)
    defined, 419
    metastatic recurrence, 245–246
    staging with, 144
coping
    with cancer, 317
    resources, 414
    skill intervention groups, 411
core needle biopsy
    defined, 134–135, 420
    MRI-guided, 135–136
    preparation for, 135
    during procedure, 135–136
    pros and cons, 136
    stereotactic, 135
    ultrasound-guided, 135
    See also biopsy procedures
CT. *See* computerized tomography
cyclophosphamide (Cytoxan), 185
cysts
    defined, 44, 420
    in fine-needle aspiration biopsy, 133
    ovarian, 278
    solid masses versus, 132
cytoplasm, 33, 40

D
death rates, 17, 32
denial
    impending death, 382, 412
    loved one in, 410
denosumab (Prolia), 345
dense breast tissue, 132
diabetes, as uterine cancer risk factor, 292–293
diagnostic mammograms, 120–121, 130, 420
DIEP flap, 208
diet
    breast cancer and, 98
    breast cancer survival and, 94–95
    fats, 93–95
    fruits/vegetables and, 95
    lignans, 96–97
    risk and, 92

as risk factor, 71
as self-help strategy, 314
soy and phytoestrogens, 95–96
survivorship, 372
vitamins and minerals, 95
See also lifestyle factors; prevention
dietary supplements
black cohosh, 359
cancer and, 358–359
flaxseed, 359
ginseng, 359
green tea, 359
vitamin C, 359
vitamin D, 359–360
vitamin E, 359
See also complementary and alternative
therapies
dilation and curettage (D&C)
defined, 297, 420
illustrated, 298
procedure, 297–299
DNA, 58, 420
do-not-resuscitate (DNR) status, 393–394
doxorubicin, 185
drug therapy
local recurrence after lumpectomy, 240
visual guide, 40
drug tolerance, 385
ductal carcinoma *in situ* (DCIS), 153–160
age and, 155
cell structure, 155
defined, 48, 153–154, 420
diagnosis, 154
diagnosis rates, 54–56
invasive cancer and, 156
key factors, 154–155
pathologic margins, 154
in pathology report, 140
radiation treatment option, 157
recurrent, risk of, 157
stories of, 158–159
surgery treatment option, 155–157
tamoxifen, 159
treatment, 153
treatment decision, making, 160
treatment factors, 154–155
treatment options, 155–157
tumor grade, 155
tumor size, 154–155
ducts, 45

E
eating, during chemotherapy, 326
education, 311–312
educational intervention groups, 411
emotional support, partners, 402–403
endometrial hyperplasia, 291–292, 421
endometrioid (type I) cancer, 288–289
environmental factors
alcohol consumption, 72
as breast cancer cause, 53–54
diet, 71
exercise, 71
occupational exposures, 72
pesticides and environmental pollution, 72
radiation exposure, 72
risk factors, 70–72
weight, 71
See also risk factors
epidemiologic studies, 27–28
epirubicin (Ellence), 185
Español (Spanish) resources, 414
estrogen, 191, 421
estrogen therapy, 292, 344
excess body weight, 54
excessive alcohol use, 54
exemestane (Aromasin), 152
exercise
with cancer, 373
in osteoporosis prevention/treatment, 344
as risk factor, 71
as self-help strategy, 312–314
for sleep, 375
survivorship, 372–374
external beam radiation, 39, 421
external beam radiation therapy
defined, 173, 421
team members, 173–174
after treatment, 174
before treatment, 174
during treatment, 174
See also radiation therapy
external factors, 24, 421

F
family and friends
communicating with, 315–322
responses to cancer, 316
support, 307
family disagreements, supportive care,
383

family history
hereditary breast cancer versus, 75
mapping, 82
as risk factor, 26, 68
fatigue
accepting, 324–325
causes of, 323–324
self-help strategies, 325
See also side effects
fats
classification of, 93
negative results, 93
omega-3/omega-6 fatty acids, 93–94
research on, 92–93
See also diet
fears
coping with, 368
managing, 366–368
recurrence, 366–367
sharing, 368
fertility treatments, 51
fibroadenomas, 44–45, 422
fibrocystic breast changes, 44, 422
fibrocystic breasts, 104
financial resources, 414
fine-needle aspiration biopsy
defined, 133
illustrated, 134
image guidance, 133
pros and cons, 134
See also biopsy procedures
FISH test, 142–143
flaxseed, 359
fluorescent *in situ* hybridization (FISH),
142–143
fluorouracil, 186
follow-up care, 228–232
blood tumor markers, 231–232
cancer survivor continuation with, 376
imaging tests, 232
key studies, 231
mammography, 229–230
medical history and, 229
newer options, 230
nonrecommended tests, 230–231
physical exam, 229
purpose of, 228
recommended tests, 229–230
research, 231–232
uncertainty and, 232–234

whole self, 234
free TRAM flap surgery, 206
friends. *See* family and friends
frozen section analysis, 168–169
fruits and vegetables, 95
fulvestrant (Faslodex), 256

G
Gail model, 66–67, 422
Gayle's story, 391–392
gene expression signature tools, 184
gene therapy, 422
genes
BRCA, 77–79
breast cancer, search for, 78
defined, 22, 422
mismatch repair, 23
oncogenes, 23, 51
tumor suppressor, 23, 50–51
genetic counseling
elements of, 83–86
questions to ask, 83
genetic factors, 50–52
genetic mutations, inheriting, 79–80
genetic testing
approach, 82
benefits of, 81
BRCA-negative families, 83
candidates for, 82–83
cost of, 86–87
decision to undergo, 87–90
defined, 422
negative results, 90
positive results, 87–90
unclear results, 86
genetic versus inherited, 26
geneticists, 81
genetics, 22, 422
genomics, 31, 423
Geraldine's story, 158
ginseng, 359
glossary, 417–432
green tea, 359
grieving, partners, 409–410
guided imagery, 356
gynecologic anatomy, 272

H
hair loss
preventing with scalp freezing, 329

process of, 329
self-help strategies, 329–330
See also side effects
health care
eating well, 372
follow-up care, 376
healthy weight, 374–375
physical activity, 373–374
sleep and rest, 375
See also survivorship
healthy weight, 374–375
helping others, 371
HER2 medications
lapatinib (Tykerb), 260–261
pertuzumab, 261
trastuzumab (Herceptin), 259–260
See also advanced breast cancer
HER2 protein, 60, 259, 423
HER2 status
additional treatment decision and, 184
as advanced breast cancer prognosis factor, 248–249
pathology report, 142–143
HER2-negative breast cancer, 198
HER2-positive breast cancer, 197, 198
herbal products, 360
Herceptin. *See* trastuzumab (Herceptin)
hereditary breast cancer
BRCA genes, role of, 77–79
BRCA1, 77
BRCA2, 77
clues, 76
decision to test, 87–90
defined, 423
family history versus, 75
family story, 88–89
genetic counseling and testing, 81–87
hallmarks, 50
risk, 51–52
statistics, 51, 77
hereditary nonpolyposis colorectal cancer (HNPCC), 275
high-risk women
defined, 99
groups, 113
issues faced by, 99–100
options, 100, 107
prevention and, 99–109
prevention medicines, 106–109
proactive steps, 100

prophylactic mastectomy, 100–102
prophylactic oophorectomy, 102–106
screening for ovarian cancer, 281
Hodgkin disease survivors
breast cancer risk and, 215
treatment, 215–216
See also second cancer
homeopathy, 361
hope, maintaining, 381–383
hormonal and reproductive factors
hormone replacement therapy (HRT), 70
menstrual history, 69
oral contraceptives, 69–70
pregnancy and breast-feeding, 69
types of, 52
hormone receptor status
as advanced breast cancer prognosis factor, 248
defined, 191
ER or PR positive, 142
hormone replacement therapy (HRT)
defined, 70
after prophylactic oophorectomy, 104
as risk factor, 70
for vaginal dryness, 338
hormone therapy
aromatase inhibitors, 193–194
decision to use in metastatic breast cancer, 254
defined, 423
goal of, 189
local recurrence after mastectomy, 242
ovarian ablation, 192–193
postmenopausal women, 254–257
pregnancy and breast cancer, 222
premenopausal women, 250–254
tamoxifen, 190–192
withdrawal phenomenon, 255
See also adjuvant systemic therapy
hospice care
beginnings of, 390
defined, 389, 423
do-not-resuscitate status, 393–394
eligibility, 393
partners and, 409
resources, 413
services, 390–393
See also supportive care
hot flashes
defined, 337

hot flashes continued
    medications for, 337–339
    relief from, 337–339
    self-help strategies, 337
    See also sudden menopause
hyperplasia
    defined, 34, 423
    as risk factor, 73
hypnosis, 356
hysterectomy, 423

I
imaging tests
    benefit of, 130
    diagnostic mammography, 130
    follow-up care, 232
    metastatic recurrence, 245–246
    results, interpreting, 131
    ultrasound, 130–132
    in uterine cancer extent determination, 299
    See also breast cancer diagnosis
immunohistochemistry tests, 142
immunotherapy, 423
implants
    defined, 423
    evaluating breasts with, 132
    in reconstructive surgery, 207
infections, 45
infertility, 338
inflammatory breast cancer, 212–213, 424
information-gathering checklist, 400–401
inherited versus genetic, 26
intercourse, painful, 341–342
internal radiation therapy, 175, 179, 424
intraductal radiation, 424
invasive breast cancer
    additional treatment, 179
    additional treatment decision factors, 183–184
    anti-HER2 therapy and, 197–199
    chemotherapy and, 185–188
    clinical trials, 199–202
    defined, 424
    ductal carcinoma *in situ* (DCIS) and, 156
    frequency, 57
    hormone therapy and, 188–196
    locoregional therapy, 162
    lumpectomy, 163–164
    lymph node removal, 165–168
    mastectomy, 164–165
    in pathology report, 140
    prevention medications, 152
    stories, 180–182, 200–202
    surgery, 162–171
    systemic therapy, 162
    therapy options, 184–199
    time for weighing options, 162
    treatment, 162–202
    treatment options, 162
invasive cancer
    in cancer development, 35
    illustrated, 47
    types of, 47–48
invasive ductal carcinoma (IDC), 47–48
invasive lobular carcinoma (ILC), 48

J
Jane's story, 201–202, 266–267
Janice's story, 105
Jan's story, 180–181
Jeanne's story, 320–321
Join the Journey, 370
joint aches/pains
    aromatase inhibitor arthralgias, 346–347
    post-chemotherapy rheumatism, 346
    See also side effects
journey, the
    absorbing the diagnosis, 306–307
    adjustment disorder, 308–309
    anxiety level, 307–308
    communication with family, 315–317
    going through the treatment, 307–309
    handling decisions, 306–307
    making, 305–311
    positive attitude, 311
    sadness, 308–309
    searching for meaning, 310
    self-help strategies, 311–315
    spirituality, 310–311
    story, 320–321
    tips for, 311–315
    treating the whole person, 315
    after treatment, 309–311

K
Karen's story, 369
Kegel exercises, 342

L
lapatinib (Tykerb), 198, 260–261

latissimus flap surgery, 206
laughter, 313
Laura's story, 221
lifestyle factors
    alcohol consumption, 97
    diet, 92–97
    physical activity, 97–99
    weight control, 94
    See also prevention
lifetime cancer risk, 424
lignans, 96–97
Lisa's story, 103
liver ultrasound, 246
lobes, 46, 425
lobular carcinoma *in situ* (LCIS)
    defined, 48, 73, 151, 425
    illustrated, 151
    in pathology report, 141
    as precancerous condition, 151–152
    as risk factor, 73–74
local recurrence, 238–242
    chemotherapy and hormone therapy, 242
    defined, 226, 236
    drug therapy, 240
    after lumpectomy, 238–241
    after mastectomy, 241–242
    prognosis, 240–241, 242
    prognostic factors, 238
    radiation therapy, 240, 242
    signs and symptoms, 239, 241
    surgery, 240, 242
    tests, 239–240, 241
    treatment, 240–241, 242
    See also breast cancer recurrence
locally advanced breast cancer
    occurrence of, 212–213
    statistics, 212
    surgery, 214
    treatment, 213–214
    tumor characteristics, 212
locoregional therapy, 162, 425
loss, dealing with, 14–15
lumpectomy
    as DCIS treatment option, 156–157
    defined, 156, 163
    duration, 170
    for invasive breast cancer, 163–164
    local recurrence after, 238–241
    mastectomy decision versus, 176–177
    as not the right choice, 163

pros and cons, 178
radiation therapy after, 163–164, 171–172
roles, 163
See also surgery
lymph nodes
    axillary dissection, 167–168
    cancer spread to, 166
    defined, 45, 165–166, 425
    dissection, 167–168
    removal, 165–168
    removal side effects, 168
    sentinel node biopsy, 166–168
    sentinel nodes, identification and removal,
        166–167
    unknown primary cancers and, 216–217
    See also surgery
lymph vessels, 45
lymphedema
    burn avoidance, 335–336
    defined, 333–334
    medication and, 335
    risk reduction, 334–335
    tips for, 335
    treating, 335–336
    See also side effects
lymphoma, breast, 218

M
magnetic resonance imaging (MRI)
    defined, 126, 425
    metastatic recurrence, 246
    staging with, 144
male breast cancer
    diagnosis, 223
    prognosis, 224
    risk factors, 223
    staging, 223
    statistics, 222
    treatment, 223–224
malignant tumors, 425
mammograms
    breast compression during, 122
    day of the test, 122–123
    dense areas on, 123
    diagnostic, 120–121, 130
    instructions before, 122
    preparing for, 121–122
    procedure, 122–123
    questionable findings, evaluating, 132
    radiation from, 124

mammograms continued
   results, understanding, 123
   screening, 120, 430
   tumor discovery with, 124
   tumor images, 125
   where to get, 124–126
mammography
   abnormalities prompting addition testing,
      123
   advantage, 113
   defined, 426
   drawbacks, 124
   facilities, 126
   false-negatives, 124
   false-positives, 124
   follow-up care, 229–230
   illustrated views, 121
   limitations of, 123–124
   performance of, 120
   trials, 112–113
Margaret's story, 233, 267–268
margins
   defined, 165, 426
   negative, 426
   pathologic, 154
   positive, 165
Mary's story
   being proactive, 16
   a changed life, 15
   choices and decisions, 14
   dealing with loss, 14–15
   fear and uncertainty, 13
   support and strength, 16
massage, 357–358
mastectomy
   as DCIS treatment option, 155–156
   defined, 155, 164
   duration, 170
   local recurrence after, 241–242
   lumpectomy decision versus, 176–177
   modified radical, 165
   partial, 164
   pros and cons, 178
   radiation therapy after, 172–173
   radical, 164–165
   simple, 165
   See also surgery
meaning, searching for, 310
medical history
   in breast cancer diagnosis, 128–129

   follow-up care and, 229
   information, 129
medications
   acting on cell membrane, 40
   HER2, 259–261
   hot flash, 337–339
   nausea, 325–326
   ovarian suppression, 252
   pain, 385–387
   See also prevention medications
meditation, 355
menstrual history, 69
metaplastic breast cancer, 217–218
metastasis, 426
metastatic breast cancer. *See* advanced breast
      cancer
metastatic recurrence
   biopsy, 245
   defined, 227, 236, 244
   imaging tests, 245–246
   laboratory tests, 245
   prognosis, 246
   signs and symptoms, 244–245
   treatment, 246
   See also breast cancer recurrence
microcalcifications, 138–139, 426
mind-body techniques, 355–357
miscarriage, 51
mismatch repair genes, 23
mitotic inhibitors, 256
modified radical mastectomy, 165, 426
molecular breast imaging (MBI), 230
MRI-guided core needle biopsy, 135–136
Musa's story, 233
music therapy, 356–357

N
Nancy's story, 200–201
National Cancer Act, 26
naturopathy, 361
nausea
   anticipatory, 327
   medications, 325–326
   self-help strategies, 326–327
   supportive care, 389
   See also side effects
negative margins, 426
negative test results, 90
neoplasia, 426
neuropathy

acute pain syndrome, 345
    defined, 345
    peripheral, 345–346
    See also side effects
night sweats, 337, 339
nipple reconstruction, 208, 209
nonhereditary disease, 76–77
noninvasive cancer
    in cancer development, 35
    defined, 427
    illustrated, 47
    in pathology report, 140–141
nonsteroidal anti-inflammatory drugs
        (NSAIDs), 109
normal cells, 18–19, 21, 34
nuclear grade, 141
nuclear medicine studies, 126, 427
nucleotide, 22
nucleus, 22, 33, 40

O

obesity, as uterine cancer risk factor, 290–291
occupational exposures, as risk factor, 72
omega-3/omega-6 fatty acids, 93–94
oncogenes, 23, 51, 427
oncology, 427
online support groups, 411
opioids, 386–387
oral contraceptives, as risk factor, 69–70
organization, this book, 12
orgasm, difficulty reaching, 342
osteoporosis
    defined, 344
    prevention and treatment, 344–345
    See also side effects
ovarian ablation
    defined, 192–193
    side effects, 192
    trials, 193
ovarian cancer, 271–286
    birth control pills and, 276
    CA 125, 278–279
    characteristics of, 273–274
    defined, 273
    diagnosis, 283–284
    early warning signs, 281–282
    high-risk women, screening, 281
    incidence of, 274
    nonspecific symptoms, 281–282
    pelvic exam, 280

pelvic ultrasound, 279
    preventing, 275–277
    prophylactic oophorectomy and, 104,
        276–277
    risk factors, 275
    screening methods, 277–281
    screening recommendations, 279–281
    screening research, 279
    signs and symptoms, 281
    spread illustration, 284
    spread of, 282
    stages, 283
    statistics, 274
    story, 285–286
    surgery, 284
    treatment, 283–284
    as uterine cancer risk factor, 292
ovarian cysts, 278
ovarian suppression
    aromatase inhibitors and, 253–254
    defined, 251
    medications, 252
    oophorectomy, 251
    radiation therapy, 252
    tamoxifen and ovarian suppression, 252–253
ovaries
    defined, 271, 427
    functions, 273
    hormone production, 291
    illustrated, 272
    removal of, 276–277

P

p53 protein, 60
Paget's disease
    defined, 48, 219, 427
    prognosis, 220
    signs and symptoms, 219
    treatment, 220
pain
    acute, 384
    addiction and, 385
    assessing with doctor, 384–387
    chronic, 384
    controlling through relaxation, 387
    medications, 385–387
    opioids and, 386–387
    rating, 384
    recording, 384–385
    See also supportive care

palliative care
  benefits, 388
  defined, 427
  elements of, 388
  See also supportive care
Pap test, 280, 428
partners, 395–412
  adjustments to daily life, 397
  balance, finding, 407–408
  caring for yourself, 407–408
  challenges of, 395–396
  communication with loved one, 403–405
  concerns, 396–398
  dealing with loved one's diagnosis, 396–398
  educating yourself, 402
  emotional support, 402–403
  emotions and feelings, 396
  emotions from loved one, 398
  expectations from loved one, 397–398
  fearing cancer, 396
  grieving, 409–410
  hospice care, 409
  how to help, 398–403
  information-gathering checklist, 400–401
  inner strength, 408
  knowing how to offer support, 397
  loved one in denial and, 410
  practical support, 403
  professional help, 404
  resources, 410–412
  sexual intimacy, maintaining, 405–407
  support groups, 410–412
  supportive care, 408–410
  time of growth, 412
pathologic margins, 154
pathology report
  cancer details, 139–143
  defined, 139, 428
  explanations, 139
  HER2 status, 142–143
  hormone receptor status, 142
  tumor grade, 141–142
  type of cancer, 140–141
pathology results, discussing, 170–171
patient safety, clinical trials, 31
Pat's story, 285–286
pedicle TRAM flap surgery, 206
peer support groups, 411
pelvic exam
  defined, 428
  illustrated, 280
  in uterine cancer diagnosis, 295–296
pelvic ultrasound, 279
peripheral neuropathy, 345–346
personal stories
  Agnes's story, 159
  Carol's story, 264–266
  Cathy's story, 158–159
  Colleen's story, 181–182
  Gayle's story, 391–392
  Geraldine's story, 158
  Jane's story, 201–202, 266–267
  Janice's story, 105
  Jan's story, 180–181
  Jeanne's story, 320–321
  Karen's story, 369
  Laura's story, 221
  Lisa's story, 103
  Margaret's story, 233, 267–268
  Mary's story, 13-16
  Musa's story, 233
  Nancy's story, 200–201
  one family's story, 88–89
  Pat's story, 285–286
  Rosemarie's story, 182–183
  Shirley's story, 348–350
pertuzumab, 261
pesticides and environmental pollution, 72
PET. *See* positron emission tomography
physical activity
  cancer survivors, 372–374
  prevention and, 97–99
  risk and, 98–99
  types of, 97–98
  weight control and, 99
physical examination
  in breast cancer diagnosis, 129
  follow-up care, 229
  uterine cancer diagnosis, 294–295
pleural effusions, 269
positive attitude, 311
positive margins, 165, 428
positive test results
  anxiety, 87
  family relationships, 87
  guilt, 87
  health insurance discrimination concerns, 90
  risk status, knowing, 87
  See also genetic testing

positron emission tomography (PET)
defined, 428
metastatic recurrence, 246
staging with, 144–145
post-chemotherapy rheumatism, 346
postmenopausal women, 252
postmenopausal women, hormone therapy
aromatase inhibitors, 255–256
decision to use, 254
fulvestrant (Faslodex), 256–257
high-dose estrogen vs. tamoxifen, 255
treatment, 254
See also advanced breast cancer
practical support, partners, 403
precancerous conditions
atypical hyperplasia, 151
cancer-preventing medications, 152
defined, 428
lobular carcinoma *in situ* (LCIS), 151–152
options, 152
preventative surgery, 152
types of, 149
watchful waiting, 152
pregnancy
after breast cancer, 222
as risk factor, 69
pregnancy, breast cancer and
chemotherapy, 222
hormone therapy, 222
radiation therapy, 222
surgery, 221–222
treatment, 220–222
premenopausal women, hormone therapy
aromatase inhibitors and ovarian
suppression, 253–254
decision to use, 254
ovarian suppression, 251–252
tamoxifen, 252
tamoxifen and ovarian suppression,
252–253
See also advanced breast cancer
preventative surgery, 152
prevention
antioxidants and, 96–97
future directions, 109–110
high-risk women and, 99–109
lifestyle factors, 92–99
risk and, 91–92
screening and, 91
secondary, 100

weight control and, 94
prevention medications
aromatase inhibitors, 109
clinical trials, 106
defined, 106
exemestane, 152
nonsteroidal anti-inflammatory drugs
(NSAIDs), 109
raloxifene, 108–109, 152
tamoxifen, 106–108, 152
use of, 106
primary peritoneal carcinoma, 277
primary tumors, 429
prior breast cancer, 72
proactive, being, 16
progressive relaxation, 356
prophylactic mastectomy
candidates for, 101
defined, 10, 429
high-risk women and, 100–102
procedure, 101—102
risks, 102
studies, 100–101
prophylactic oophorectomy
defined, 102, 429
HRT after, 104
motivation, 104
ovarian cancer and, 276–277
procedure timing, 106
recommendation, 104
risks, 104–106
prosthetics, 209, 429
proteins, in breast cancer development, 58–60
proteomics, 31
proton therapy, 171
public events, 378
punch biopsy, 429

R
race and ethnicity, as uterine cancer risk
factor, 290
radiation exposure
as breast cancer cause, 54
mammograms, 124
as risk factor, 72
types, in cancer cause, 27
radiation therapy, 171–179
as DCIS treatment option, 157
defined, 171, 429
delivery of, 173

radiation therapy continued
  external beam radiation, 173–174
  how it works, 173–175
  internal, 175
  local recurrence after lumpectomy, 240
  local recurrence after mastectomy, 242
  after lumpectomy, 156, 157, 171–172
  after mastectomy, 172–173
  pregnancy and breast cancer, 222
  proton, 171
  sarcoma risk and, 219
  side effects, 175–179
  situations where not appropriate, 172
  survival rates and, 172
  types of, 157
  use of, 171
  uterine cancer, 300
  visual guide, 39
  ways to improve, 175
radical mastectomy, 164–165, 429
raloxifene, 108–109, 152, 344
reconstructive surgery
  decision, 203
  decision tips, 210
  defined, 418
  do's and don'ts of, 209
  estrogen therapy after menopause, 292
  free TRAM flap, 206
  immediate versus delayed, 204
  implants, 207
  issues to consider, 209–210
  latissimus flap, 206
  multiple procedures, 205
  nipple reconstruction, 208, 209
  options, 203
  pedicle TRAM flap, 206
  prosthetics, 209
  recurrence detection and, 204
  tissue expanders, 205–207
  tissue flaps, 206–209
  types of, 204–209
rectovaginal exam, 280
recurrence. *See* breast cancer recurrence
regional recurrence
  axillary node, 242
  defined, 226–227, 236, 242
  illustrated, 243
  internal mammary node, 243
  prognosis, 244
  signs and symptoms, 243–244

supraclavicular node, 243
  tests, 244
  treatment, 244
  types of, 242–243
  See also breast cancer recurrence
reiki, 362
relationship with family, 315–317
  cancer as barrier, 316–317
  drawing together, 316
  seeking help, 317
relationships, enjoying, 370–371
relative risk
  absolute risk versus, 64–65
  defined, 63
  facts, 63
  ratio, 63–64
remission, 430
reproductive risk factors
  early onset of menstruation and late
    menopause, 291
  endometrial hyperplasia, 291–292
  no pregnancy, 291
  See also uterine cancer
research
  basic, 27
  clinical trials, 28–31
  epidemiologic studies, 27–28
  as paying off, 32
  resources, 415
resources
  clinical trial information, 413
  complementary and alternative therapies,
    413–414
  coping, 414
  Español (Spanish), 414
  financial, 414
  general information, 415
  partners, 410–412
  research, 415
  specific cancers, 415–416
  survivorship, 416
  treatment, 416
rest, 375
risk assessment models
  BOADICEA, 67
  BRCAPRO, 67
  Claus, 67
  defined, 66
  Gail, 66–67
  Tyrer-Cuzick, 67

risk factors
  age, 25
  benign breast disease, 73–74
  breast density, 74
  caregiving and hospice, 413
  clinical trials and, 66
  defined, 24–25, 430
  diet and, 92
  environmental, 70–72
  external, 421
  family history, 26, 68
  hormonal and reproductive, 68–70
  identification of, 68
  male breast cancer, 223
  other, 26
  ovarian cancer, 275
  prior breast cancer, 72
  in quantifying risk, 66–67
  studies, 66
  uterine cancer, 289–293
risk statistics
  presentation of, 61–62
  understanding, 61–74
risk(s)
  absolute, 62–63, 64–65
  determination, 62
  perspective, 65–66
  in prevention, 91–92
  prophylactic mastectomy, 102
  prophylactic oophorectomy, 104–106
  quantifying, 66–67
  relative, 63–65
  screening, 113
  surgical biopsy, 138–139
  tamoxifen, 108
  things that don't increase, 74
  understanding, 62
Rosemarie's story, 182–183
routines, reconnecting with, 368–370

S
sadness, dealing with, 308–309
sarcoma, breast, 218–219, 430
screening
  awareness, 112
  clinical exam, 119
  controversies, 112–114
  defined, 430
  goal of, 100
  guide, 114
  guidelines, 91
  magnetic resonance imaging (MRI), 126
  making sense of, 114
  mammography, 120–126
  mammography trials, 112–113
  methods, 111
  nuclear medicine studies, 126
  purpose of, 111
  recommendations, 115–116
  risks, 113
  self-exam, 116–119
  ultrasound, 126
  usefulness of, 114
screening mammograms, 120, 430
second cancer
  BRCA carriers, 214–215
  Hodgkin disease survivors, 215–216
  women at high risk, 214–216
secondary prevention, 100
sedentary lifestyle, 54
self-help strategies, 311–315
  appetite problems, 326–327
  diet, 314
  education, 311–312
  exercise, 312–314
  expressing feelings, 312
  fatigue, 325
  hair loss, 329–330
  hot flashes, 337
  laughter, 313
  learning from others, 312
  staying connected, 314
  taking care of self, 312–314
  working, 314
sentinel node biopsy
  defined, 166, 430
  side effects, 167
  visual guide, 38
sentinel nodes
  defined, 38
  dissection, 167–168
  identification of, 166–167
  removal of, 167
  See also lymph nodes
sex, decreased interest
  as common problem, 342–343
  doctor communication, 343
  partner communication, 343
  testosterone and, 343
  time for romance, 343

sexual changes
　decreased interest, 342–343
　Kegel exercises and, 342
　orgasm difficulty, 342
　painful intercourse, 341–342
　See also side effects
sexual intimacy (partners)
　barriers to, 405–406
　breaks, 406
　communication, 406
　contacting cancer concern, 407
　dates, 406
　health relationship, 406–407
　loss acknowledgement, 406
　loved one as guide, 406–407
　maintaining, 405–407
　position experimentation, 407
Shirley's story, 348–350
shortness of breath, 387
side effects, 323–350
　appetite problems, 325–328
　cognitive changes, 347–348
　decreased arm/shoulder mobility, 330–333
　fatigue, 323–325
　hair loss, 329–330
　joint aches/pains, 346–347
　lymphedema, 333–336
　nausea, 325–328
　neuropathy, 345–346
　osteoporosis, 344–345
　sexual changes, 341–343
　story, 348–350
　sudden menopause, 336–341
　weight gain, 347
signs and symptoms, 128
signs and symptoms management
　　(supportive care)
　appetite problems, 387–389
　nausea and vomiting, 389
　pain, 383–387
　shortness of breath, 387
　weight loss, 387–389
simple mastectomy, 165, 430
skin-sparing mastectomy, 430
sleep, 375
solid masses
　cysts versus, 132
　in fine-needle aspiration biopsy, 133
soy and phytoestrogens, 95–96
spirituality, strengthening, 310–311

staging
　with blood tests, 143
　with bone scan, 143–144
　breast cancer grouping, 147
　with chest X-ray, 143
　classification, 145–147
　with CT, 144
　defined, 143, 431
　definitions summary, 145
　male breast cancer, 223
　with MRI, 144
　ovarian cancer, 283
　with PET, 144–145
　stage 0, 146
　stage I, 146
　stage II, 146
　stage III, 146
　stage IV, 147
　survival estimation, 147–148
　tests, 143–145
　TNM system, 145–146
　uterine cancer, 301
　See also breast cancer diagnosis
statistics
　breast cancer, 11, 43, 55–57
　cancer, 17
　cancers in women, 12
　hereditary breast cancer, 77
　locally advanced breast cancer, 212
　male breast cancer, 222
　ovarian cancer, 274
　risk, 61–74
　survival, 147–148
stereotactic core needle biopsy, 135
stories. *See* personal stories
stress, 52–53
stress reduction, 375
subcutaneous mastectomy, 431
sudden menopause
　defined, 336
　effects of, 337
　emotional changes, 337
　hot flashes, 337–339
　infertility, 338
　night sweats, 337, 339
　reasons for, 336
　vaginal dryness, 337, 339–341
　See also side effects
support
　emotional, 402–403

family and friends, 16, 307
to other breast cancer women, 367
practical, 402–403
support groups
benefits of, 376
choosing, 377
participation decision, 377
support groups (partners)
advantages, 410
coping skill intervention, 411
educational intervention, 411
finding, 411–412
online, 411
peer, 411
therapy, 411
types of, 411
supportive care
benefits of, 388
defined, 270
family disagreements, 383
hope, 381–383
hospice, 389–394
impending death denial and, 382
partners and, 408–410
signs/symptoms management, 383–389
situation acceptance, 380–381
story, 391–392
time left and, 380
transitioning to, 379–394
treatment goals, 380
surgery
after, 170–171
before, 169–170
as DCIS treatment option, 155–157
decision on what type of, 162–163
drug therapy before, 187
during, 170
as first form of treatment, 162
frozen section analysis, 168–169
hospital stays and, 170–171
for invasive breast cancer, 162–171
local recurrence after lumpectomy, 240
local recurrence after mastectomy, 242
locally advanced breast cancer, 214
lumpectomy, 163–164
lymph node removal, 165–168
mastectomy, 164–165
ovarian cancer, 284
positive margins, 165
pregnancy and breast cancer, 221–222

preventative, 152
uterine cancer, 300
visual guide, 39
what to expect, 168–171
surgical biopsy
aftercare, 138–139
defined, 136
preparation for, 136–137
procedure, 137–138
risks, 138–139
use of, 136
wire localization, 136–137
See also biopsy procedures
survival estimation, 147–148
survival rates
male breast cancer, 224
racial and ethnic differences in survival
rates, 57
radiation therapy and, 172
uterine cancer, 300
survivorship, 365–378
community and, 370
defined, 366
fear management, 366–368
health care, 372–376
helping others, 370
moving forward, 366–371
public events, 378
relationships, enjoying, 370–371
resources, 416
routines, reconnecting with, 368–370
support groups, 376–377
systemic therapy
defined, 431
uterine cancer, 300

T
tamoxifen
as advanced breast cancer treatment option,
252
aromatase inhibitors use after, 194
aromatase inhibitors versus, 194
as DCIS treatment option, 159–160
defined, 159, 190
dual role, 193
in LCIS treatment, 152
ovarian suppression and, 252–253
as postmenopausal metastatic breast cancer
treatment, 255
risk reduction, 106–108

tamoxifen continued
  risks, 108
  side effects, 108, 190–192
  studies, 106
  study follow-up results, 159–160
  use of, 190
  as uterine cancer risk factor, 292
  See also prevention medications
targeted therapies, 431
taxanes, 186
therapeutic touch, 362
therapy groups, 411
tissue expanders, 205–207
tissue flaps
  DIEP, 208
  free, 206, 208
  pedicle TRAM, 206, 207–208
  TRAM, 206–207
TNM staging system, 145–146
TRAM flaps, 206–208
trastuzumab (Herceptin)
  benefits, 260
  defined, 198, 259–260
  story of, 59
  studies, 198
  when to discontinue, 260
trauma, 45
treatment resources, 416
triple-negative breast cancer, 199
tubule formation, 141
tumor grade
  in additional treatment decision, 183–184
  in DCIS treatment, 155
  defined, 423
  mitotic activity, 141
  nuclear grade, 141
  scores, 141–142
  tubule formation, 141
tumor size
  in additional treatment decision, 183
  in DCIS treatment, 154–155
tumor suppressor genes, 23, 50–51, 431
Tyrer-Cuzick model, 67

U
ultrasound
  core needle biopsy, 135
  defined, 130, 432
  in diagnosis, 130–132
  exams, 132

liver, 246
  pelvic, 279
  in screening, 126
  transvaginal, 431
  in uterine cancer diagnosis, 296
uncertainty
  coping with, 368
  dealing with, 232–234
unknown primary cancers, 216–217
uterine cancer, 287–302
  age as risk factor, 289–290
  basics, 288–289
  biopsy, 297
  breast cancer as risk factor, 292
  causes, 289
  defined, 288, 432
  diabetes as risk factor, 292–293
  diagnosis, 294–299
  dilation and curettage, 297–299
  endometrioid (type I), 288–289
  extent determination, 299–300
  health history and, 294
  hereditary nonpolyposis colorectal cancer
      (HNPCC), 290
  imaging tests, 299
  incidence of, 289
  obesity as risk factor, 290–291
  ovarian cancer as risk factor, 292
  pelvic exam, 295–296
  physical exam, 294–295
  prevention and, 293
  race and ethnicity as risk factor, 290
  radiation therapy, 300
  reproductive risk factors, 291–292
  risk factors, 289–293
  risk perspective, 293
  screening, 294–295
  staging, 301
  surgery, 300
  surgery in determining extent, 299
  survival estimation, 300–301
  systemic therapy, 300
  tamoxifen use and, 292
  treatment options, 300–302
  type II, 289
  ultrasound, 296
  warning signs, 293–294
uterine fibroids, 432
uterus
  defined, 287–288, 432

lining (endometrium), 288
myometrium, 288

V
vaginal dryness
    defined, 337
    estrogen preparations, 340–341
    relief from, 339–340
vaginal estrogen, 340–341
vaginal exam, 280
vaginal hysterectomy, 432
vaginismus, 341
vinca alkaloids, 257
visual examination, 117
visual guide
    breast cancer stages, 36–37
    cancer biology, 33
    cancer development, 34–35
    drug therapy, 40
    radiation therapy, 39
    sentinel node biopsy, 38
    surgery, 39
vitamin C, 359
vitamin D, 359–360
vitamin E, 359
vitamins and minerals, 95
vomiting. *See* nausea

W
watchful waiting, 152, 199
weight, as risk factor, 71
weight control
    breast cancer prevention and, 94
    gain, 347
    loss, 387–389
    supportive care, 387–389
wire localization, 136–137, 432
women
    common cancers, 274
    death rates by cancer type, 32
    high risk of second cancer, 214–216
    leading new cancers in, 12
Women's Health Initiative (WHI), 64, 65

X
X-ray (ionizing) radiation, 27
X-rays, 245

Y
yoga, 355–356

Z
zoledronic acid (Zometa), 345

Visit our online store

for a wide selection of books, newsletters and DVDs developed by Mayo Clinic doctors and editorial staff.

Discover practical, easy-to-understand information on topics of interest to millions of health-conscious people like you …

➤ *Mayo Clinic Health Letter* — our award-winning monthly newsletter filled with practical information on today's health and medical news

➤ *Mayo Clinic Family Health Book* — the ultimate home health reference

➤ *The Mayo Clinic Diet: Eat Well, Enjoy Life, Lose Weight* — step-by-step guidance from Mayo Clinic weight-loss experts to help you achieve a healthy weight.

➤ *Mayo Clinic Book of Alternative Medicine* — the new approach to combining the best of natural therapies and conventional medicine

➤ *Mayo Clinic Book of Home Remedies* — discover how to prevent, treat or manage over 120 common health conditions at home

➤ *Mayo Clinic on Digestive Health* — learn how to identify and treat digestive problems before they become difficult to manage

➤ *Plus* — books on arthritis, aging, diabetes, high blood pressure and other conditions

Mayo Clinic brings you more of the
health information you're looking for!

Learn more at:

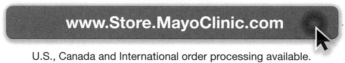

www.Store.MayoClinic.com

U.S., Canada and International order processing available.

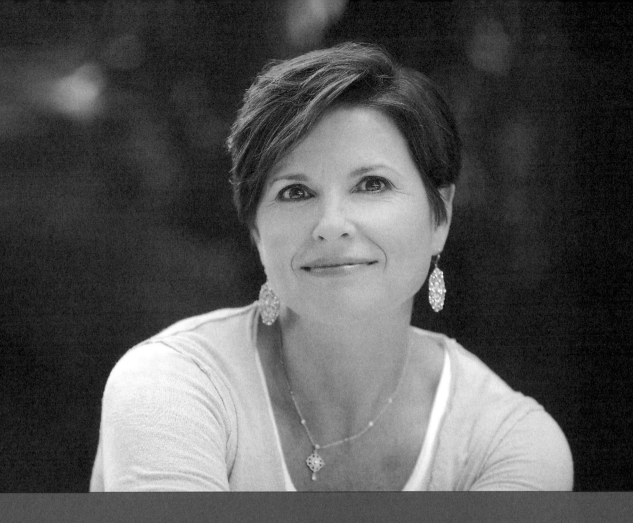

Other Books By Mayo Clinic
Available from Good Books

The Mayo Clinic Diet:

Eat well. Enjoy life. Lose weight.

by the weight-loss experts at Mayo Clinic

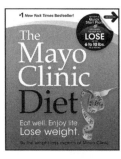

#1 *New York Times* bestseller!

From Mayo Clinic, a leading authority on health and nutrition, comes *The Mayo Clinic Diet*, designed to be the last diet you'll ever need.

Packed with encouragement—meal planners, recipes, tips for overcoming challenges, and starting an exercise plan—*The Mayo Clinic Diet* gives you everything you need in one book.

Toss out the scales and calculators and pick up the foods you love. This is the diet you've been waiting for!

**256 pages • full color throughout
$25.99 • hardcover with dust jacket**

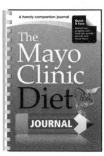

The Mayo Clinic Diet Journal:

by the weight-loss experts at Mayo Clinic

Losing weight with *The Mayo Clinic Diet* just got easier with help from *The Mayo Clinic Diet Journal*.

The *Lose It!* section helps you keep track as you add 5 habits, break 5 habits, and adopt 5 bonus habits. The *Live It!* section makes losing weight easier as you use this section to record your activity each day and keep track of your goals.

224 pages • $14.99 plastic comb binding

"Inspired by *The Mayo Clinic Diet*, I'm making changes."
—*U.S. News and World Report*

Also Available —

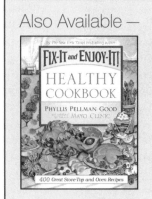

Fix-It and Enjoy-It! Healthy Cookbook:
400 Great Stove-Top and Oven Recipes
*by Phyllis Pellman Good
with nutritional expertise from Mayo Clinic*

Can you believe it? Great tasty recipes that are easy to prepare—and they're HEALTHY! Bring *New York Times* bestselling author Phyllis Pellman Good together with the prestigious Mayo Clinic, and that's what you have.

284 pages • $15.95, paperback • $18.95, plastic comb binding • $24.95, hardcover gift edition

---

To order these and other Mayo Clinic books, newsletters and DVDs—visit us online or call our toll-free number:
**Bookstore.MayoClinic.com
877-647-6397**

Available from bookstores and online booksellers, or order from the publisher:
**GoodBooks.com
800-762-7171, ext. 221**